THYROID HORMONES AND
BRAIN DEVELOPMENT

Thyroid Hormones
and
Brain Development

Edited by

Gilman D. Grave, M.D.
Medical Officer
Developmental Biology and Nutrition Branch
National Institute of Child Health
and Human Development
Bethesda, Maryland

Raven Press ▪ New York

1977

Raven Press, 1140 Avenue of the Americas, New York, New York 10036

Raven Press, New York 1977

Made in the United States of America

Library of Congress Cataloging in Publication Data
Main entry under title:

Thyroid hormones and brain development.

   Proceedings of a conference held in Elkridge,
Md., sponsored by the Growth and Development
Branch of the National Institute of Child Health and
Human Development.
   Bibliography: p.
   Includes index.
   1. Brain--Growth--Congresses. 2. Thyroxine--
Physiological effect--Congresses. 3. Brain chemistry--
Congresses. 4. Amphibians--Physiology--Congresses.
5. Mammals--Physiology--Congresses. I. Grave,
Gilman D. II. United States. National Institute of
Child Health and Human Development. Growth and
Development Branch. [DNLM: 1. Brain--Growth
and development--Congresses. 2. Hypothyroidism--
Complications--Congresses. 3. Thyroid hormones--
Physiology--Congresses. QL350 T549 1975]
QP376.T52   596'.01'88   76-52899
ISBN 0-89004-146-6

Preface

Pumpkins and princes, changelings and toads. Our myths and fairy tales tell of marvelous transmogrifications. Children and primitive people alike thrive on the magic of metamorphosis. And so do scientists.

We watch transfixed as tadpoles become frogs, but we still cannot explain how. But we do know that thyroid hormone throws the switch. Without this magic hormone no transmutation takes place. Somehow this bulky iodinated molecule affects the nuclear machinery of dividing cells and makes them differentiate.

This special property of thyroid hormone controls the postnatal development of the brain. Actively multiplying cerebellar neurons and glia throughout the developing brain require thyroid hormone at critical times to convey the message to stop dividing and start migrating, or stop dividing and start myelinating. Without such precisely timed messages, portions of the brain grow into tangled masses of poorly insulated, poorly connected neuropil.

Too much thyroid hormone, on the other hand, accelerates dramatically the tempo of neurophysiologic development, and too many connections are created and fixed too soon. The resulting hyperthyroid brain is deprived of plasticity and modulated response.

The contributors to this book have all been enchanted by the magic of thyroid hormone. They have at one time or another produced stunning chimeras in their laboratories and have amazed their colleagues with phenomenologic freaks. Now they seek to understand what they have wrought at cellular and molecular levels. Somehow thyroxine controls the flow of genetic information released by the primordial cells of the developing brain. In this book the contributors have presented many ingenious models in an attempt to unveil the mechanisms behind this profound control of brain development.

The tragedy of sporadic cretinism persists, made all the more insidious by the false sense of security engendered by the successful eradication of endemic cretinism in medically sophisticated countries of the world. Next year in the United States of America about 450 sporadic cretins will be born, but only some of them will be recognized at birth. Those who are not will be on their way to permanent mental retardation, as their postnatal cerebral development goes daily more awry without enough thyroid hormone.

The contributors to this book gathered at Belmont, the conference facility of the Smithsonian Institution in Elkridge, Maryland, in April 1975, to address many aspects of this puzzling problem of thyroid hormone and brain development. The conference was sponsored by the Growth and Development

Branch of the National Institute of Child Health and Human Development. The 21 chapters collected in this volume and the discussions that follow represent the latest thoughts and experiments on the problem of aberrant development of the brain in dysthyroid states.

Gilman D. Grave, M.D.

Contents

Contributors

Joseph Altman
Department of Biology and Physiology
Purdue University
Lafayette, Indiana 47970

Robert Balázs
MRC Developmental Neurobiology
Unit
Medical Research Council Labora-
tories
Carshalton, Surrey SM5 4EF, England

Norman H. Bass
Department of Neurology
University of Virginia School of
Medicine
Charlottesville, Virginia 22901

Ingrid Bennet
Hunter College
New York, New York 10028

John F. Burkart
Department of Biology
State University of New York at
Farmingdale
Farmingdale, New York 11735

Leon Cintra
Department of Physiology
Instituto de Investigaciones Bio-
médicas
Universidad Nacional Autónoma de
México
Mexico 20 D.F., Mexico

Eva B. Cramer
Department of Anatomy
Downstate Medical Center
State University of New York
Brooklyn, New York 11203

Sofia Diaz
Department of Physiology
Instituto de Investigaciones Bio-
médicas
Universidad Nacional Autónoma de
México
Mexico 20 D.F., Mexico

Beatriz H. Duvilanski
Departamento de Química Biológica
Facultad de Farmacia y Bioquímica
Universidad de Buenos Aires
Buenos Aires, Argentina

Norman L. Eberhardt
Department of Biochemistry
University of California Medical
School
San Francisco, California 94720

Donald H. Ford
Department of Anatomy
Downstate Medical Center
State University of New York
Brooklyn, New York 11203

Howard Frankfort
Department of Biology
City College of New York
New York, New York 10031

Edward Geller
Neurobiochemistry Laboratory
Brentwood Veterans Administration
Hospital
and
Department of Psychiatry and Brain
Research Institute
UCLA School of Medicine
Los Angeles, California 90073

Carlos J. Gómez
Departamento de Química Biológica
Facultad de Farmacia y Bioquímica
Universidad de Buenos Aires
Buenos Aires, Argentina

Amos G. Gona
Department of Anatomy
College of Medicine and Dentistry of
  New Jersey
Newark, New Jersey 07103

Gilman D. Grave
Developmental Biology and Nutrition
  Branch
National Institute of Child Health and
  Human Development
Bethesda, Maryland 20014

Alicia E. R. de Guglielmone
Departamento de Química Biológica
Facultad de Farmacia y Bioquímica
Universidad de Buenos Aires
Buenos Aires, Argentina

Max Hamburgh
Department of Biology
City College of New York
New York, New York 10031
and
Department of Anatomy
Albert Einstein College of Medicine
Bronx, New York 10461

Mariel A. Harris
Department of Pathology
The University of Chicago
Chicago, Illinois 60637

Susan L. Harris
Department of Pathology
The University of Chicago
Chicago, Illinois 60637

Kenneth Hogreff
Department of Biology
City College of New York
New York, New York 10031

Ronald Kahn
Department of Biology
City College of New York
New York, New York 10031

Young So Kim
Center for Biomedical Education
City College of New York
New York, New York 10031

Jerry J. Kollros
Department of Zoology
University of Iowa
Iowa City, Iowa 52242

Leon Krawiec
Departamento de Química Biológica
Facultad de Farmacia y Bioquímica
Universidad de Buenos Aires
Buenos Aires, Argentina

Paul Krupa
Department of Biology
City College of New York
New York, New York 10031

Jean M. Lauder
Department of Biobehavioral Sciences
University of Connecticut
Storrs, Connecticut 06268

Michael J. Malone
Geriatric Research Educational and
  Clinical Center
Veterans Administration Hospital
Bedford, Massachusetts 01730

Lorenzo A. Mendoza
Department of Neurology
Vargas Hospital
Caracas, Venezuela

Carlos A. Montalbano
Departamento de Química Biológica
Facultad de Farmacia y Bioquímica
Universidad de Buenos Aires
Buenos Aires, Argentina

Sally Oklund
Department of Anatomy
University of Colorado Medical Center
Denver, Colorado 80220

E. Williams Pelton, II
Department of Neurology
The Albany Medical College of Union
  University
Albany, New York 12208

Irwin Pesetsky
Department of Anatomy
Albert Einstein College of Medicine
Bronx, New York 10461

Helen Robinson
Department of Biological Sciences
Dartmouth College
Hanover, New Hampshire 03755

N. Paul Rosman
Departments of Pediatrics and Neu-
  rology (Pediatric Neurology)
Boston University School of Medicine
Boston City Hospital
Boston, Massachusetts 02118

Manuel Salas
Department of Physiology
Instituto de Investigaciones Bio-
  médicas
Universidad Nacional Autónoma de
  Mexico
Mexico 20 D.F., México

Louis Sokoloff
Laboratory of Cerebral Metabolism
National Institute of Mental Health
U.S. Department of Health, Educa-
  tion, and Welfare
Public Health Service
Bethesda, Maryland 20014

Dorothy Breslin Spangenberg
Department of Molecular, Cellular,
  and Developmental Biology
University of Colorado
Boulder, Colorado 80302

Paola S. Timiras
Department of Physiology-Anatomy
University of California at Berkeley
Berkeley, California 94720

Theony Valcana
Chair of Human and Animal Physi-
  ology
School of Natural Sciences and Math-
  ematics
University of Patras
Patras, Greece

Morton E. Weichsel, Jr.
Division of Pediatric Neurology
Department of Pediatrics
Harbor General Hospital
UCLA School of Medicine
Torrance, California 90509

Ting-Wa Wong
Department of Pathology
The University of Chicago
Chicago, Illinois 60637

Elizabeth Young
Department of Neurology
University of Virginia School of
  Medicine
Charlottesville, Virginia 22901

Introduction

Most of us have been introduced to the effects of thyroid hormones by the profoundly altered and dramatic states of hypothyroidism and hyperthyroidism. The toadlike, sluggish stupor of myxedema and the excitable, tremulous activity of hyperthyroidism are characteristic and unmistakable. The cerebral effects of these altered thyroid states may range from apathy to coma and from anxiety to frank psychosis. Fortunately, these metabolic disorders, even at their most florid, when present in adults are reversible, as are their accompanying states of aberrant mentation.

A hypothyroid state present at birth, however, if allowed to go unrecognized and untreated, results in the tragedy of cretinism, an irreversible misfortune. In this case, the altered mental state is one of permanent retardation. Unless florid, the condition of neonatal hypothyroidism may be readily missed, particularly in this country where endemic goiter has been virtually eliminated. Because sporadic cretinism appears only once in every 7,000 live births, a low level of suspicion prevails in most newborn nurseries (Dussault, Coulombe, Laberge, Letarte, Guyda, and Khoury, 1975). These undiagnosed cases constitute the greatest tragedy, for it is at this period in their lives, while their brain cells are actively differentiating, that their disease is most amenable to intervention with exogenous thyroxine.

Within the past several years, it has become much easier to diagnose neonatal hypothyroidism accurately and quickly by radioimmunoassays for thyroid-stimulating hormone and for serum free thyroxine (Klein, Augustin, and Foley, 1974; Dussault et al., 1975). I was fortunate recently to have the opportunity to include sporadic hypothyroidism in bill no. S-1614, introduced by Senator Hubert Humphrey, which makes testing for several aminoacidopathies mandatory in newborn nurseries of federally related health care facilities. Although not exactly an aminoacidopathy, the problem of altered thyroid states fits nicely into the package of diseases for which screening is intended. The iodinated phenolic structure of thyroxine so overshadows the rest of the molecule that we often forget that the hormone really is an amino acid. Thinking of it as such may help in accounting for its many apparently disparate effects.

Sterling (1975) has suggested that thyroxine may act as a neurotransmitter like another phenolic amino acid, dihydroxyphenylalanine. Instead of augmenting the actions of catecholamines, it may actually substitute for them. This possible action as a neurotransmitter could account for the range of bizarre mental states associated with too much or too little of this iodinated amino acid. Its striking enhancement of protein synthesis (see Chapter 5) may similarly be related to its amino acid structure. This hypothesis offers an appealing approach to the problem of accounting for the myriad effects of this remarkable hormone.

Beyond its effects on cerebration, oxygen consumption, mitochondrial respiration, and uncoupling of oxidative phosphorylation, thyroid hormone has even more dramatic effects on differentiation. The metamorphosis of tadpole to frog is one of the most startling examples, and the poor axolotl, with no thyroid gland at all, remains a perpetual larva. No more persuasive argument could be mustered to emphasize the importance of this molecule and its strength as a prime mover in cellular differentiation. Without thyroid hormone, the axolotl remains just that, the tadpole fails to become a frog, and the jellyfish polyp cannot change into a medusa (see Chapter 10). And without thyroid hormone, the human brain is arrested at a primitive level in which axons are poorly myelinated, and neurons display rudimentary dendritic arborization. The cretin brain is feeble in many other ways, some of which are explored in the chapters that follow. Most of the papers in this book, however, are not about the cretin brain but instead address the problem of the mechanism of action of thyroid hormone and its effects on the developing brain.

The developing brain is affected by hypothyroidism more profoundly than any other organ. The liver, kidneys, lungs, gut, muscles, blood, and reticuloendothelial system of the cretin continue to function with a strong semblance of normality. The brain, however, is crippled beyond possible recovery. At some time in its development, the brain becomes a critical target organ for thyroid hormone. The precise role of this crucial hormone in brain development remains unknown, although the papers in this book bring us closer to an understanding of its mechanism of action. Undoubtedly, the hormone plays a permissive role and may play an initiating role in the release of the flow of genetic information contained in the neurons and glia of the developing brain and in the multitudinous synthetic and organizational events that follow.

A theme that runs through many of the chapters in this volume concerns the effects of dysthyroid states on protein synthesis. The specific activities of many cerebral enzymes are decreased in hypothyroidism (Chapters 1 and 4). Activities of some cerebral enzymes can be augmented in hyperthyroidism or can be induced to appear earlier in the maturational process than they would normally (Chapters 18 and 20). The rate of protein synthesis has been shown to decrease in hypothyroidism (Chapter 16) and to accelerate in hyperthyroidism (Chapter 5). Thyroid hormones function in at least four basic ways during transcription and translation: (1) by affecting RNA polymerase II which assembles messenger RNA (Chapter 19); (2) by affecting tRNA sulfurtransferase which confers codon specificity onto transfer RNA (Chapter 21); (3) by affecting release of nascent polypeptide chains from ribosomes (Chapter 5); and (4) by affecting the activity of thymidine kinase (Chapter 20) and other enzymes which assemble nucleotides.

No evidence was adduced by anyone reporting in this volume to indicate that thyroid hormones act at levels of cellular hierarchy more basic than the assembly and functioning of the three kinds of RNA. Whether thyroxine or triiodothyronine exert even more basic an influence on the genome (e.g., in a manner akin to the steroid hormones) during brain development remains unknown. Rather than stimulating the initial release of encoded genetic information, it appears now that thyroid hormones act to control the rates of several critical enzymatic steps in the flow of that information from storage in DNA to expression in structural and enzymatic proteins. This early exertion of control of reaction speed accounts for its startling metamorphic and chronotropic properties.

The host of cerebral structural abnormalities that appear in dysthyroid states must follow from alterations of such basic transcriptional and translational events. Because not all reaction rates are slowed or accelerated equally by thyroid hormones, the brain develops asynchronously. The grotesqueries produced by ill-timed axonal myelination and a multitude of erroneous synaptic connections can be visualized in the microarchitecture of the cerebral (Chapter 12) and the cerebellar (Chapter 14) cortices.

This book presents the compiled and edited proceedings of a conference of the same title held at the Belmont Conference facility of the Smithsonian Institution. The conference was sponsored by the Growth and Development Branch of the National Institute of Child Health and Human Development. The purpose of the conference was to elucidate the mechanism of action of thyroid hormone by examining various experimental models that seek to explain its role in normal and abnormal neurophysiologic development. A glance at the Contents of this volume will show how varied these models are, yet each has its own compelling rationale. Participants at the conference witnessed some confrontations and some harmonious agreements. Among other accomplishments, the confounding roles played by other trophic hormones and by proper nutrition in brain development were dissected away from thyroid hormone's role as prime mover in cerebral differentiation.

This volume is the product of many erudite and skilled contributors. I wish at this time to thank especially Sharon Swinburne and Anne Schmid who did a superb job in making the transcripts of the clamorous discussions readable and enlightening.

REFERENCES

Dussault, J. H., Coulombe, P., Laberge, C., Letarte, J., Guyda, H., and Khoury, K. (1975): Preliminary report on a mass screening program for neonatal hypothyroidism. *J. Pediatrics,* 86:670–674.

Klein, A. H., Augustin, A. V., and Foley, J. P., Jr. (1974): Successful laboratory screening for congenital hypothyroidism. *Lancet,* 2:77–79.

Sterling, F. (1975): Letter to the editor. *N. Engl. J. Med.,* 293:309.

Gilman D. Grave

Thyroid Hormones and Brain Development,
edited by Gilman D. Grave. Raven Press,
New York, 1977.

Developing Nervous System in Relation to Thyroid Hormones

Donald H. Ford and Eva B. Cramer*

An awareness of a relationship between the thyroid gland and brain development has been evident since at least the middle of the nineteenth century (Fagge, 1871), particularly in relation to the mental retardation associated with cretinism. However, beyond this observation, attempts to understand further the role of thyroid hormones in brain development were seldom undertaken despite an increasing accumulation of data indicating a powerful role for these hormones in many cellular functions. An extensive review of these mechanisms from the Russian literature (Turakulov, Gol'ber, Gagel'gans, Kandror, Salakhova, Mirakhmedov, and Gaidina, 1972) has appeared in translation. Although this report is concerned primarily with the effect of the thyroid hormone on tissues other than brain in the adult, it also delineates its significant role in cell respiration and metabolism, which applies equally to the nervous system.

The interest in neuroendocrinology so prevalent today probably represents a part of the overall upsurge in investigations of the nervous system which started after World War II. In the three postwar decades, a virtual revolution in technology has made extensive advances possible in every field. New histological techniques have markedly extended our knowledge of the anatomical organization of the brain, and the electron microscope has advanced our understanding of neuronal and glial cell structure and their interrelationships. Neurochemistry and neuropharmacology have become separate disciplines from chemistry, and neuroendocrinology has evolved as an almost entirely new venture in the neurosciences. The emergence of the hypothalamus as the site for control of the endocrine system has occurred almost completely in this period, so that today it is generally accepted that there are small groups of cells in the hypothalamus wherein each group is capable of initiating or preventing the release of one of the adenohypophyseal hormones. Another principle in neuroendocrinology pertains to the observations that these same pituitary hormones, as well as the hormones secreted by the glands whose activity is controlled by the pituitary, will themselves have a role in regulating the hypothalamus via long- and short-feedback loops. Furthermore, these hormones have general effects throughout the

---

* Department of Anatomy, Downstate Medical Center, State University of New York, Brooklyn, New York 11203.

entire nervous system which influence excitability and various metabolic functions.

Investigations dealing with the effects of hormone deficiencies or excesses in relation to the central and peripheral nervous system have been performed on both adult and maturing animal forms of many species. In the adult one may observe how these hormones influence neuronal function chemically and physiologically; in prenatal and postnatal animal forms data of an entirely different character have emerged which indicate that thyroidal, gonadal, and adrenal hormones are all necessary for the normal differentiation of the nervous system. Deficiencies or excesses of any hormone lead to disturbances in brain development which have severe consequences as the animal matures to adulthood, assuming that the condition permits survival.

Numerous experimental models have been used to evaluate the effects of thyroid hormones, as well as the other hormones, on the developing brain, at both the *in vivo* and *in vitro* levels, by anatomical, physiological, biochemical, and behavioral methods.

TABLE 1. *Effect of altered thyroid states on growth of brain or neurons in neonatal animals*

Observations	Animal	Reference
Hypothyroid		
Hypoplasia of cerebral cortex with decrease of size of Betz cells in man	Man	Lotmar, 1933
Brain weight lower than in controls	Rabbit	Cuaron et al., 1963
Hypoplasia of cerebral cortical neurons and neuropil	Rat	Eayrs, 1953, 1960, 1961
Hypoplasia of Purkinje cells and slowed migration of external granule cell layer	Rat	Legrande, 1965, 1967
Slowed diminution of external granule cell layer and continued DNA synthesis	Rat	Hamburgh and Bunge, 1964; Hamburgh et al., 1964, 1971; Hamburgh 1968, 1969
Regression of Mauthner cells linked to decrease in thyroid hormone at metamorphosis	Frog	Pesetsky, 1962, 1966
Decrease in size of cortical neurons with retarded differentiation at 16 days (few ribosomes on endoplasmic reticulum, which is less developed)	Rat	Mitskevich and Moskovkin, 1971
Dry weight of cortex decreased, cortical thickness decreased with no change in water content compared with controls Impaired gliogenesis or impairment of glial differentiation and migration	Rat	Bass and Young, 1973
Hyperthyroid or thyroid hormone treated		
Regression of Mauthner cells	Anuran	Weiss and Rossetti, 1951
Accelerated eye opening	Rat	Eayrs and Lishman, 1955; Schapiro, 1968
Development of external granule layer of cerebellum and massive migration of granule cells	Frog	Gona, 1973

The literature pertaining to these studies is voluminous. The information on thyroid hormones pertaining to rats has been briefly summarized in Tables 1 through 7 and indicates their significant effects on neuronal differentiation and growth. Specifically, thyroid hormones affect tissue respira-

TABLE 2. *Effect of altered thyroid states on protein and nucleic acid synthesis in neonatal rat*

Observations	Reference
Hypothyroid	
Increase in DNA concentration and decrease in RNA/DNA ratio	Geel and Timiras, 1967*a*
Decrease in cortical nuclear and cytoplasmic RNA/unit wet wt DNA	
Reduced RNA content associated with increased turnover without change in net synthesis	Balázs and Cocks, 1967
Decrease in RNA and protein synthesis in cerebral cortex and cerebellum accompanied by increase in DNA	Pasquini, et al., 1967
DNA μg atom P/g increased in cerebrum, RNA μg atom P/g minimally affected, RNA/DNA increasingly depressed with age. Protein/DNA depressed. Similar results in cerebellum for all parameters	Balázs et al., 1968
Severe hypothyroidism during critical period did not damage brain polysomes	Nievel et al., 1968
Decreased brain levels of glutamic and aspartic acid	Marcucci and Airoldi, 1969
Depressed protein synthesis based on relative specific activity of brain tissues after injection of [^{3}H]phenylalanine	Szijan et al., 1971
Reduced RNA in ribosomal fraction with increased incorporation of [^{14}C]orotic acid	Geel and Timiras, 1971; Geel and Valcana, 1971
Decreased conversion of ^{14}C from leucine into proteins and lipids and increase in ^{14}C in amino acids associated with tricarboxylic cycle. Normal age-dependent increase in glutamate/glutamine specific activity retarded; relating hormone to maturation of metabolic compartmentation	Patel and Balázs, 1971
Depressed incorporation of [^{3}H] leucine into mitochondrial, microsomal, and synaptosomal protein; restored by thyroxine treatment	Jarlstedt and Norstrom, 1972
Hyperthyroid or thyroid hormone treated	
Increased incorporation of ^{35}S after injection of [^{35}S]-methionine in 10-day-old animals	Schneck et al., 1965
Increased incorporation of [^{14}C]leucine	Gelber et al., 1964
Stimulation of protein synthesis in neonates dependent on mitochondria	Sokoloff and Kaufman, 1961; Sokoloff et al., 1962; Sokoloff, 1964; Sokoloff and Roberts, 1971
Stimulation of protein synthesis *in vitro* and *in vivo*	Geel and Timiras, 1967*b*
Decreased time after birth for proliferation of small neurons & induced differentiation	Hamburgh et al., 1971
Reduced brain size associated with permanent reduction in cell proliferation, as revealed by decrease in DNA	Balázs, et al., 1971*b*

TABLE 3. *Effect of altered thyroid states on development of CNS enzymes in the rat*

Observations	References
Hypothyroid	
Succinic dehydrogenase activity depressed	Hamburgh and Flexner, 1957
Succinic dehydrogenase and aspartate aminotrans-	Pasquini et al., 1967
ferase activity depressed in brain homogenates,	
oxidative phosphorylation depressed	
Glutamic acid decarboxylase and GABA	García Argiz et al., 1967
transaminase and ATPase depressed	
Acetylcholinesterase activity depressed	Geel and Timiras, 1967*b*
No change in alanine aminotransferase and	Balázs et al., 1968
lactate dehydrogenase, glutamate dehydrogenase;	
glutamate decarboxylase depressed	
Neuronal G6PD depressed, neuronal acid	Robinson and Eayrs, 1968
phosphatase and MAO in nerve fibers depressed,	
glial acid phosphatase increased	
Succinic dehydrogenase and GABA-T in cerebrum	Krawiec et al., 1969
and cerebellum depressed	
Decrease in activity of Na,K-ATPase	Valcana and Timiras, 1969
Reduction in cerebral acetylcholinesterase 22 and	Valcana, 1971
29 days after birth, most evident in nuclei and	
mitochondria + lesser reduction in myelin and	
synaptosomal fraction; microsomal fraction showed	
increased activity; cholineacetyltransferase activity	
increased; cerebellar acetylcholinesterase activity	
increased after 29 days, decreased in cerebral cortex	
Cerebral and cerebellar cortical	Mitskevich and Moskovkin,
succinic dehydrogenase depressed;	1971
α-glycerophosphate	
dehydrogenase—no change, but depressed in	
cerebellum; NADPH-diaphorase depressed in	
cerebral and cerebellar cortex; NADH in	
cerebral cortex—no change, depressed in	
cerebellum	
Development of normal levels of acetylcholinesterase	Clos, 1972
activity reduced	

tion, cell division, the synthesis of RNA and protein, and the maturation of various enzyme systems. Inasmuch as not all enzyme systems are influenced in the same way by thyroid hormone stimulation, there is apparently some degree of selectivity in the proteins which respond to the hormone. Further, the observations of Sokoloff and co-workers (Sokoloff and Kaufman, 1961; Sokoloff, Kaufman, and Campbell, 1962; Sokoloff and Roberts, 1971) on mitochondrial-dependent protein synthesis by the neonatal rat brain may be of particular significance in relation to the maturation of the respiratory enzyme systems associated with mitochondria. From the data summarized in these tables, multiple effects of thyroid hormones on the developing nervous system are evident. Undoubtedly, the hormones secreted by other endocrine glands may interact with those from the thyroid

TABLE 4. *Effect of altered thyroid states on myelinization and brain lipids in the neonatal rat*

Observations	Reference
Hypothyroid	
Transient decrease in phospholipids and cholesterol concentration at 23 days of age after neonatal thyroidectomy. Decrease in cerebrosides, total phospholipids, and cholesterol at 35 days of age, reduction in myelinization and myelin lipids	Balázs et al., 1969
Reduction in cerebrosides, sulfatides, and cholesterol which, to some degree, was maintained when treated with thyroid hormone after the 18th day	Walravens and Chase, 1969
Hyperthyroid or thyroid hormone treated	
Stimulation of myelinization in organ culture by addition of thyroid hormone	Hamburgh, 1968
Triiodothyronine stimulated brain sulfatide formation	Walravens and Chase, 1969
Triiodothyronine accelerated some processes preceding deposition of cerebroside in myelin	Balázs et al., 1971c
Increased incorporation of malonyl-CoA into fatty acids	Grippo and Menkes, 1971

TABLE 5. *Effect of altered thyroid states on tissue respiration in the neonatal rat*

Observations	Reference
Hypothyroid	
Oxygen utilization, lactate formation and glucose uptake depressed; oxygen utilization and lactate formation becomes normal by day 20, whereas glucose uptake becomes normal by day 30 (in cortical slices)	Ghittoni and Gómez, 1964
Oxygen consumption decreased in cortical slices	Fazekas et al., 1951
Hyperthyroid or thyroid hormone treated	
Oxygen utilization increased	Fazekas et al., 1951
Increased oxygen consumption in cerebral cortex, cerebellum, and medulla	Hamburgh et al., 1964
Facilitates electron transport; general role in tissue respiration reviewed in relation to oxidative phosphorylation, etc., in numerous species	Turakulov et al., 1972

gland during this period, so that the resultant mature brain depends ultimately on the summation of all these factors.

In consideration of the rapid changes in brain RNA, protein, enzyme activities, electrolyte levels, glial populations, and myelinization, the developing brain differs literally from day to day, both anatomically and biochemically. Thus, among the known changes there could be some which influence the accumulation and degradation of thyroid hormones by the brain. Changes in accumulation could be related to the decrease in the extracellular space known to occur during maturation (Vernadakis and

TABLE 6. *Effect of altered thyroid states on electrical activity in CNS and related factors in the neonatal animal*

Observations	Animal	References
Hypothyroid		
Diminished amplitude of EEG and evoked potentials with behavioral alterations.	Rat	Bradley et al., 1960; Eayrs, 1966
Slow α-rhythm in young hypothyroid children	Man	Andersen, 1966, 1971
Retardation of normal EEG in sleep in some hypothyroid children	Man	Schultz et al., 1967
Retardation of transcallosal response	Rat	Hatotani and Timiras, 1967
Na^+ and Cl^- elevated; K^+ and Mg^{2+} depressed	Rat	Valcana and Timiras, 1969
Electroshock seizure threshold depressed, indicating higher brain excitability	Rat	Meisami et al., 1970
Duration of maximal electroshock seizure response depressed for flexion and increased for extension with a prolongation of recovery time	Rat	Meisami et al., 1970
Increased latency and duration of the surface-negative component of the recruiting response and reduction in amplitude	Rat	Bradley et al., 1960
Hyperthyroid or thyroid hormone treated		
Thyroxine acceleration of evoked cortical responses to visual, auditory, and sciatic nerve stimuli	Rat	Salas and Schapiro, 1970

Woodbury, 1962; Bondareff and Pysh, 1968). These could lead to a decrease in accumulation of thyroid hormone if its uptake into the brain is purely by passive diffusion. However, because there is evidence indicating that at least a part of the hormone accumulation is dependent on active (enzyme-mediated) transport (Ford, 1971), there could be changes in uptake during the maturational period which are influenced by the development of this pathway. There may be changes in the enzymatic degradation of thyroid hormone which depend on the development of the deiodinase enzyme system, generally accepted as being responsible for the breakdown of thyroid hormones. Paradoxically, the development of these enzyme systems may themselves depend on the capability of thyroid hormones to stimulate protein synthesis, particularly in the neonatal brain. Finally, the level of accumulation of thyroid hormones achieved by brain tissue may depend on the synthesis of binding sites within cells. This, too, may be influenced by the hormone, inasmuch as such receptors are believed to be proteins. Because more [131I]triiodothyronine (T_3) is accumulated in neurons than in the surrounding neuropil (Ford and Rhines, 1967), it would be logical to conclude that there are more of such receptors in the neurons

TABLE 7. *Effect of altered thyroid states on behavior in the neonatal animal*

Observations	Animal	Reference
Hypothyroid		
More frequent errors in a simple T maze and in other tests as adult when hypothyroidism was induced at time of birth	Rat	Eayrs and Lishman, 1955
Delay in appearance of startle reflex	Rat	Eayrs, 1964
Increased learning time in a water escape response in 20-day-old rats	Rat	Hamburgh et al., 1964
Delayed acquisition of sensorimotor maze escape response	Mouse Rat	Essman et al., 1968
Hyperthyroid or thyroid hormone treated		
No lasting effect on learning in 20-day-old rat; however, 28-day-old rats learned more slowly	Rat	Hamburgh et al., 1964
Younger response to startle reflex and an increase in motor activity induced by thyroxine treatment	Rat	Schapiro, 1968
Learn to avoid electric shock sooner after thyroxine treatment, but make more errors later, suggesting that excess hormone levels at ontogenetically inappropriate times may compromise the development of certain adaptive or survival mechanisms	Rat	Schapiro, 1968
Maturation of swimming ability accelerated	Rat	Schapiro et al., 1970

than the glia. In view of the differences between male and female neonatal rats in relation to the brain RNA base ratios (Soriero and Ford, 1971) and the incorporation of [^{3}H]lysine into brain protein (Kartzinel, Ford, and Rhines, 1971), it seems likely that there may be sex-induced differences in the accumulation of the thyroid hormone by neonatal rat brain.

[^{131}I]T$_3$ ACCUMULATION IN NEONATAL RAT BRAIN

Bleecker, Ford, and Rhines (1971) investigated the possibility that there might be age- and sex-related differences in the accumulation of T$_3$ in the brain. Young male and female Wistar rats were injected intravenously with a tracer dose (0.5 μg/kg) of [^{131}I]T$_3$ and killed at various time intervals thereafter at either 2, 4, or 8 weeks of age. Samples of various areas of the central nervous system (CNS) were removed and fixed in 10% neutral formalin and then counted in a scintillation counter (Nuclear Chicago). Other samples were extracted with ammoniacal absolute ethanol (pH 8.5) to remove T$_3$-free iodide and the various iodinated compounds that may be derived from T$_3$ (Cohan, Ford, and Rhines, 1967). These extracts were concentrated (at 50°C under reduced pressure) to a few drops, which were applied to thin-layer cellulose chromatogram sheets (Kodak); the labeled materials were separated chromatographically in a Kodak chromatogram sandwich chamber using a butanol-dioxane-ammonia solvent system.

Appropriate nonlabeled compounds were also applied to the sheets to provide for carriers which could be subsequently identified after separation by ninhydrin spray (amino compounds) or palladium chloride (iodine). After drying, the chromatograms were cut into sections corresponding to the distribution of identifiable compounds and the radioactivity in the sections determined by scintillation counting. From the data obtained, the percent was determined of the ^{131}I activity associated with free iodide, T_3, thyroxine (T_4 — as a small contaminent obtained with the original material), monoiodotyrosine (MIT), and diiodotyrosine (DIT). Knowing the total cpm in the sample per gram and the percent of activity associated with T_3 and the cpm per unit weight of hormone, the amount of hormone accumulated per unit weight of tissue was then calculated for animals killed at 0.5, 1, 2, 4, and 7 hr after injection of the hormone. For each tissue an uptake curve was plotted. Maximal accumulation in the CNS gray matter occurred at 2 hr; thereafter there was a loss, presumably due to replacement of labeled hormone by endogenous nonlabeled hormone and loss of hormone not bound to receptor sites through degradation (Tata, 1964). In constructing the curves used for Fig. 1, only the level of accumulation present 2 hr after injection of the hormone has been utilized. Similar curves for the amount of hormone accumulated would be observed at other time intervals. The cerebral white and gray matter are not readily separable at

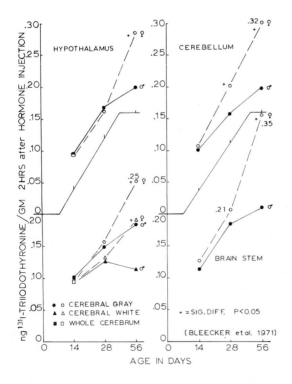

FIG. 1. [^{131}I]T_3 accumulation in the hypothalamus, cerebellum, cerebral gray and white matter, and in the brainstem of male and female rats at various ages 2 hr after intravenous injection of the hormone.

2 weeks of age; therefore, the data on T_3 accumulation in 2-week-old rats are those obtained for the whole cerebrum.

The data presented in Fig. 1 demonstrate a significant increase in the amount of T_3 accumulated in different areas of brain with increasing age. Similar data were obtained for the thalamus. Only white matter in male animals failed to show a significant increase in accumulation with increasing age. Also, there are sex differences in T_3 accumulation after puberty (4 weeks of age). The cerebellum was the only tissue in which prepubertal sex differences in T_3 accumulation occurred. Conceivably this could be related to the greater degree of immaturity of the cerebellum at birth compared with the rest of the brain. Note further that there are slight differences in the total amount of T_3 accumulated in the hypothalamus, cerebellum, cerebral gray and white matter, and brainstems from female rats at the age of 56 days, which were not noted in the male brains, except for the cerebral white matter. The pattern of accumulation of T_3 into the white matter from male rats related to age is quite different from that observed in the females, which suggests a different maturational pattern in relation to uptake, binding, and degradation. This sex difference in accumulation in the various brain areas is maintained until the animals are 2 years old, when the male levels of accumulation approach those of the female (Ford and Rhines, 1970). Further, because the levels of $[^{131}I]T_3$ in the plasma from both male and female rats available for uptake are equivalent, the sex differences in brain hormone accumulation seem to be intrinsically dependent on factors within the CNS itself.

In view of the sex differences in T_3 accumulation, an additional investigation was undertaken to determine the effect of neonatal gonadectomy on day 3 on accumulation of hormone by the brain at 8 weeks of age (Bleecker et al., *unpublished data*). Three-day-old male and female rats were anesthetized by cold and gonadectomized. They were allowed to regain consciousness and returned to their mothers. At 8 weeks of age they were injected intravenously with $[^{131}I]T_3$ as in the previous study, and the tissues were processed in a similar manner. The effect of neonatal gonadectomy was to reduce significantly the accumulation of T_3 in the cerebral cortex and cerebellum during the first half hour in both sexes (Fig. 2). However, after this early period, the effect on T_3 uptake depended on the area of brain examined, as well as on the sex.

In the cerebral cortex, there was no difference in T_3 accumulation after the first half hour in the male group, whereas in the female group the level of hormone accumulation during the entire experimental period was significantly below control levels. In the cerebellum, the level of T_3 accumulation in male rats after the first half hour exceeded that observed in unoperated controls through the 1- and 2-hr periods, then began to decrease to below control levels. These differences were not significant, however, due to the degree of variability between animals. In the cerebellar tissue

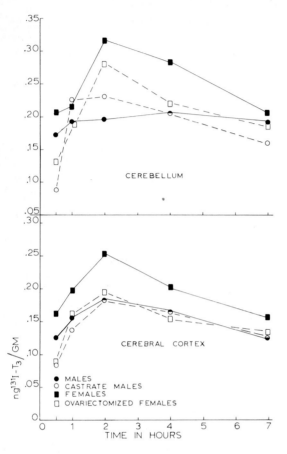

FIG. 2. Effect of gonadectomy on the third day of life on accumulation of $[^{131}]T_3$ in the cerebellum and cerebral cortex at various time intervals after intravenous injection in male and female rats at 8 weeks of age.

from female rats, T_3 accumulation in the ovariectomized group was lower for the entire group at all time intervals when compared with controls. Although the differences at individual time intervals were not significant, the difference between the groups, considering all time intervals together, was significant. In the hypothalamus of the male rats, there were no significant differences in T_3 accumulation between the castrate and intact group. In the hypothalamic tissue from female animals (Fig. 3), T_3 accumulation was significantly depressed in the ovariectomized group during the first hour and was comparable to intact female tissue thereafter. The sex difference in $[^{131}I]T_3$ accumulation indicated in Fig. 1, at 2 hr after $[^{131}I]T_3$ injection, is present throughout the duration of the experimental period in 56-day-old rats. These observations suggest that there may be a greater effect of estrogenic hormones on T_3 accumulation in postpubertal rats than of androgens, at least in those parts of the brain examined. The effects in the male animals were considerably less and generally limited to the first half hour after injection of the hormone.

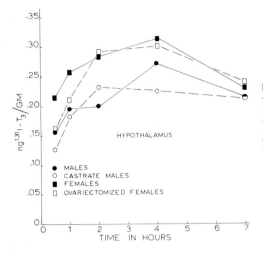

FIG. 3. Effect of gonadectomy on the third day of life on accumulation of $[^{131}I]T_3$ in the hypothalamus at various time intervals after intravenous injection in male and female rats at 8 weeks of age.

VARIATIONS IN T_3 DEGRADATION IN RELATION TO AGE

Studies of the presence of enzyme systems or their functional activities (Ford, 1974) in the rat demonstrate that many essential systems are developed at birth and then show rapid changes in activity during the first month of life. In view of the variety of enzyme systems involved in these changes, it is not unreasonable to suppose that there might be parallel changes in the activity of the enzymes involved in degradation of the thyroid hormones. The observations of Cohan et al. (1967) in developing rats are germane. Among the variables of measurement was an evaluation of the percent of the injected ^{131}I present in the plasma and brain at the time of death of the animals which was still bound to the thyronine molecule, and of how much appeared to be associated with monoiodotyrosine (MIT), diiodotyrosine (DIT), or present as free iodide. Although data were collected throughout a 7-hour period from injection of $[^{131}I]T_3$ until killing, only those obtained at the end of the longest time interval will be presented to demonstrate the final distribution of degradation products.

Six animals were used for each age group. Using the same chromatographic procedures described, Cohan et al. (1967) demonstrated that there were surprisingly high levels of MIT and DIT in the plasma obtained from the 7-day-old rat (Fig. 4). This was surprising inasmuch as it has generally been conceded that thyroid hormone was degraded primarily by deiodination (Pitt-Rivers and Tata, 1959; Tata, 1964). Further, the amount of radioactivity still associated with T_3 was remarkably high compared with adult levels in plasma at the end of a 7-hr experimental period, whereas free iodide levels were somewhat lower than anticipated. Both of these observations suggested that the hormone metabolism had not followed the adult pattern. Examination of the plasma at 1, 2, 3, and 4 weeks of age demon-

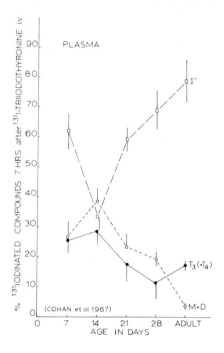

FIG. 4. ^{131}I-labeled compounds in the plasma of male rats injected intravenously with [^{131}I]T_3 at various ages. I⁻ = iodide; T_3 (+T_4) = triiodothyronine (plus a 3 to 4% contamination of thyroxine which was also present in the injected labeled hormone); M = MIT; D = DIT. Data are expressed in percent of total radioactivity present. Vertical lines indicate the SEM. The sum of the percent of radioactivity present at any single age for T_3 (+T_4), I⁻, and M + D does not equal 100% because there were other bands of radioactivity not associated with these compounds. Some of these labeled bands, which constituted only a very small fraction of the total radioactivity, had migrational Rf values comparable to the acetic and propionic acid metabolites of T_3.

strated that there was a trend toward attainment of an adult distribution of metabolites by 4 weeks, which was not complete until 3 months, when the major peak of radioactivity in the plasma of animals receiving [^{131}I]T_3 was associated with iodide and the activity associated with MIT and DIT was very low.

Examination of the distribution of ^{131}I-labeled compounds in the brain (Fig. 5) demonstrates relatively low levels of free iodide at all ages except at 14 days of age. This corresponds to the time when plasma levels of iodide showed a sudden drop, instead of continuing to increase with increasing age. The significance of this reciprocal change is unknown. Muscle tissue also shows a high level of free iodide between 14 and 21 days in relation to other iodinated compounds. At 1 week of age there is a very high percentage of the labeled material present in the brain as MIT and DIT, which drops nearly to adult levels within the next week, as also observed in skeletal muscle. The levels of T_3 in brain increase rapidly during the first 3 weeks to an adult level and then remain constant, presumably bound to appropriate receptor sites.

These observations of Cohan et al. (1967) suggest that in the postnatal period there is a significant amount of thyroid hormone which is not degraded along the generally accepted pathway of deiodination. The appreciable amounts of [^{131}I]MIT and DIT observed in both the plasma and brain imply that the thyronine molecule is being broken at the ether bond. Whether this is accomplished by an "etherase" enzyme or through other mechanisms

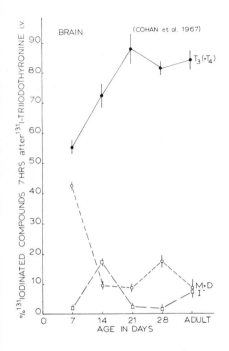

FIG. 5. ^{131}I-labeled compounds in the cerebral cortex of male rats injected intravenously with [^{131}I]T$_3$ at various ages. See legend for Fig. 3 for other details.

is not known and warrants further investigation. In conjunction with the findings of Bleecker et al. (1971), these observations indicate that there are well-defined differences in T$_3$ accumulation and degradation which change with advancing age. The degree to which these changes can be related to an effect of the hormone itself on the synthesis of enzymes involved with transport or degradation, or to changes in intracellular affinity because of an increase in specific protein binding sites, is not known at this time. However, because thyroid hormones appear to play a significant role in protein synthesis, some of the proteins which respond to thyroid stimulation might be those associated with the transport, degradation, or binding of the hormone to the tissue. It would be important in future investigations to determine further how the hormone may influence its subsequent fate in relation to the synthesis of these proteins.

The observations of a sex difference in accumulation of T$_3$ during this early postnatal period is of interest because of the possible interaction between hormones, and because of the varied roles which the three hormones play in hypothalamic differentiation and subsequent adult behavioral manifestations. This seems of particular relevance in view of the post-pubertal differences in accumulation of [³H]lysine (Kartzinel et al., 1971) by male and female cerebral cortex and of the difference in the RNA base ratios, particularly in the hypothalamus.

Thus, there are numerous well-known effects of thyroid hormones on the growth and differentiation of neurons, the functional enzyme systems within the tissues of the nervous system, and effects on myelin formation. There are also changes in thyroid hormone accumulation and degradation which may be directly or indirectly associated with the role the hormones play in protein synthesis and differentiation. Further, the final response of the cells of the CNS to thyroid hormone may be influenced by an interaction with the gonadal hormones as evidenced by the sex differences in $[^{131}I]T_3$ accumulation and the effects of gonadectomy. In this regard, the ovarian hormones seem to exert a greater postpubertal influence than androgens. In view of such potential interactions, it may be difficult to define what aspects of neuronal or glial growth and differentiation are precisely related to thyroid hormones and what aspects depend on one of the other hormones, or to an interaction between several of the hormones: e.g., the prolongation of postnatal cell division in the CNS as influenced by corticosterone in rats, compared with the shortening of the proliferative phase in favor of a differential phase caused by thyroid hormone (Balázs, Brookbank, Patel, Johnson, and Wilson, 1971a; Hamburgh, Mendoza, Burkart, and Weil, 1971; Schapiro, 1968; Schapiro, Salas, and Vukovich, 1970).

REFERENCES

Andersen, H. J. (1966): Congenital hypothyroidism. *Sandoz J. Med. Sci.,* 7:210–219.

Andersen, H. J. (1971): Prenatal damage in hypothyroidism. In: *Hormones and Development,* edited by M. Hamburgh and E. J. W. Barrington, pp. 558–566. Appleton-Century-Crofts, New York.

Balázs, R., Brookbank, B. W. L., Davidson, A. N., Eayrs, J. T., and Wilson, D. A. (1969): The effect of neonatal thyroidectomy on myelination in the rat brain. *Brain Res.,* 15:219–232.

Balázs, R., Brookbank, B. W. L., Patel, A. J., Johnson, A. L., and Wilson, D. A. (1971a): Incorporation of (^{35}S) sulfate into brain constituents during development and the effects of thyroid hormone on myelination. *Brain Res.,* 30:273–293.

Balázs, R., and Cocks, W. A. (1967): RNA metabolism in subcellular fractions of brain tissue. *J. Neurochem.,* 14:1035–1055.

Balázs, R., Cocks, W. A., Eayrs, J. T., and Kovacs, S. (1971b): Biochemical effects of thyroid hormones on the developing brain. In: *Hormones in Development,* edited by M. Hamburgh and E. J. Barrington, pp. 357–379. Appleton-Century-Crofts, New York.

Balázs, R., Kovacs, S., Cocks, W. A., Johnson, A. L., and Eayrs, J. T. (1971c): Effect of thyroid hormone on the biochemical maturation of rat brain: Postnatal cell formation. *Brain Res.,* 25:555–570.

Balázs, R., Kovacs, S., Teichgräber, P., Cocks, W. A., and Eayrs, J. T. (1968): Biochemical effects of thyroid deficiency on the developing brain. *J. Neurochem.,* 15:1335–1349.

Bass, N., and Young, E. (1973): Effects of hypothyroidism on the differentiation of neurons and glia in developing rat cerebrum. *J. Neurol. Sci.,* 18:155–173.

Bleecker, M. L., Ford, D. H., and Rhines, R. K. (1971): Accumulation of ^{131}I-L-triiodothyronine in the rat brain: Effect of age and sex. In: *Influence of Hormones on the Nervous System,* edited by D. H. Ford, pp. 231–239. S. Karger, Basel.

Bondareff, W., and Pysh, J. J. (1968): Distribution of the extracellular space during postnatal maturation of rat cerebral cortex. *Anat. Rec.,* 160:773–780.

Bradley, P. B., Eayrs, J. T., Glass, A., and Heath, R. W. (1961): The maturational and metabolic consequences of neonatal thyroidectomy upon the recruiting response in the rat. *Electroenceph. Clin. Neurophysiol.,* 13:577–586.

Bradley, P. B., Eayrs, J. T., and Schmalbach, K. (1960): The electroencephalogram of normal and hypothyroid rats. *Electroenceph. Clin. Neurophysiol.,* 12:467–477.

Clos, J. M. (1972): Etude histochemique et biochemique de la deficience thyroidienne et de la thyroxine sur le dévelopment de l'activité cholinestérasique dans le cervelet du jeune rat. *C. R. Acad. Sci. (Paris),* 275:2917–2920.

Cohan, S., Ford, D. H., and Rhines, R. K. (1967): The effect of age on the uptake and degradation of thyroid hormone by the brain and skeletal muscle. *Acta Neurol. Scand.,* 43:11–32.

Cuaron, A., Gamble, J. A., Myant, N. B., and Osario, C. (1963): The effect of thyroid deficiency on the growth of the brain and the deposition of brain phospholipids in foetal and newborn rabbits. *J. Physiol.,* 168:613–630.

Eayrs, J. T. (1953): Thyroid hypofunction and the development of the central nervous system. *Nature,* 172:403–405.

Eayrs, J. T. (1960): Influence of the thyroid on the central nervous system. *Br. Med. Bull.,* 16:122–127.

Eayrs, J. T. (1961): Age as a factor determining the severity and reversibility of the effects of thyroid deprivation in the rat. *J. Endocrinol.,* 22:409–419.

Eayrs, J. T. (1964): Endocrine influence on cerebral development. *Arch. Biol.,* 75:529–565.

Eayrs, J. T. (1966): Thyroid and central nervous development. In: *Scientific Basis of Medicine Annual Reviews,* pp. 317–339. University of London Athlone Press, London.

Eayrs, J. T., and Lishman, W. A. (1955): The maturation of behaviour in hypothyroidism and starvation. *Br. J. Anim. Behav.,* 3:17–24.

Essman, W. B., Mendoza, L. A., and Hamburgh, M. (1968): Critical periods of maze acquisition development in euthyroid and hypothyroid rodents. *Psychol. Rep.,* 23:795–800.

Fagge, C. H. (1871): On sporadic cretinism occurring in England. *Br. Med. J.,* 1:279.

Fazekas, J. F., Graves, F. B., and Alman, R. W. (1951): The influence of the thyroid on cerebral metabolism. *Endocrinology,* 38:169–174.

Ford, D. H. (1971): (^{131}I) Triiodothyronine transport into rat cerebral cortex slices. *J. Neurol. Sci.,* 14:107–117.

Ford, D. H. (1974): Thyroid hormones in relation to development of the nervous system. In: *Drugs and the Developing Brain,* edited by A. Vernadakis and N. Weiner, pp. 451–471. Plenum Press, New York.

Ford, D. H., and Rhines, R. K. (1967): Accumulation of ^{131}I-triiodothyronine in neurons and other tissues following intravenous injection of the labeled hormone. *Brain Res.,* 6:481–488.

Ford, D. H., and Rhines, R. K. (1970): Effect of age on the accumulation of (^{131}I) triiodothyronine in male and female rat brains and other tissues. *Brain Res.,* 21:265–274.

Garcia Argiz, C. A., Pasquini, J. M., Kaplún, B., and Gómez, C. J. (1967): Hormonal regulation of brain development. II. Effect of neonatal thyroidectomy on succinate dehydrogenase and other enzymes in developing cerebral cortex and cerebellum of the rat. *Brain Res.,* 6:635–646.

Geel, S. E., and Timiras, P. S. (1967a): The influence of neonatal hypothyroidism and of thyroxine on the ribonucleic acid and desoxyribonucleic acid concentration of rat cerebral cortex. *Brain Res.,* 4:135–142.

Geel, S. E., and Timiras, P. S. (1967b): Influence of neonatal hypothyroidism and of thyroxine on the acetylcholinesterase and cholinesterase activities in the developing central nervous system of the rat. *Endocrinology,* 80:1069–1074.

Geel, S. E., and Timiras, P. S. (1971): The role of thyroid and growth hormone on RNA metabolism in the immature brain. In: *Hormones in Development,* edited by M. Hamburgh and E. J. W. Barrington, pp. 391–402. Appleton-Century-Crofts, New York.

Geel, S. E., and Valcana, T. (1971): Cerebral RNA metabolism and thyroid function in early life. In: *Influence of Hormones on the Nervous System,* edited by D. H. Ford, pp. 165–173. S. Karger, Basel.

Gelber, S., Campbell, P. L., Deibler, G. E., and Sokoloff, L. (1964): Effects of L-thyroxine on amino acid incorporation into protein in mature and immature rat brain. *J. Neurochem.,* 11:221–229.

Ghittoni, N. E., and Gómez, C. J. (1964): Respiration and aerobic glycolysis in rat cerebral cortex during postnatal maturation. Influence of hypothyroidism. *Life Sci.,* 3:979–986.

Gona, A. G. (1973): Effects of thyroxine, thyrotropin, prolactin, and growth hormone on the maturation of the frog cerebellum. *Exp. Neurol.,* 38:494–501.

Grippo, J., and Menkes, J. H. (1971): Effect of thyroid on fatty acid biosynthesis in brain. *Pediatr. Res.,* 5:466–471.

Hamburgh, M. (1968): An analysis of the action of thyroid hormones on development based on *in vivo* and *in vitro* studies. *Gen. Comp. Endocrinol.,* 10:198–213.

Hamburgh, M. (1969): The role of thyroid and growth hormones in neurogenesis. In: *Current Topics in Developmental Biology,* Vol. 4, pp. 109–148. Academic Press, New York.

Hamburgh, M., and Bunge, R. P. (1964): Evidence for a direct effect of thyroid hormone on maturation of nervous tissue grown *in vitro. Life Sci.,* 3:1423–1430.

Hamburgh, M. and Flexner, L. B. (1957): Biochemical and physiological differentiation during morphogenesis. XXI. Effect of hypothyroidism and hormone therapy on enzyme activities of the developing cerebral cortex of the rat. *J. Neurochem.,* 1:279–288.

Hamburgh, M., Lynn, E., and Weiss, E. P. (1964): Analysis of the influence of thyroid hormone on prenatal and postnatal maturation of the rat. *Anat. Rec.,* 150:147–161.

Hamburgh, M., Mendoza, L. A., Burkart, J. F., and Weil, F. (1971): Thyroid-dependent processes in the developing nervous system. In: *Hormones in Development,* edited by M. Hamburgh and E. J. W. Barrington, pp. 403–415. Appleton-Century-Crofts, New York.

Hatotani, N., and Timiras, P. S. (1967): Influence of thyroid function on the postnatal development of the transcallosal response in the rat. *Neuroendocrinology,* 2:147–156.

Jarlstedt, J., and Norstrom, A. (1972): Effect of neonatal hypothyroidism and hyperthyroidism on amino acid incorporation into proteins of subcellular fractions from developing brain tissue. *Exp. Neurol.,* 34:51–63.

Kartzinel, R., Ford, D. H., and Rhines, R. K. (1971): Lysine accumulation in the protein-containing fraction of the rat brain. The effect of age, sex and neonatal castration. In: *Influence of Hormones on the Nervous System,* edited by D. H. Ford, pp. 296–305. S. Karger, Basel.

Krawiec, L., García Argiz, C. A., Gómez, C. J., and Pasquini, J. M. (1969): Hormonal regulation of brain development. III. Effects of triiodothyronine and growth hormone on the biochemical changes in the cerebral cortex and cerebellum of neonatally thyroidectomized rats. *Brain Res.,* 15:209–218.

Legrande, J. (1965): Influence de l'hypothyroidisme sur la maturation du cortex cerebelleux. *C. R. Acad. Sci. (Paris),* 261:544–547.

Legrande, J. (1967): Analyse de l'action morphogenetique des hormones thyroidiennes sur le cervelet du jeune rat. *Arch. Anat. Microsc. Morphol. Exp.,* 56:205–244.

Lotmar, F. (1933): Histopathologische Befunde in Gehirnen von endemischen Kretinismus, Thyreoalasie, und Kachexia thyreopriva. *Z. Ges. Neurol. Psych.,* 146:1–53.

Marcucci, F., and Airoldi, L. (1969): Postnatal changes in brain aspartic and glutamic acid content of normal and hypothyroid suckling rats. *J. Neurochem.,* 16:673–674.

Meisami, E., Valcana, T., and Timiras, P. S. (1970): Effects of neonatal hypothyroidism on the development of brain excitability in the rat. *Neuroendocrinology,* 6:160–167.

Mitskevich, M. S., and Moskovkin, G. N. (1971): Some effects of thyroid hormone on the development of the central nervous system in early ontogenesis. In: *Hormones in Development,* edited by M. Hamburgh and E. J. Barrington, pp. 437–452. Appleton-Century-Crofts, New York.

Nievel, J. G., Robinson, N., and Eayrs, J. T. (1968): Protein synthesis in the brain of rats thyroidectomized at birth. *Experentia,* 24:677–678.

Pasquini, J. M., Kaplún, B., García Argiz, C. A., and Gómez, C. J. (1967): Hormonal regulation of brain development. I. The effect of neonatal thyroidectomy upon nucleic acids, protein and two enzymes in developing cortex and cerebellum of the rat. *Brain Res.,* 6:621–634.

Patel, A. J., and Balázs, R. (1971): Effect of thyroid hormone on metabolic compartmentation in the developing rat brain. *Biochem. J.,* 121:469–481.

Pesetsky, I. (1962): The thyroxine stimulated enlargement of Mauthner's neuron in anurans. *Gen. Comp. Endocrinol.,* 2:229–235.

Pesetsky, I. (1966): The role of the thyroid in the development of Mauthner's neuron. A karyometric study in thyroidectomized anuran larvae. *Z. Zellforsch.,* 75:138–145.

Pitt-Rivers, R., and Tata, J. R. (1959): *The Thyroid Hormones.* Pergamon Press, New York.

Robinson, N., and Eayrs, J. T. (1968): Histochemical study of the cerebral cortex in rats thyroidectomized at birth. *Brain Res.,* 9:351–362.

Salas, M., and Schapiro, S. (1970): Hormonal influences upon the maturation of the rat brain's responsiveness to sensory stimuli. *Physiol. Behav.,* 5:7–11.

Schapiro, S. (1968): Some physiological, biochemical and behavioural consequences of neonatal hormone administration: Cortisol and thyroxine. *Gen. Comp. Endocrinol.*, 10:214–228.

Schapiro, S., Salas, M., and Vukovich, K. (1970): Hormonal effects on ontogeny of swimming ability in the rat: Assessment of central nervous system development. *Science*, 168:147–150.

Schneck, L., Ford, D. H., and Rhines, R. K. (1965): The uptake of S^{35}-L-methionine into the brain of euthyroid and hyperthyroid neonatal rats. *Acta Neurol. Scand.*, 40:285–290.

Schultz, M. A., Schultz, F. J., and Parmale, A. H. (1967): Schilddrüsenhorman und hirnentwicklung. *Monatsschr. Kinderheilkd.*, 115:284–285.

Sokoloff, L. (1964): The action of thyroid hormones on protein synthesis, as studied in isolated preparations and in the whole rat. *Proc. Sec. Int. Cong. Endocrinol. Excerpta Med. Int. Cong. Series*, 83:87–94.

Sokoloff, L., and Kaufman, S. (1961): Thyroxine stimulation of amino acid incorporation into protein. *J. Biol. Chem.*, 236:795–803.

Sokoloff, L., Kaufman, S., Campbell, P. L., Francis, C. M., and Gelboin, H. V. (1962): Thyroxine stimulation of amino acid incorporation into protein. Localization of stimulated step. *J. Biol. Chem.*, 238:1432–1437.

Sokoloff, L., and Roberts, P. (1971): Biochemical mechanisms of the action of thyroid hormones in nervous and other tissues. In: *Influence of Hormones on the Nervous System*, edited by D. H. Ford, pp. 213–230. S. Karger, Basel.

Soriero, O., and Ford, D. H. (1971): Age and sex: The effect on the composition of different regions of the neonatal rat brain. In: *Influence of Hormones on the Nervous System*, edited by D. H. Ford, pp. 322–333. S. Karger, Basel.

Szijan, I., Chepelinsky, A. B., and Piras, M. M. (1971): Effect of neonatal thyroidectomy on enzymes in subcellular fractions of rat brain. *Brain Res.*, 20:313–318.

Szijan, I., Kalbermann, L. E., and Gómez, C. J. (1971): Hormonal regulation of brain development. IV. Effect of neonatal thyroidectomy upon incorporation *in vivo* of (^{3}H) phenylalanine into proteins of developing rat cerebral tissue. *Brain Res.*, 27:309–318.

Tata, J. R. (1964): Distribution and metabolism of thyroid hormones. In: *The Thyroid Gland*, edited by R. Pitt-Rivers and W. R. Trotter, pp. 163–186. Butterworths, London.

Turakulov, Y. K., Gol'ber, L. M., Gagel'gans, A. I., Kandror, V. I., Salakhova, N. S., Mirakhmedov, A. K., and Gaidina, G. A. (1972): *The Thyroid Hormones*. Fan. Tashkent.

Valcana, T. (1971): Effect of neonatal hypothyroidism on the development of acetylcholinesterase and choline acetyltransferase activities in the rat brain. In: *Influence of Hormones on the Nervous System*, edited by D. H. Ford, pp. 174–184. S. Karger, Basel.

Valcana, T., and Timiras, P. S. (1969): Effect of hypothyroidism on ionic metabolism and Na-K activated ATP phosphohydrolase activity in the developing rat brain. *J. Neurochem.*, 16:935–943.

Vernadakis, A., and Woodbury, D. M. (1962): Electrolyte and amino acid changes in rat brain during maturation. *Am. J. Physiol.*, 203:748.

Walravens, P., and Chase, H. P. (1969): Influence of thyroid on formation of myelin lipids. *J. Neurochem.*, 16:1477–1484.

Weiss, P., and Rossetti, F. (1951): Growth responses of opposite sign among different neuron types exposed to thyroid hormone. *Proc. Natl. Acad. Sci. (USA)*, 37:540–556.

DISCUSSION

Lauder: Do you see any differences in the time course of uptake in the hippocampus vs. cerebellum?

Ford: We did not determine uptake in the hippocampus. More recently, we have studied RNA and protein synthesis in hippocampus compared with hypothalamus. There are developmental differences which are sex-related. However, we did not investigate the effect of thyroid hormone on this phenomenon.

Valcana: Have you studied the uptake of thyroxine by the brain in animals thyroidectomized at birth? In other words, if this increased uptake was related to T_4 receptors or to the development of such receptors, it could, in turn, be regulated by the availability of T_4.

Ford: Possibly, but we have not studied that yet. It would be exciting to study the development of receptors.

Sokoloff: Might not the uptake into the tissues be influenced by the development of the plasma proteins which have such a strong binding effect on thyroid hormones, and thereby influence the free levels which are available for diffusion or transport into the tissues? The plasma protein-binding capacity for thyroid hormones is continually altered during this developmental period.

Ford: Yes, but an increase in plasma proteins would depress uptake, whereas we saw an increase. The plasma proteins which are synthesized in that early period might not be the binding proteins for thyroid hormones.

Balázs: Have you any information on the specificity of thyroid hormone uptake in the cells in the brain? Is there any indication that a specific binding process may be involved in your case?

Ford: No.

Balázs: This question has become important with respect to the mechanism of the action of thyroid hormone, since it has been demonstrated that specific binding proteins for thyroid hormone, especially for T_3, occur in various tissues, including brain.

Ford: We have speculated that this is related to a development of a specific thyroid-binding protein, but we have not done any studies on it yet.

Bass: I am also curious to know why you used T_3 rather than T_4, since the major circulating thyroid hormone, in terms of quantity, is T_4.

Ford: At one time we did a comparison study on the relative uptakes of T_4 versus T_3 into brains of several species of animals. T_3 is taken up about three to five times more readily than T_4 by brain. This reflects the proportionately lowered binding to plasma protein. Initially we wondered whether there was a blood-brain barrier to T_4 and not to T_3. We concluded that their differential uptake relates to their degree of binding to plasma protein. Since we used relatively small tracer doses (0.5 μg/kg), we selected T_3 since it would be taken up more readily by the brain than T_4.

Bass: By the same token, though, T_3 is degraded about three times faster than T_4.

Ford: T_3 is degraded three times faster because it is taken up three to five times more readily. Its catabolism also reflects its capacity to bind to plasma proteins because this determines how much hormone is available to be taken up and degraded.

Bass: Do you think that T_3 is the important biologic component of circulating thyroid hormone, especially in regard to brain development?

Ford: At one time we thought that. However, it is difficult to say flatly that such is the whole truth. Since T_3 is taken up more readily than T_4, one would think it might be more biologically active because of its availability. Since both compounds are taken up, however, perhaps they are active in proportion to their circulating free levels in plasma. Their relative contributions to biological activity would then have to be calculated in relation to their uptakes. I do not know if there is a transport mechanism for T_4 as there is for T_3.

Sokoloff: People have been saying for years that T_4 itself is not the active molecule because of its long latent period of action; it must be converted to something else first. When T_3 was first discovered simultaneously by Pitt-Rivers and by Roche, everyone thought they had found the active form of T_4. For various reasons, this idea went out of fashion until recently. The issue has now been brought up again by the evidence that in peripheral tissues there are mechanisms for converting T_4 to T_3. Oppenheimer's group, in particular, advocates the concept that T_4 must be converted to T_3 in the tissues before any biological activity ensues. This question remains open, and I am not prepared to take sides.

Thyroid Hormones and Brain Development,
edited by Gilman D. Grave. Raven Press,
New York, 1977.

Ultrastructural Changes in the Hypothalamo-Hypophyseal Axis in Rats Thyroidectomized at Birth

Eva B. Cramer and Donald H. Ford*

When thyroid deficiency occurs in humans early in life, it causes the mental retardation associated with cretinism. Attempts to study the effects of thyroid deficiency on brain development have led investigators to study animals such as the rat, which show a significant degree of brain development after birth (Balàzs, Cocks, Eayrs, and Kovacs, 1971). In rats made hypothyroid soon after birth, those parts of the neuraxis that mature late, such as the cerebral cortex and the cerebellar cortex, do not develop normally, and hypoplasia of the neurons and neuropil occurs (Eayrs and Taylor, 1951; Eayrs, 1955; Legrand, 1967). There also are abnormalities in the vascularity of the cerebral cortex (Eayrs, 1954). Recent evidence now indicates that the hypothalamo-hypophyseal axis also continues to mature after birth with pituitary thyroid-stimulating hormone (TSH) and hypothalamic thyrotropin-releasing factor (TRF)-like activity reaching adult levels in the first and second postnatal weeks, respectively (Conklin, Schindler, and Hull, 1973). The anterior pituitary plasma flow in the hypothalamic-pituitary portal system reaches adult levels by the fourth postnatal day, but blood flow does not reach adult levels until 25 days (Florsheim and Rudko, 1968). With this in mind, we studied the ultrastructural effects of neonatal hypothyroidism on the development of the hypothalamus and anterior pituitary. Because the medial basal hypothalamus in the region of the arcuate nucleus and median eminence has been shown to concentrate labeled thyroid hormone (Ford, Kontounis, and Lawrence, 1959), we centered our investigation in this area of the hypothalamus.

MATERIALS AND METHODS

Animals

Pregnant Sprague-Dawley rats (second or third litters) were obtained from Charles River Breeding Laboratories. Within 24 hr of birth, the pups were

---

* Department of Anatomy, Downstate Medical Center, State University of New York, Brooklyn, New York 11203.

removed from their mothers and grouped together by sex. From these groups, 4 female and 4 male pups were selected randomly and returned to the mothers. The litters were scrambled in this manner in an attempt to eliminate any normal differences which might occur between litters. Six litters were established in this manner.

Treatment

Pups were injected intraperitoneally with a single dose of either physiological saline or 210 μCi Na ^{131}I as described by Goldberg and Chaikoff (1949). Control animals were kept in separate litter groups to prevent contamination by [131]I. Animals were weighed at weekly intervals and were killed at 1, 14, 28, and 41 days of age. Only 2 of the hypothyroid animals survived 41 days. At the time of death the endocrine organs were removed and weighed. By 28 days, significant differences in body and endocrine weights were apparent, and tissue from the pituitary and medial basal hypothalamus was processed for electron microscopy. Gross and histological examination of the thyroid region of the trachea of these animals revealed no visible thyroid tissue.

Electron Microscopy

Hypothalamic and pituitary tissues were prepared for electron microscopy by different procedures. If the rats were to be used to study the CNS, the animals were pretreated with heparin, anesthetized with ether, and perfused with phosphate-buffered glutaraldehyde-paraformaldehyde (Sotelo and Palay, 1968; modified by Cohen and Pappas, 1969). The brains were removed after perfusion, and the median eminence arcuate region was cut into 1-mm blocks of tissue and kept in fixative for 2 to 3 hr. These small blocks were rinsed, stored in 0.1 M phosphate buffer overnight, then postfixed in 1% OsO_4 in 0.1 M phosphate buffer for 1 hr, dehydrated, and embedded in Epon. Thin sections were cut, stained with uranyl acetate and lead citrate, and then examined with a Philips 300 electron microscope.

If the pituitary tissue was to be examined, the animals were decapitated and the pituitary quickly removed. The anterior was separated from the posterior pituitary, fixed in 2% glutaraldehyde in 0.1 M phosphate buffer for 4 hr, and then processed in a manner similar to that from the median eminence arcuate region.

RESULTS

Body and Endocrine Weight

Neonatal hypothyroidism caused a marked impairment in body growth (Fig. 1). By 26 days, both male and female rats were significantly smaller

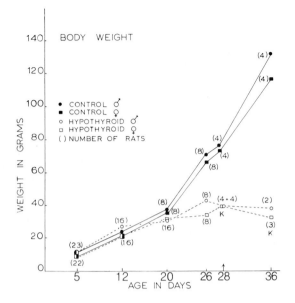

FIG. 1. Graphic representation of change in body weight of control and hypothyroid male and female rats.

than their controls, with impairment in the growth of endocrine organs (Table 1). The absolute weights of the testes, ovaries, and adrenals were significantly smaller than corresponding controls. However, because body weights of the experimental animals were significantly lighter than controls, the endocrine gland weights were compared in relation to body weight; then, only the testes weighed significantly less than controls.

Anterior Pituitary

By 28 days, the cells of the anterior pituitary of control animals were well granulated (Fig. 2) and acidophils and basophils were distinguishable. Mitotic figures were seen frequently and occurred more often in male than female rats. The dividing cells were differentiated, granulated pituitary cells. Somatotrophs were the most common cell type seen undergoing mitosis (Fig. 4), but examples of gonadotrophs (Fig. 5), thyrotrophs (Fig. 6), and follicular cells (Fig. 7) were also observed.

In hypothyroid animals the pituitary cells appeared less granulated (Fig. 3) because of a decrease in the number of granules in somatotrophs. Many cells in various stages of transformation into "thyroidectomy" cells were seen, recognized by the presence of the characteristic granules and the dilated rough endoplasmic reticulum. In some of these cells, the enlarged rough endoplasmic reticulum also contained spherical electron-dense structures which looked like secretory granules. In these animals, the number of mitotic figures was three to four times fewer than that of controls. As in control animals, more mitotic figures were seen in male than in female rats.

TABLE 1. Endocrine gland weights in control and newborn thyroidectomized rats at 28 days of age

| | Testes ($n = 4$) | | Ovary ($n = 4$) | | Adrenal ($n = 8$) | |
	Mean weight (g) ± SEM	Percent weight	Mean weight (g) ± SEM	Percent weight	Mean weight (g) ± SEM	Percent weight
Control	437.0 ± 31.84	0.557 ± 0.018	18.00 ± 1.61	0.024 ± 0.002	17.96 ± 1.13	0.023 ± 0.003
Hypothyroid	59.3 ± 7.60[a]	0.148 ± 0.017[a]	8.20 ± 1.22[b]	0.023 ± 0.004	11.40 ± 1.21[b]	0.029 ± 0.001

[a] $p < 0.001$.
[b] $p < 0.005$.

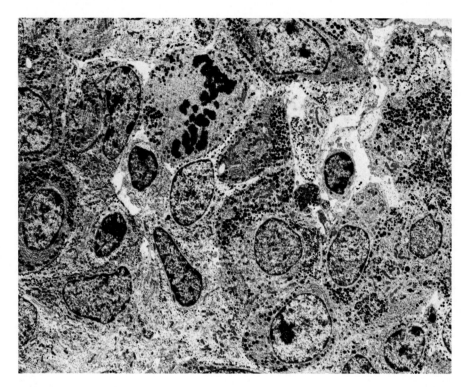

FIG. 2. Adenohypophysis of control 28-day-old female rat. The cells are well differentiated and mostly somatotrophs. Note the relative granularity of the cells and the somatotroph undergoing mitosis. × 2,200.

The cells in mitosis were mostly thyrotrophs or nongranulated cells; relatively few were somatotrophs.

Hypothalamus

Examination of the medial basal hypothalamus in the region of the arcuate nucleus of 28-day-old hypothyroid and control rats disclosed two differences. We noted a small glial cell in both controls and experimental animals, which had an oval nucleus (5 to 6 μm) containing clumped chromatin and a nucleolus, a dense cytoplasm with many ribosomes and a few dense bodies. Although Rinne (1966) considered this cell to be an oligodendroglia, it also fits the description of a microglial cell of Mori and Leblond (1969). While it is common for the oligodendroglia or microglia to contain dense bodies, in our experiment it appeared that the small glial cell of the experimental animals contained more dense bodies (Fig. 8) than those of the control animals.

The second and perhaps more striking difference between experimental

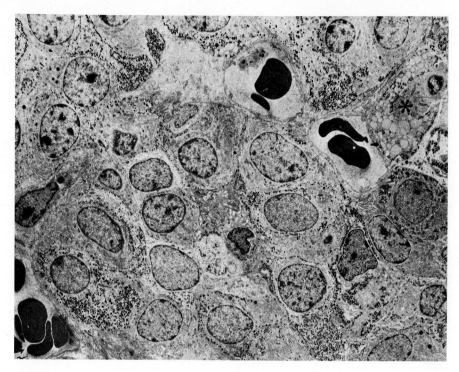

FIG. 3. Adenohypophysis of hypothyroid 28-day-old male rat. Although the cells are differentiated, they appear relatively degranulated. Note the "thyroidectomy" cell (∗) with its dilated endoplasmic reticulum. × 1,500.

and control groups was in the perikaryon of the neurons of the arcuate nucleus. The arcuate neurons of thyroidectomized animals contained more whorled formations of closely apposed concentric cisternae of smooth endoplasmic reticulum (ratio approximately 7:1) (Fig. 9). The outermost cisternae of the whorls had ribosomes on the outer membranes and were continuous with the cisternae of rough endoplasmic reticulum. The whorled bodies appeared in slightly different variations; the intercisternal distances were not always uniform, nor were the outer cisternae always completely wrapped around the whorl but sometimes formed semicircular incomplete outer rings. Clear vesicles were frequently found in the center of the whorls. In all cases, the whorled bodies occurred singly in the perikaryon.

DISCUSSION

At 28 days, the gross effects of neonatal hypothyroidism were evident. The animals were significantly smaller in size and appeared stunted, and their endocrine weights were significantly reduced. Of particular interest

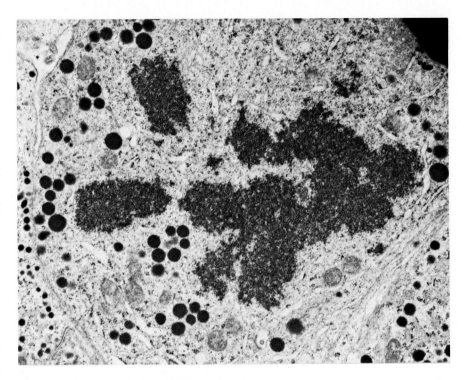

FIG. 4. Somatotroph of a control 28-day-old female rat undergoing mitosis. × 9,800.

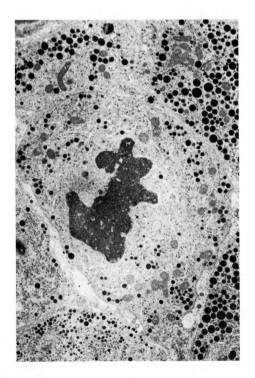

FIG. 5. Basophil (presumably gonado-troph) of a control 28-day-old female rat in telophase. × 6,800.

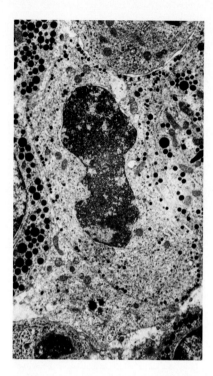

FIG. 6. Basophil (presumably thyrotroph) of a control 28-day-old female rat in telophase. × 6,800.

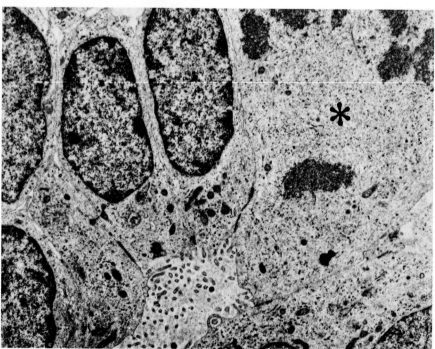

FIG. 7. Follicular cells of anterior pituitary of a control 28-day-old female rat. One cell (✱) surrounding the follicular lumen is undergoing mitosis. × 6,800.

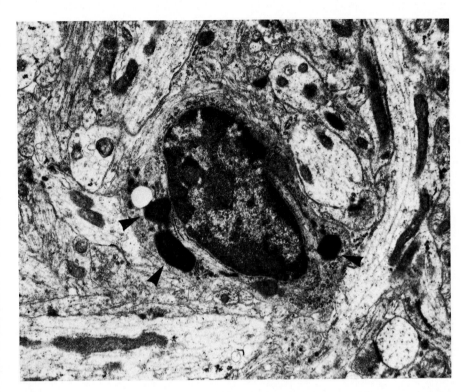

FIG. 8. Small glial cell from median eminence arcuate region of hypothyroid 28-day-old female rat. The cell contains an oval nucleus with clumped chromatin and a nucleolus. The cytoplasm is dark with many free ribosomes and dense bodies (*arrow*). ×13,600.

were the very small testes in the 28-day-old hypothyroid rats. The effects of hypothyroidism on the developing gonads persist into adulthood, because perinatal treatment with propylthiouracil (PTU) results in delayed puberty (as indicated by a delay in vaginal openings), and there is an interference in normal cyclicity (as revealed by a significant lengthening of estrous cycles) (Bakke, Gellert, and Lawrence, 1970). However, Kikuyama, Nagasawa, Yanai, and Yamanouchi (1974) report that if PTU treatment is stopped on day 20, testis weight returns to normal by day 60. In contrast to neonatal hypothyroidism, induction of chronic hypothyroidism in adult male rats significantly decreases pituitary luteinizing hormone (LH) and follicle-stimulating hormone (FSH) but does not modify testicular function or weight (Vilchez-Martinez, 1973).

The effects of neonatal hypothyroidism on the developing pituitary gland are in many ways similar to the effects of chronic hypothyroidism on the adult gland. Cytological changes in this experiment and in the adult pars distalis (Purves and Griesbach, 1946; Farquhar and Rinehart, 1954) con-

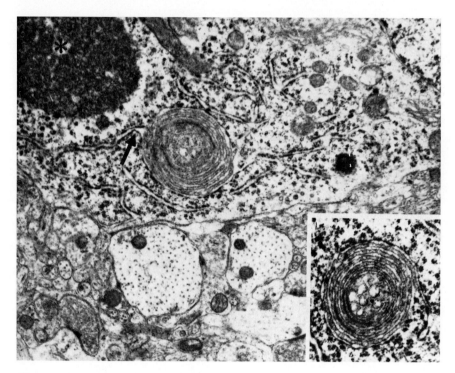

FIG. 9. Portion of cell body of an arcuate neuron [containing the characteristic "chromatoid body" (∗)] from a hypothyroid 28-day-old female rat. The rough endoplasmic reticulum is continuous (*arrow*) with a whorled body. The outermost membrane of the whorl is studded with ribosomes, whereas the inner cisternal membranes are free of ribosomes. ×13,600. The cytoplasmic core of the whorled body contains vacuoles. (*inset*) ×15,300.

sist essentially of the development of numerous thyroidectomy cells and a degranulation of acidophils. These cytological changes seen during development corroborate physiological experiments with 20-day-old rats of PTU-treated mothers. The anterior pituitary glands of these pups contain significantly less growth hormone (GH) and prolactin than those of normal controls (Kikuyama et al., 1974).

The results of this study indicate that neonatal hypothyroidism reduces the number of pituitary cells undergoing mitosis in the developing pituitary gland and causes a shift in the type of mitotic cells (from predominantly somatotrophs to fewer somatotrophs and more thyrotrophs). This shift resembles the response of pituitary cells in the adult. Mitosis is infrequent in the adult pituitary gland (Leblond and Walker, 1956). However, using high-resolution autoradiography in normal adult male rat anterior pituitary glands, Stratmann, Eznn, Sellers, and Simon (1972) observed tritiated thymidine label over some pituitary cells. Most of the labeled cells were somatotrophs. In PTU-treated adult animals the number of labeled cells decreased and, of those labeled, a greater number belonged to thyrotropin-producing cells (Stratmann et al., 1972). There is a similarity in the response of the neonatal and adult pituitary gland to thyroid deficiency. Although the neonatal hypothalamic pituitary axis is neither physiologically (Conklin et al., 1973) nor structurally (Florsheim and Rudko, 1968) mature, the neonatal pituitary gland responds to thyroidectomy like that of the adult.

Arcuate neurons in neonatal thyroidectomized rats exhibit one obvious difference from normal animals: an increase in whorled bodies. The response of these neonatal cells to thyroidectomy is similar to the response of the adult arcuate neuron cells to castration. Brawer (1971) reported whorled bodies in arcuate nuclei, as many as five in a single cell. Whether the fewer number of whorled bodies per cell in this experiment reflects a normal difference in physiological response or a less mature cell is unclear. It is interesting that neurons of the arcuate nucleus respond to a loss of negative feedback from different target organs in a similar manner. In this experiment and in Brawer's castration experiments, not all the neurons developed whorls. Brawer (1971) deduced, therefore, that the arcuate nucleus comprises a heterogenous population of nerve cells; this experiment supports his idea.

The role of the arcuate nucleus in the neuroendocrine control of the pituitary is unknown. Both thyroid hormone (Ford et al., 1959) and estradiol (Stumpf, 1968; Attramadal, 1970) concentrate in this region in the rat. Yet, localization of luteinizing hormone-releasing hormone (LHRH) occurs in the peripheral region of the median eminence of the rat (Baker, Dermody, and Reel, 1974), and the exact site of thyrotropin-releasing factor (TRF) formation is not known (Schally, Arimura, and Kastin, 1973).

The significance of the whorled body is uncertain. It is seen in other areas, such as testicular interstitial cells (Christensen and Fawcett, 1966), and the ductus deferens (Hamilton, Jones, and Fawcett, 1969). When observed in neurons of the median eminence arcuate region, as in mature female rats during diestrus, or in castrate female rats (King, Williams, and Gerrall, 1973), in male castrates (Brawer, 1971), or in male rats after morphine (Ford, Voeller, Callegari, and Gresik, 1974), it is postulated to be a sign of enhanced synthetic activity. Whereas the rough endoplasmic reticulum in the arcuate nuclei responds to neonatal hypothyroidism by developing whorls of smooth endoplasmic reticulum, the rough endoplasmic reticulum in the thyroidectomy cells of the anterior pituitary gland dilate and coalesce. In both cases the morphologic appearance of the endoplasmic reticulum is altered by either the direct or indirect effect of loss of thyroid hormone.

ACKNOWLEDGMENT

The authors express their thanks to Dr. Nathan Solomon and the Division of Radiation Therapy of the Department of Radiology of the State University Kings County Medical Center for their cooperation in providing Na[131]I whenever needed for this study. We also wish to thank Mr. Jack Illari for his photographic assistance and Mrs. Ida Muntner for her secretarial help in preparing the manuscript.

REFERENCES

Attramadal, A. (1970): Cellular localization of ^{3}H-oestradiol in the hypothalamus. *Z. Zellforsch.*, 104:572–581.

Baker, B. L., Dermody, W. C., and Reel, J. R. (1974): Localization of LHRH in the mammalian hypothalamus. *Am. J. Anat.*, 139:129–34.

Bakke, J. L., Gellert, R. J., and Lawrence, N. L. (1970): The persistent effects of perinatal hypothyroidism on pituitary, thyroidal, and gonadal functions. *J. Lab. Clin. Med.*, 76:25–33.

Balá;zs, R., Cocks, W. A., Eayrs, J. T., and Kovacs, S. (1971): Biochemical effects of thyroid hormones on the developing brain. In: *Hormones in Development*, edited by M. Hamburgh and E. J. Barrington, pp. 357–379. Appleton-Century-Crofts, New York.

Brawer, J. R. (1971): The role of the arcuate nucleus in the brain pituitary-gonad axis. *J. Comp. Neurol.*, 143:411–446.

Christensen, A. K., and Fawcett, D. W. (1966): The fine structure of testicular interstitial cells in mice. *Am. J. Anat.*, 118:551–572.

Cohen, E. B., and Pappas, G. D. (1969): Dark profiles in the apparently normal central nervous system: A problem in the electron microscopic identification of early antegrade axonal degeneration. *J. Comp. Neurol.*, 136:375–395.

Conklin, P. M., Schindler, W. J., and Hull, S. F. (1973): Hypothalamic thyrotropin releasing factor. Activity and pituitary responsiveness during development in the rat. *Neuroendocrinology*, 11:197–211.

Eayrs, J. T. (1954): The vascularity of the cerebral cortex in normal and cretinous rats. *J. Anat. (Lond.)*, 88:164–174.

Eayrs, J. T. (1955): The cerebral cortex of normal and hypothyroid rats. *Acta Anat. (Basel)*, 25:160–183.

Eayrs, J. T., and Taylor, S. H. (1951): The effect of thyroid deficiency induced by methyl thiouracil on the maturation of the central nervous system. *J. Anat. (Lond.)*, 85:350–358.

Farquhar, M. G., and Rinehart, J. F. (1954): Cytologic alterations in the anterior pituitary gland following thyroidectomy: An electron microscope study. *Endocrinology*, 55:857–876.

Florsheim, W. H., and Rudko, P. (1968): The development of portal system function in the rat. *Neuroendocrinology*, 3:89–98.

Ford, D. H., Kantounis, S., and Lawrence, R. (1959): The localization of I[131] labeled triiodothyronine in the pituitary and brain of normal and thyroidectomized male rats. *Endocrinology*, 64:977–991.

Ford, D. H., Voeller, K., Callegari, B., and Gresik, E. (1974): Changes in neurons of the median eminence-arcuate region of rats induced by morphine treatment: An electron microscopic study. *Neurobiology*, 4:1–11.

Goldberg, R. C., and Chaikoff, I. L. (1949): A simplified procedure for thyroidectomy of the newborn rat without concomitant parathyroidectomy. *Endocrinology*, 45:64–70.

Hamilton, D. W., Jones, A. C., and Fawcett, D. W. (1969): Cholesterol biosynthesis in the mouse epididymis and ductus deferens. A biochemical and morphological study. *Biol. Reprod.*, 1:167–184.

Kikuyama, S., Nagasawa, H., Yanai, R., and Yamanouchi, K. (1974): Effect of perinatal hypothyroidism on pituitary secretion of growth hormone and prolactin in rats. *J. Endocrinol.*, 62:213–223.

King, J. C., Williams, T. H., and Gerrall, A. A. (1973): Ultrastructural transformations in rat arcuate neurons during the estrous cycle. *Anat. Rec.*, 175:358.

Leblond, C. P., and Walker, B. E. (1956): Renewal of cell populations. *Physiol. Rev.*, 36:255–276.

Legrand, J. (1967): Analyse de l'action morphogenetique des hormones thyroidiennes sur le cervelet du jeune rat. *Arch. Anat. Microsc. Morphol. Exp.*, 56:205–244.

Mori, S., and Leblond, C. P. (1969): Identification of microglia in light and electron microscopy. *J. Comp. Neurol.*, 135:67–80.

Purves, H. D., and Griesbach, W. E. (1946): Observations on the acidophil changes in the pituitary in thyroxine deficiency states. I. Acidophil degranulation in relation to goitrogenic agents and extrathyroid synthesis. *Br. J. Exp. Pathol.,* 27:170–179.

Rinne, V. K. (1966): Ultrastructure of the median eminence of the rat. *Z. Zellforsch.* 74:98–122.

Schally, A. V., Arimura, A., and Kastin, A. J. (1973): Hypothalamic regulatory hormones. *Science,* 179:241–350.

Sotelo, C., and Palay, S. L. (1968): The fine structure of the lateral vestibular nucleus in the rat. I. Neurons and neuroglial cells. *J. Cell Biol.,* 36:151–179.

Stratmann, I. E., Eznn, C., Sellers, E. A., and Simon, G. T. (1972): The origin of thyroidectomy cells as revealed by high resolution radioautography. *Endocrinology,* 90:728–734.

Stumpf, W. E. (1968): Estradiol concentrating neurons: topography in the hypothalamus by dry-mount autoradiography. *Science,* 162:1001–1003.

Vilchez-Martinez, J. A. (1973): Study of the pituitary testicular axis in hypothyroid adult male rats. *J. Reprod. Fertil.,* 35:123–126.

DISCUSSION

Gona: One of my colleagues has been studying the effect of chronic hypoxia in rats, and he finds very similar lamellar bodies in cells of the cerebral and cerebellar cortices.

Ford: I suspect that the development of a whorl or lamellar body is somewhat nonspecific. However, the degree of response in certain cells might be specific. The recent report of Cragg showed lamellar bodies, but they were different from ours. I have always interpreted what he describes as being myelin figures. There is no doubt that in the hypothyroid or in the morphine study these whorls are associated with endoplasmic reticulum, while Cragg's (1970) report does not show any relation to endoplasmic reticulum.

Balázs: My other question relates to your finding that certain mitotic cells in the anterior pituitary seem to be fully differentiated, in terms of the ultrastructural appearance of the production and packaging of specific proteins. These results argue strongly against my prejudice that differentiated cells do not divide.

Cramer: We, too, were surprised. We thought that perhaps they had divided as chromophobes and then became chromophils; it was obvious that granulated cells were dividing.

Ford: We were rather surprised to see the degree of cell division in the control animals, which are presumably, at least biochemically, mature at 4 weeks of age. Had they been younger animals, we might not have been so surprised.

Cramer: Interestingly, this phenomenon was more prevalent in male than in female rats.

Pesetsky: Do you think the cells of the hypothalamus could have been damaged by the levels of radioiodine that you used to thyroidectomize?

Ford: That is possible, because the level we used is very high, 150 to 200 μCi/pup. On the other hand, the brain does not accumulate iodine. If you inject sodium iodide, or iodine itself, there is little uptake by the brain until iodine becomes organified. Thus, the site of iodine organification gets badly battered by the dose which is given. There seems to be no significant effect on the brain.

Pesetsky: When you give the radioiodine, you are producing labeled thyroid hormone for a brief period of time which could be concentrated in the median arcuate area, because rather high concentrations of thyroid hormone occur in this zone compared with other areas of the brain. This might be significant in terms of your observation of the many lysosomes in the microglia.

Ford: Initially, it appeared as if there were a degradative process or some pathologic response in the hypothyroid rat brains; then we started to find them in the controls as well. There are, certainly, more lysosomes in the microglia in hypo-thyroid brains. Why we see so many microglia in a neonatal animals is another question. In adults we seldom see them. In the brains of 15 adult animals, I have seen only one microglial cell in the median arcuate area.

It has often been stated in the literature that neonatal and adult brain is resistant to high levels of radioactivity. Despite that, we have demonstrated that exposing the head of the neonatal rats to 200 r causes a significant effect on thyroid hormone up-take and degradation. Therefore, I question the whole philosophy about radioresis-tance. The level of radioactivity obtained, if one injects 200 μCi of thymidine, ap-proaches 500 r in a dividing cell. This is a great deal of radiation to be focused at a single point. We may have produced some radiation damage.

Bass: Certainly, the cerebral cortex of a 4-week-old rat is far from mature. In fact, the thyroid-pituitary axis is only mature at 25 days in terms of circulating blood levels of thyroxine and TSH. So I am not surprised that you see mitotic figures. Al-though you might say a cell is postmitotic because of its apparent differentiation, it might not be irreversibly differentiated. Even undifferentiated cells may have com-plicated cytoplasmic architecture and yet divide very rapidly.

The cytoplasmic bodies that you call whorls have been found in other diseases as well as in states of hormonal imbalance. These whorls remind me of the cyto-plasmids found in Tay-Sachs disease: membranous cytoplasmic bodies known to be lysosomally produced. So I wonder if those whorls are not actually products of a dying cell, in which lysosomal release has caused lipid-protein aggregates which you see as membranous cytoplasmic configurations, unrelated to myelin.

DISCUSSION REFERENCE

Cragg, B. G. (1970): Synapses and membranous bodies in experimental hypothyroidism. *Brain Res.*, 18:297–307.

Thyroid Hormones and Brain Development,
edited by Gilman D. Grave. Raven Press,
New York, 1977.

Influences of Thyroid Levels in Brain Ontogenesis *In Vivo* and *In Vitro*

Sally Oklund and Paola S. Timiras**

The study of so-called critical periods represents a favorite pursuit of developmental biologists. Out of this interest, we have identified periods or ages of accelerated growth and/or development that are characterized by increased vulnerability to internal and external environmental influences.

In humans, the critical period during which thyroid hormones influence brain development has been delineated as encompassing the last trimester of fetal development and the first postnatal year. In rats, the corresponding period is telescoped to postnatal days 10 to 12 (Timiras, 1972; Sokoloff and Kennedy, 1973). In both species, this critical period is associated with rapid myelinogenesis, intense proliferation of dendritic and axonal processes and synaptogenesis, and the continuing division of neuroblasts in some brain areas (e.g., the cerebellum) together with the rapid proliferation of glial cells (Timiras, Vernadakis, and Sherwood, 1968). Attempts to determine fetal sensitivity to thyroid hormones in rats have not been successful; thus, studies such as those of Hamburgh, Legrand, and their associates suggest that thyroid activity may not contribute to total body growth and CNS development in the rat fetus (Hamburgh, Lynn, and Weiss, 1964; Legrand, 1969; Clos, Crépel, Legrand, Legrand, Rabié, and Vigouroux, 1974).

Another aspect of thyroid/brain relationships that remains unsolved is whether thyroid hormones regulate brain development through direct action on brain tissue or through generalized metabolic effects. Evidence in support of a direct action has been provided by the experiments of Hamburgh, who has shown that thyroid hormones added *in vitro* to rat cerebellar explants influence both myelination and cell maturation (Hamburgh and Bunge, 1964; Hamburgh, 1969). On the other hand, according to Tata and associates, hypothyroidism does not affect the rate of protein synthesis in brain slices and cell-free systems (Andrews and Tata, 1971), observations which contradict the generally accepted view that thyroid hormones, *in vivo* and *in vitro,* influence protein and nucleic acid metabolism in several tissues, including brain (Gelber, Campbell, Deibler, and Sokoloff, 1964; Geel and Timiras, 1970; Geel and Valcana, 1972; Geel and Gonzales, 1975).

* Department of Anatomy, University of Colorado Medical Center, Denver, Colorado 80220.
** Department of Physiology-Anatomy, University of California at Berkeley, Berkeley, California 94720.

33

The purpose of the present experiments is twofold: (1) to investigate the effect of hypothyroidism in the rat during fetal and early postnatal development; (2) to compare the incorporation of precursors into protein and RNA in explants of cerebral cortex, cerebellum, and hypothalamus from control and hypothyroid animals, with and without addition of thyroxine (T_4) to the medium.

BODY AND ORGAN GROWTH AND MATURATION

Hypothyroidism was induced in the pregnant rat by dietary administration of propylthiouracil (PTU) at conception, day 8 (coincident with rapid brain organogenesis), day 15 (when the thyroid gland begins to develop), and during lactation. Controls were maintained on a standard diet. Pilot experiments indicate that a concentration of 0.2% PTU is effective in producing hypothyroidism without interfering with the success of pregnancy nor the postnatal viability of the offspring.

Body growth was significantly impaired in the offspring of PTU-treated mothers compared with those of controls (Fig. 1). Fetuses of animals treated with PTU at the beginning of gestation were most affected; body weights show significant reduction as early as the 16th gestational day. (Fig. 1; Table 1). The hypertrophy of the thyroid at birth indirectly con-

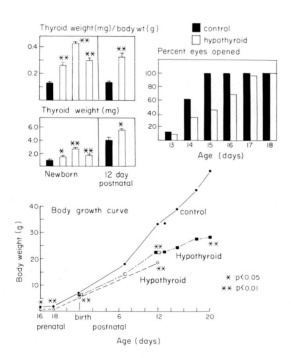

FIG. 1. Effects on growth and development of progeny when dietary PTU is administered to pregnant rats. Growth curve: ●———● = control progeny; ○———○ = progeny of mothers receiving PTU (0.2% since conception); ■———■ = progeny of mothers receiving PTU (0.2% from day 15 of pregnancy); □———□ = progeny of mothers receiving PTU (0.1% from day 15 of pregnancy). Differences between control and hypothyroid groups were determined by Student's *t*-test.

TABLE 1. *Total body and cerebral hemisphere weights in control and hypothyroid rats*

Treatment 0.2% PTU	Total body weight (g)			Cerebral hemisphere weight (mg)		
	Neonatal	Prenatal 18 days	16 days	Neonatal Wet	Neonatal Dry	Prenatal 18 days Wet
Control	6.8 ± 0.1	1.4 ± 0.1	0.77 ± 0.01	145.5 ± 8.5	16.8 ± 2.1	31.0 ± 2.6
Hypothyroid (gestational day 15)	6.5 ± 0.1	Not measured		117.4 ± 3.6 $p < 0.05$	13.8 ± 0.5	24.8 ± 1.5
Hypothyroid (gestational day 8)	6.4 ± 0.1	Not measured		Not measured		
Hypothyroid (gestational day 0)	5.7 ± 0.1 $p < 0.001$	1.0 ± 0.1 $p < 0.002$	0.74 ± 0.01 $p < 0.025$	85.1 ± 2.7 $p < 0.001$	9.7 ± 0.4 $p < 0.05$	Not measured

PTU = propylthiouracil.
Differences between control and hypothyroid groups were determined by Student's *t*-test and *p* values given when the differences were significant.

firmed that the offspring of treated animals were hypothyroid during fetal life. Thyroid weight in the young hypothyroid continued to be elevated until day 12. The development of the hypothyroid pups was retarded; for instance, eye opening occured at day 15 in controls but not until day 18 in the hypothyroid rats (Fig. 1).

The significant reduction of body weight in 16- and 18-day-old fetuses and in newborns of mothers receiving PTU treatment from the beginning of gestation suggests that thyroid hormones play a role in regulating growth, both pre- and postnatally. Although hypothyroidism in the mother exerts general metabolic effects that may implicate nutritional factors in the findings reported, it should be noted that weight gain during pregnancy was similar in control and treated animals, and that decreases in neonatal weight have been observed only when maternal malnutrition is severe (Allen and Zeman, 1971; McLeod, Goldrick, and Whyte, 1972; Zamenhof, van Marthens, and Gravel, 1971*a,b*).

In addition to reduced body growth, the weight of cerebral hemispheres in the hypothyroid newborns was also less than controls, suggesting that hypothyroidism had already impaired brain development during fetal life (Table 1). That hormones can influence growth of the fetal brain has been reported with respect to growth hormone (Zamenhof, van Marthens, and Gravel, 1971*b;* Sara, Lazarus, Stuart, and King, 1974). Neither Hamburgh (1964) nor Legrand (1969) found neonatal growth to be affected by hypothyroidism when PTU treatment is initiated late in pregnancy, but when hypothyroidism is induced earlier in fetal development, the effects of thyroid hormones on body and brain growth are manifest by the last fetal week.

[¹⁴C] LEUCINE INCORPORATION INTO PROTEINS

In order to assess the direct action of T_4 on brain tissue and to minimize environmental (e.g., circulatory, metabolic) influences, experiments were conducted *in vitro* using organ culture techniques. In our laboratory and in others, brain tissues have been kept viable for 24 hr or longer when incubated exclusively in a chemically defined medium. Histological examination has confirmed that tissues so treated remain in good condition.

Explants were prepared from control and hypothyroid rats at day 16 and 18 of gestation, at birth, and at 12 days postnatally (Fig. 2). [¹²⁵I]T_4 (specific activity 725 mCi/mg) was added to the medium to a final concentration of 0.083 μCi/ml and radioactivity measured after an 18-hr incubation. T_4 was incorporated by all tissues, both in the acid-soluble fraction (supernatant) and in the macromolecular fraction (pellet) (Fig. 3). Differences between control and hypothyroid slices were minimal in all tissues at all ages, although cortical incorporation of T_4 was greater in control than in hypothyroids at fetal day 18 and greater in the hypothyroids at day 12 postnatally.

The incorporation of radioactive leucine was measured by adding [¹⁴C]L-leucine (specific activity 312 mCi/mM) to achieve a concentration of 0.2

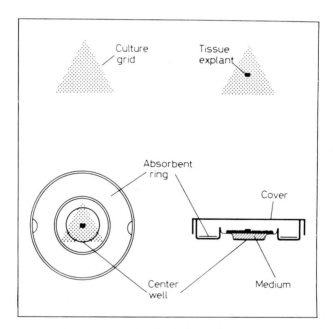

FIG. 2. Organ culture method: excised tissues are placed on a metal grid (upper portion) and positioned over the central well of a Falcon organ culture dish (lower left) so that the explant is in contact with the incubation medium (Eagle's Basic Medium). Sterile distilled water is placed in the surrounding trough to ensure adequate humidity. The covered dish (lower right) is placed in an incubator and maintained at 37°C in an atmoshpere of 95% $O_2 = 5\%$ CO_2. (From Vernadakis and Gibson, 1974.)

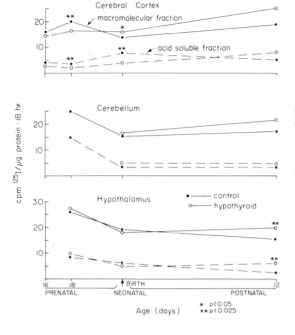

FIG. 3. $[^{125}I]T_4$ uptake in the acid-soluble and macromolecular fraction of brain slices (cerebral cortex, cerebellum, and hypothalamus) incubated for 18 hr in the presence of T_4 from rats of four different ages. Differences between control and hypothyroid groups were determined by Student's *t*-test.

μCi/ml in the medium. Fetal and newborn explants were incubated first for 18 hr, with or without T_4 as indicated previously, transferred to fresh medium containing the radioactive isotope, then incubated for 2 hr. Because the incorporation of $[^{14}C]$L-leucine decreases considerably with age, slices from 12-day-old animals were incubated immediately for 18 hr in a medium containing labeled leucine with or without T_4. Na^+ L-thyroxine $\cdot$ $5H_2O$ was dissolved in 1 N NaOH and added to the medium to a final concentration of 2 μg/ml, with the pH adjusted to 7.4.

Tissues were sonified, and the acid-soluble nucleic acid and protein fractions were recovered using differential extraction methods (Schneider, 1945; Shibko, Koivistoinen, Tratnyek, Newhall, and Friedman, 1967). Aliquots were taken from each fraction, suspended in 10 ml of Aquasol, and counted in a Beckman LS-100 scintillation counter. In addition to $[^{14}C]$leucine, tritiated uridine was added to the incubation medium, and the appropriate calculations were made to determine the amount of radioactivity attributable to ^3H and ^{14}C (Kobayashi and Maudsley, 1970).

Specific activity of the acid-soluble and protein fractions is expressed as dpm per microgram of protein and that of the nucleic acid fraction as dpm per microgram of RNA. Protein was determined according to Lowry's method (Lowry, Rosebrough, Farr, and Randall, 1951) and RNA by the orcinol reaction (Ceriotti, 1955).

We used the two-way analysis of variance for the statistical analysis of differences among the four experimental conditions (controls; controls with T_4; hypothyroid; and hypothyroid with T_4).

An age comparison of leucine incorporation into proteins in the cerebral cortex did not show any effect of hypothyroidism in fetal tissues, but a significant increase in newborn tissue (Fig. 4). No such increase was apparent in 12-day-old explants incubated for 18 hr; however, when incubation was limited to 2 hr, as in another experiment not illustrated here, incorporation in the 12-day-old tissue was also significantly increased (40%) by hypothyroidism. The addition of T_4 resulted in increased incorporation, detected as early as the 18th fetal day.

In the acid-soluble fraction, radioactivity was increased only in 12-day-old tissue from hypothyroid animals (Fig. 4). Because leucine is rapidly metabolized by brain tissue *in vivo* (Roberts and Morelos, 1965), and its metabolism is accelerated by hypothyroidism (Patel and Balázs, 1971), the increase in radioactivity of the acid-soluble fraction may represent an increase of leucine and its metabolites rather than leucine alone.

When values are expressed as a function of age, the resultant developmental curve shows the classical chronologic decline in protein synthesis with age; in addition, we see a peak in radioactivity associated with the protein fraction at day 18 in control and in hypothyroid, cultured in the presence or absence of T_4. This peak is followed by a sharp fall at birth and

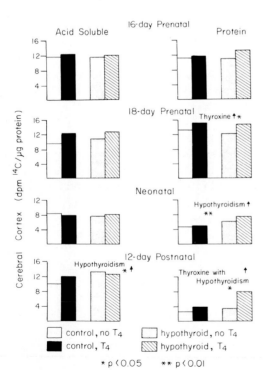

FIG. 4. Age-related effects of hypothyroidism and T_4 administration *in vitro* on the incorporation of [^{14}C]leucine in the acid-soluble and protein fractions from cerebral cortical slices (incubation with [^{14}C]leucine = 2 hr, except day 12 = 18 hr). Statistical significance was determined by the two-way analysis of variance (*). The effective treatment is written above the bar graph and direction of change shown by arrows.

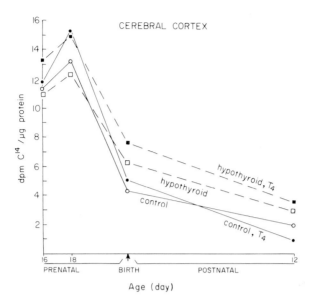

FIG. 5. Developmental changes in ^{14}C incorporation into protein by cerebral cortical slices (incubation time with [^{14}C]leucine = 2 hr).

a continuing but slower decline to day 12 (Fig. 5). In comparing the levels of radioactivity among the various groups, the control and the hypothyroid with T_4 show the highest levels at 18 days prenatally; at birth and postnatally, the hypothyroid and hypothyroid receiving T_4 were higher than controls.

When leucine incorporation is measured in cerebellum and hypothalamus, two brain regions chosen not only for their specific functional significance, but also for their different timetables of development, hypothyroidism significantly increases incorporation of leucine in the cerebellum at 12 days postnatally, and in the hypothalamus at 18 days prenatally (Fig. 6). In addition, at 12 days, T_4 markedly increases the incorporation of leucine in the cerebellum, a structure undergoing rapid maturation at this time. If we compare the developmental patterns of these three areas of brain, specific age- and region-dependent differences emerge. The hypothalamus, which matures early in fetal development, is sensitive to thyroid hormones at an early fetal age; the cerebral cortex, with a rate of maturation between that of hypothalamus and cerebellum, becomes susceptible to thyroid hormones neonatally; and the cerebellum, which matures last, responds to thyroid hormones postnatally.

[^{3}H]URIDINE INCORPORATION INTO RNA

Incorporation of [^{3}H] uridine into RNA was measured by adding uridine-(5[^{3}H]) (specific activity 28 Ci/mM) to the medium to achieve a concentra-

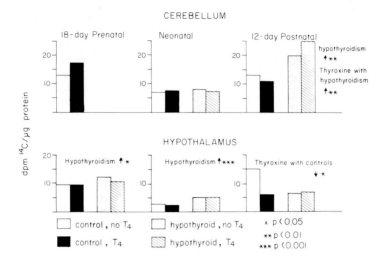

FIG. 6. Age- and region-specific effects of hypothyroidism and T₄ administration on *in vitro* ¹⁴C incorporation into protein by cerebellar and hypothalamic slices taken from 18-day fetuses, neonatal, and 12-day postnatal rats. Statistical significance determined by the two-way variance (*). Effective treatment is written above the bar graph and direction of change shown by arrows.

tion 1 μCi/ml. All techniques of tissue collection, processing, culturing, and counting were the same as described for [¹⁴C]leucine.

Hypothyroidism increases [³H]uridine incorporation in the cerebral cortex in an age-dependent manner (Fig. 7). No effects are observed in tissues from 16-day-old fetuses; on the other hand, in tissues from 18-day-old fetuses, hypothyroidism significantly decreases incorporation into RNA, whereas adding T₄ to both control and hypothyroid tissue increases incorporation. These findings are in contrast to our observation of amino acid incorporation which, at this age, responds only to T₄. Whereas at later ages hypothyroidism always increases incorporation of the precursor, whether [¹⁴C]leucine or [³H]uridine, hypothyroidism at this fetal stage significantly decreases uridine incorporation. In the tissues from the neonatal and postnatal animals, hypothyroidism plus T₄ increase incorporation of uridine both into the nucleic acid and the acid soluble fraction (Fig. 7).

When values are expressed as a function of age, the developmental pattern is similar to that delineated for leucine incorporation into protein (Fig. 8). Again, a peak occurs at the 18th prenatal day in controls, followed by a sharp decline which continues to the 12th postnatal day. In the hypothyroid, a slower increase in levels of radioactivity occurs which reaches a peak at birth. The shift in the time of peak activity supports our postulate that a major effect of hypothyroidism is to delay the maturational processes, and that thyroid hormones influence brain development prenatally.

Regional differences in ³H incorporation are similar to those reported

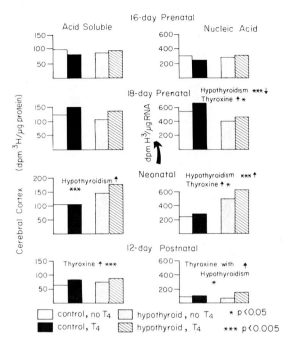

FIG. 7. Age-related effects of hypothyroidism and T_4 administration *in vitro* on the incorporation of [³H]uridine in the acid-soluble fraction and into RNA from the cerebral cortical slices (incubation with [³H]uridine = 2 hr, except day 12 = 18 hr). Statistical significance was determined by the two-way analysis of variance (*). Effective treatment is written above the bar graph and direction of change shown by arrows.

for ¹⁴C. The cerebellum shows significant effects of hypothyroidism neonatally and postnatally but not prenatally, and the hypothalamus shows more marked effects prenatally than postnatally (Fig. 9). The hypothalamus continues to be sensitive to T_4 even by the 12th postnatal day, at which time the hypothalamic-pituitary-thyroid axis becomes functional (Cons, Umezu, and Timiras, 1975).

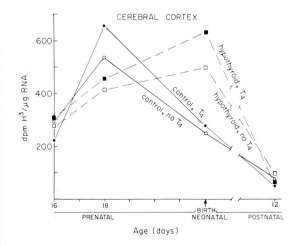

FIG. 8. Developmental changes in ³H incorporation into RNA by cerebral cortical slices (incubation time with [³H]uridine = 2 hr). The horizontal scale is expanded on the prenatal side of birth in order to emphasize the delay in the prenatal peak associated with hypothyroidism.

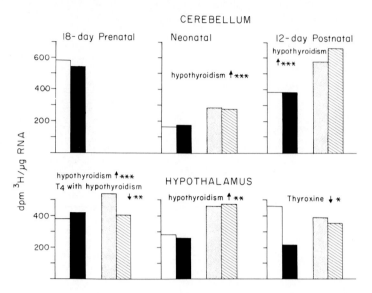

FIG. 9. Age- and region-specific effects of hypothyroidism and T_4 administration on *in vitro* ^3H incorporation into RNA by cerebellar and hypothalamic slices taken from 18-day fetuses, neonatal, and 12-day postnatal rats. Statistical significance determined by the two-way variance (*). Effective treatment is written above the bar graph and the direction of change shown by arrows.

DISCUSSION AND CONCLUSIONS

Our study indicates that thyroid hormones influence the growth and development of the entire animal and of the brain, not only during critical periods postnatally but also during fetal development. With respect to brain development, we report that: (1) thyroid hormones influence the incorporation of labeled precursors into protein and RNA of brain slices in culture; (2) this influence becomes manifest during fetal development and continues postnatally; (3) this influence is both age- and region-dependent, e.g., the cerebral cortex, the cerebellum, and the hypothalamus each has its specific schedule of maturation and susceptibility to thyroid hormones; and (4) the general increase associated with hypothyroidism in the incorporation of precursors into protein and nucleic acid is consistent with findings from numerous studies conducted *in vivo*.

The role of hormones in the fetus is still not well established. Although the action of sex hormones, e.g., in regulating differentiation and growth of the gonads and sex organs, is well recognized, the role of growth hormone in promoting fetal growth is still questionable. Our studies explore the role played by thyroid hormones in fetal life, and suggest that they may have an organizational action on the early development of the brain. Our data identify individual timetables of maturation in specific areas, and suggest that thyroid hormones may play a role in determining the ultimate competence of specific neuroendocrine functions (Umezu, Cons, and Timiras, 1976).

Finally, although our observations on leucine and uridine incorporation into protein and RNA are compatible with our earlier suggestion that thyroid hormones affect transport mechanisms, the question of *whether* and *how* they regulate protein synthesis in the brain remains unresolved.

ACKNOWLEDGMENTS

This work was supported by research grants USPHS GM-1021, NS-08989, and HD-07340, and by the Chancellor's Patent Fund for Graduate Student Research, University of California, Berkeley.

REFERENCES

Allen, L. H., and Zeman, F. J. (1971): Influence of increased postnatal food intake on body composition of progeny of protein-deficient rats. *J. Nutr.,* 101:1311–1318.

Andrews, T. M., and Tata, J. R. (1971): Protein synthesis by membrane-bound and free ribosomes of the developing rat cerebral cortex. *Biochem. J.,* 124:883–889.

Ceriotti, G. (1955): Determination of nucleic acids in animal tissue. *J. Biol. Chem.,* 214:59–70.

Clos, J., Crepel, F., Legrand, C., Legrand, J., Rabié, A., and Vigouroux, E. (1974): Thyroid physiology during postnatal period in the rat: A study of the development of thyroxine with special reference to cerebellar maturation. *Gen. Comp. Endocrinol.,* 23:178–192.

Cons, J. M., Umezu, M., and Timiras, P. S. (1975): Developmental patterns of pituitary and plasma TSH in the normal and hypothyroid female rat. *Endocrinology,* 97(1):237–240.

Geel, S. E., and Gonzales, L. R. (1975): *In vitro* studies of cerebral cortical RNA and nucleotide metabolism in hypothyroidism. *J. Neurochem.,* 25:377–385.

Geel, S. E., and Timiras, P. S. (1970): Influence of growth hormone on cerebral cortical RNA metabolism in immature hypothyroid rats. *Brain Res.,* 22:63–72.

Geel, S. E., and Valcana, T. (1972): Synthesis of free and membrane-bound ribosomal RNA from cerebral cortex in hypothyroid rats during development. *Neurobiology,* 2:21–30.

Gelber, S., Campbell, P. L., Deibler, G. E., and Sokoloff, L. (1964): Effects of L-thyroxine on amino acid incorporation into protein in mature and immature rat brain. *J. Neurochem.,* 11:221–229.

Hamburgh, M. (1969): The role of thyroid and growth hormone in neurogenesis. In: *Current Topics in Developmental Biology,* Vol. 4, edited by A. A. Moscona and A. Monroy, pp. 104–148. Academic Press, New York.

Hamburgh, M., and Bunge, R. P. (1964): Evidence for a direct effect of thyroid hormone on maturation of nervous tissue grown *in vitro. Life Sci.,* 3:1423–1430.

Hamburgh, M., Lynn, E., and Weiss, E. P. (1964): Analysis of the influence of thyroid hormone on prenatal and postnatal maturation of the rat. *Anat. Rec.,* 150:147–162.

Kobayashi, Y., and Maudsley, D. V. (1970): Practical aspects of double isotope counting. In: *Current Status of Liquid Scintillation Counting,* edited by E. D. Bransome, Jr. Grune Stratton, New York.

Legrand, C. (1969): Influence de l'hypothyroidisme sur la croissance en longueur et la differentiation histologique chez la foetus de rat en fin de gestation. *Arch. Anat. Microsc. Morphol. Exp.,* 58:291–310.

Lowry, O. H., Rosebrough, N. J., Farr, A. L., and Randall, R. J. (1951). Protein measurements with the Folin phenol reagent. *J. Biol. Chem.,* 193:265–275.

McLeod, K., Goldrick, R. B., and Whyte, H. M. (1972). The effects of maternal malnutrition on the progeny in the rat. Studies on growth, body composition and organ cellularity in first and second generation progeny. *Aust. J. Exp. Biol. Med. Sci.,* 50:435–446.

Patel, A. J., and Balázs, R. (1971): Effect of thyroid hormone on metabolic compartmentation in the developing brain. *Biochem. J.,* 121:469–481.

Roberts, S., and Morelos, B. S. (1965): Regulation of cerebral metabolism of amino acids. IV. Influence of amino acid levels on leucine uptake and utilization and incorporation into protein *in vivo. J. Neurochem.,* 12:373–387.

Sara, V. R., Lazarus, L., Stuart, M. C., and King, T. (1974). Fetal brain growth: Selective action by growth hormone. *Science,* 186:446–447.

Schneider, W. W. (1945): Phosphorous compounds in animal tissues. I. Extraction and estimation of desoxypentose and pentose nucleic acid. *J. Biol. Chem.,* 161:293–303.

Shibko, S., Koivistoinen, P., Tratnyek, C. A., Newhall, A. R., and Friedman, L. (1967): A method for sequential quantitative separation and determination of protein, RNA, DNA. lipid and glycogen from a single rat liver homogenate or from a subcellular fraction. *Anal. Biochem.,* 19:514–528.

Sokoloff, L., and Kennedy, C. (1973): The action of thyroid hormones and their influence on brain development and function. In: *Biology of Brain Dysfunction,* Vol. 2, edited by G. E. Gaull. Plenum Press, New York.

Timiras, P. S. (1972): *Developmental Physiology and Aging,* chap. 9. Macmillan, New York.

Timiras, P. S., Vernadakis, A., and Sherwood, N. (1968): Development and plasticity of the nervous system. In: *Biology of Gestation,* Vol. 2, edited by N. S. Assali, pp. 261–319. Academic Press, New York.

Umezu, M., Cons, J. M., and Timiras, P. S. (1976): Developmental patterns of follicle-stimulating, luteinizing and thyroid-stimulating hormones in the hypothyroid female rat. *Ann. Biol. Anim. Bioch. Biophys.,* 16(3):385–394.

Vernadakis, A., and Gibson, D. A. (1974): Role of neurotransmitter substances in neural growth. In: *Perinatal Pharmacology,* edited by J. Dancis and J. C. Hwang. Raven Press, New York.

Zamenhof, S., van Marthens, E., and Gravel, L. (1971*a*): DNA (cell number) and protein in neonatal rat brain: Alteration by timing of maternal dietary protein restriction. *J. Nutr.,* 101:1265–1270.

Zamenhof, S., van Marthens, E., and Gravel, L. (1971*b*): Prenatal cerebral development: Effects of restricted diet reversal by growth hormone. *Science,* 174:954–955.

DISCUSSION

Weichsel: Do you know whether the composition of milk changes in the PTU-treated mothers? If so, the offspring of these mothers may not receive proper nourishment.

Timiras: I do not know of any compositional change in the milk of the PTU-treated mothers, but effects of PTU treatment are found in the offspring before lactation is initiated.

Weichsel: When you treated mothers at 18 days gestation, you did not produce changes in birth weight.

Timiras: We started at day 0, or at 8 or 15 days, but not at 18 days of gestation. At 15 days, we later found a neonatal weight loss. Prenatal changes manifested at day 16 or 18 of gestation occurred only when the treatment was started at conception.

Balázs: Before conclusions are drawn from *in vitro* experiments on the effects of thyroid hormone on the rate of cerebral protein synthesis, it must be considered that during normal development a remarkable difference is observed, depending on whether the rate is determined *in vitro* or *in vivo* (Balázs and Richter, 1973). *In vivo,* the rate is relatively high in the first postnatal weeks, and it starts to decrease toward the adult level only after about day 21. In contrast, the incorporation rate of amino acids into brain proteins in all the *in vitro* preparations hitherto tested — (slices, homogenates, microsomes, ribosomes) — decreases dramatically immediately after birth, and by day 21 it is only approximately 10% of the rate at the time of birth. Thus, the situations *in vivo* and *in vitro* are completely different, and thyroid hormones may influence *in vivo* a rate-limiting reaction which is no longer the rate-limiting step *in vitro*. Therefore, your interesting experiments, Dr. Timiras, still leave the basic question open concerning the effect of thyroid hormone on protein synthesis rates in the developing brain.

I am also slightly confused with respect to the effect of thyroid hormone in tissue culture, since the incorporation rate is depressed at day 12. The major question here evidently relates to the intactness of the tissue culture preparations. The maintenance of the integrity of the preparations is greatly dependent on age and also culture time, especially since certain cell types are more vulnerable than others.

Timiras: When you incubate for 2 hr only, there is a marked increase in incorporation. We have to distinguish between a *tissue* culture which can go on for several weeks from the *organ* culture presented here, in which the tissue is maintained *in vitro* for a short period of time. One has to be aware of changes which might occur in the general viability of the tissue. We always checked for morphological changes and within this short period of time, found no significant decrements in the general structure of the cell.

Lauder: When did you start the replacement therapy with T_4 in the hypothyroid animals? Could you comment on similar effects in hypothyroid animals and animals which receive such replacement?

Timiras: This was not replacement therapy, since T_4 was not administered to the animal; it was added to the culture. To classical endocrinologists it is somewhat shocking that deficiency and excess of the hormone would have the same effect. The only interpretation at the moment is that even though the effect is the same, the mechanisms may be different. The increased incorporation in hypothyroid tissue is because the tissue is physiologically younger. In other words, tissue of 18 days is comparable to normal tissue of perhaps 16 days, so that we see the greater incorporation characteristic of that age. When T_4 was added, we found an increase in incorporation, perhaps owing to an enhanced metabolic activity induced by the hormone. Consequently, while the results manifestly are the same, the mechanisms by which they occur are perhaps different. But, this interpretation is only tentative.

Krawiec: These results differ from ours. We observe a higher incorporation in cerebral RNA *in vitro* at 10 days of age in the normal, compared with the hypothyroid animals. At 30 days there are no differences. Thus, it is difficult for me to compare these results with the *in vitro* experiments in which you have less incorporation in normal animals at the 13th day of age compared with the hypothyroid.

Timiras: The point brought up by Dr. Balázs is valid; we cannot always compare *in vivo* and *in vitro* findings. Dr. Balázs suggests that the results of the *in vitro* experiments may be less valid than those from *in vivo* experiments. In my view, all experimentation has shortcomings and advantages. Despite the problems presented by the situation *in vitro*, we have demonstrated an effect of thyroid hormones. We should, of course, recognize the differences from the situation *in vivo*.

Sokoloff: One obvious difference is that *in vitro* the various proteins are not being synthesized at their normal physiological rates. If you measure the incorporation of precursors into the total RNA, you get a different weighting factor than *in vivo*. Some proteins may not even be synthesized *in vitro*. You really cannot compare the time courses of gross incorporation into total protein *in vivo* and *in vitro;* they do not bear on each other. Your explants were incubated for 18 hr before you gave any labeled precursor. Now, biochemists are generally concerned when they must resort to a long incubation, because of the dangers of contamination with yeast or bacteria which carry on their own biochemical processes. What precautions have you taken? Sometimes the precautions you take to avoid bacterial growth require chemical agents which also affect the chemical process you are trying to study.

Timiras: In fact, in fetal tissues the chances of bacterial contamination, assuming you take the tissue in very sterile conditions, are very rare, because the fetal brain has not been exposed very much to contamination. We do this work under aseptic conditions, and have had very little contamination with bacteria within this short period of time. We take these special precautions because we are very much concerned with the point you raise.

Pesetsky: I would like to comment on Dr. Weichsel's question: "Is the milk of the mother of the PTU-treated rat altered in any way?" Most of us who have raised rats treated with PTU have had the experience of litters becoming dehydrated and dying off. Recently, I had occasion to look at the mothers of some of these animals; one finds that their breasts are often hard and dry. It seems possible that the breasts of these lactating mothers might be damaged in some way by PTU.

Timiras: We have thought of this question, particularly because we do not generally use PTU to produce hypothyroidism. For these studies, however, we felt it was preferable. At the University of California at Berkeley we have an animal colony started in 1911 by Dr. Evans. Our animals are Long-Evans rats, and the husbandry conditions are excellent. Finally, we use a dose in which the growth of the mother and of the fetus is maximal. We have not found any apparent changes in the nipples, at least up to 12 days, and lactation seems to have proceeded well, although we have not analyzed the composition of the milk.

Bass: Do you really measure a thyroid effect in the fetus when you transmit PTU across the placenta? The rat fetus does not have a thyroid gland, and the fetal thyroid develops quite late in the rat compared to man. You may be producing maternal hypothyroidism which in turn affects placental implantation. Therefore you may be observing the effects of intrauterine malnutrition rather than a direct effect of thyroid hormone on the developing fetus.

Timiras: I dissociate the roles played by thyroid and malnutrition. In the rat, thyroid function starts on the 15th prenatal day; by the 18th prenatal day, the fetal thyroid is already very sensitive to TSH, and it is already functioning well. The fact that the fetal rats were hypothyroid is best illustrated by the marked thyroid hypertrophy observed at birth. This shows that the thyroid tissue was responding to the goitrogen.

Bass: That happens to the human, too. But what is happening when you give PTU at onset of gestation? You are making a hypothyroid mother and thereby affecting placental size.

Timiras: Yes, that is right. However, I have combed the literature for effects of malnutrition on fetal growth and on other variables such as brain development and eye opening. Malnutrition must be very severe before such effects are seen. The fact that hypothyroid mothers gained as much weight during pregnancy as the controls suggests that the hypothyroid mothers were not suffering from malnutrition.

Bass: Are there any differences between the placentas of the normal mothers and those of the hypothyroid mothers?

Weichsel: We, like you, Dr. Timiras, have been lucky with our mothers, and the suckling rats do beautifully. I asked the question about the milk because we have some data which should prove interesting.

Ford: I would like to make a comment on work which was done in Dr. W. C. Young's laboratory. When I was a graduate student there, we induced hypothyroidism in pregnant guinea pigs in the same fashion as you. When we gave the guinea pigs PTU during the first trimester, there were no litters; they either were resorbed or aborted. If we gave PTU after the first trimester, we got litters which showed a marked hypertrophy of the thyroid gland.

In relation to the comment about milk, we have been studying the effects of morphine and methadone on litters of rats when the drugs were given to the mothers during the last trimester of pregnancy. If we gave a dose of 0.5 mg/ml of morphine in the water, the mothers who accepted this in their drinking water bore litters which died, largely because the mother did not lactate. There appeared to be a complete failure of the mammary glands to develop. The methadone-treated mothers tended to show the same response, and most of their litters died.

We observed several years ago that, in tissue culture or incubation procedures with brain, after an hour's incubation in an appropriate medium, the cells in rat cerebral cortex became disrupted, and nuclei were extruded. This was after only an hour of incubation. Further, we examined the cortex from mice and found that after half an hour of incubation one could hardly recognize the tissue as cortex; it looked more like a peritoneal smear. I wonder what morphological pictures you have of the cortex after 18 hr.

Timiras: The cytoarchitecture of the cortex under these optimal conditions shows very little change up to almost 36 hr. At 24 hr, the tissue is in perfect condition, thus, within the period of 18 hr, there is no detectable cytoarchitectural disruption of any type.

DISCUSSION REFERENCE

Balazs, R., and Richter, D. (1973): In: *Biochemistry of the Developing Brain*, edited by W. Himwich. Marcel Dekker, New York.

Thyroid Hormones and Brain Development,
edited by Gilman D. Grave. Raven Press,
New York, 1977.

Some Unresolved Questions of Brain-Thyroid Relationships

Max Hamburgh,*,** Lorenzo A. Mendoza,† Ingrid Bennett,*† Paul Krupa,* Young So Kim,‡ Ronald Kahn,* Kenneth Hogreff,* and Howard Frankfort*

The special interest which the cretinoid syndrome holds for the neurobiologist is that it provides one of the few experimental approaches to the problem of mental deficiency. When the cretinoid syndrome was first introduced as a proper object of scientific research almost 30 years ago, it was hoped that it would serve as a perfect model to study not only mental retardation, but the related question of the neural substrate of learning, mental activity, and the physical and chemical changes that accompany or cause loss of such functions. These hopes have not been realized, although these years of rather concentrated investigation into the brain-thyroid relationship have unearthed multiple pathology.

The extent of the learning deficit in hypothyroid animals has been reinvestigated recently by Davenport and Dorcey (1972). Everything seems to go wrong in brains of animals rendered prematurely hypothyroid. Neuronal cell population is reduced (Balázs, Kovacs, Cocks, Johnson, and Eayrs, 1971*a;* Clos and Legrand, 1972; Nicholson and Altman, 1972*a,b;* Rebière, Bout, and Legrand, 1972). Synaptic interaction is decimated (Nicholson and Altman, 1972*a,b;* Cragg, 1970); protein synthesis is depressed (Klee and Sokoloff, 1964; Geel and Timiras, 1970*a;* Szigan, Kalbermann, and Gomez, 1971; Dainat and Legrand, 1971; Clos and Legrand, 1972). RNA synthesis is depressed (Geel and Timiras, 1967, 1970*b,* 1971), myelin is deficient (Walravens and Chase, 1969; Balázs, Brooksbank, Davison, Eayrs, and Wilson, 1969*a;* DeRaveglia, Gómez, and Ghittoni, 1972); and a spectrum of enzymes in neuronal and glial cells fails to form in adequate concentrations (Hamburgh and Flexner, 1957; Balázs, Kovacs, Teichgraber, Cocks, and Eayrs, 1969*b;* Pesetsky and Model, 1969; Szigan, Chepelinsky and Piras, 1970; Gomez, 1971; Pesetsky, 1973; Holt, Cheek, and Kerr, 1973; for reviews of earlier work see

* Department of Biology, City College of New York, New York 10031; ** Department of Anatomy, Albert Einstein College of Medicine, Bronx, New York 10461; † Department of Neurology, Vargas Hospital, Caracas, Venezuela; ‡ Center for Biomedical Education, City College of New York, New York, New York 10031; and *† Hunter College, New York, New York 10028.

Balázs, Kovacs, Teichgraber, Cocks, and Eayrs, 1971; Hamburgh, 1969; Eayrs, 1971).

The mere description of additional structural targets, metabolic processes, and biochemical reactions within the developing nervous system that are influenced by neonatal or early postnatal thyroid manipulation does not seem to hold much promise for an understanding of the behavioral and mental defects correlated with higher activity. The concentrated study of the cretinoid syndrome carried out for almost 30 years by dedicated investigators has yielded little information that bears directly on this problem. This is perhaps due to the fact that thyroid deprivation leads to a spectrum of subtle changes, most of which may not be relevant to functional integrity, such as mental capacity or neuromuscular behavior.

Two problems recommend themselves as particularly deserving of further study before the search for the mechanisms of action of thyroid hormone in neurogenesis is continued. (1) Does thyroid hormone affect brain maturation by direct action on the target cells, or are most of the effects indirect? (2) Where direct action can be demonstrated, is the physiologically active substance identical with or different from T_4 or T_3, or an as yet unidentified intermediate substance? It seems to us that these questions have never been unequivocally answered.

Our experiments were undertaken in order to obtain at least some preliminary clues.

EXPERIMENT I

DIRECT VERSUS INDIRECT EFFECTS OF T_4 ON THE MATURING BRAIN

The Influence of T_4 on Maternal Care

This series of experiments was undertaken to reinvestigate the suggestion that the maturational defect in the developing brain of hypothyroid animals is a secondary effect. Insufficiency of pituitary function, reduction of vascular supply, and inanition are said to be consequences of lack of thyroid hormone which may account for the neuropathology found in cretinoid animals (Eayrs, 1954; Eayrs and Horn, 1955; Eayrs and Lishman, 1955; Gómez, Ghittoni, and Delacha, 1966; Hamburgh, 1968; Balázs, 1972).

The bulk of evidence accumulated so far has shown that the neuropathology of cretinoid brains is sufficiently different from that found in brains of starved animals or of animals with hypopituitary function or deficient vascular supply to argue against the proposition that one is mediated through the other. (Balázs, 1972; Rebière et al., 1972; Reier and Hughes, 1972*a,b;* Clos, Rebière, and Legrand, 1973; Gourdon, Clos,

Coste, Dainat, and Legrand, 1973; Rabié and Legrand, 1973; Rastogi and Singhal, 1974). We were interested in investigating the possibility that maternal care may be less than optimal in a mother in which the titer of circulating thyroid hormones may be diminished, or one with a hypothyroid litter. The efficacy of maternal care was measured by two tests, the nest rating and the nursing tests, designed by Seitz (1958) and modified by Turkewitz (1974). Control mothers with litters raised on PTU diet, and mothers maintained on PTU diet the litters of which were given thyroid replacement therapy were scored on these tests.

Materials and Methods

Pregnant rats of the Charles River Breeding Laboratories cesarean-derived (CD) strain were used for all experiments. Animals were housed individually in an air-conditioned room and provided with a Rockland mouse diet (ground) and water *ad libitum.*

Hypothyroidism was induced through administration of PTU begun during intrauterine life and continued until weaning. Treatment was initiated during the last week of gestation by offering to pregnant rats a goitrogenic diet containing 0.2% PTU mixed into powdered Rockland mouse diet starting on day 15 of pregnancy and continued until weaning or beyond. Day 15 was chosen because available evidence suggests that, in the rat, the fetal thyroid does not mature functionally before the 18th day of fetal age, but that during the third trimester of gestation maternal thyroxine passes the placental barrier.

Controls consisted of pregnant rats maintained on an unsupplemented diet and which received daily injections of 0.9% saline from birth until weaning.

Thyroid replacement therapy was provided by daily injection of L-thyroxine starting at birth to rats maintained on a diet containing powdered PTU since the 15th day of gestation: 1 μg from birth to 7 days; 2 μg from 7 to 14 days; 4 μg from 14 to 21 days; and 5 μg above 21 days of age. This concentration was established as the maximum nonlethal dose for young rats. The hormone was injected in 0.05 to 0.25 ml of fluid, held to a minimum in order to prevent any interference with osmotic equilibrium in the young animals.

Nesting test: Twenty-four to 48 hr before nest rating, approximately half of the nest shavings were removed and replaced with fresh shavings, then evenly distributed over the cage floor. On the morning of testing, the nests in the maternity cages were rated according to the following scale (Seitz, 1958): 0 — no nest; 1 — shavings trampled down in one corner; 2 — shavings pushed aside to make bare spot in corner; 3 — low ring of shavings around bare spot in corner; 4 — all shavings in cage piled into high ring around bare spot in corner.

Nursing test: Two 10-min observations divided into 15-sec intervals were made of each animal on each test day. The nursing behavior of each animal was observed at approximately the same time each day within 40 15-sec intervals. The mother was considered to be in a nursing position if at least 2 pups were beneath her or suckling beside her, and if she was not engaged in any other behavior, such as eating, drinking, or nest building. A mother which had spent all 40 intervals nursing was given a score of 100, whereas a mother which had nursed only during 20 intervals received a score of 50.

Results

The extent of maternal care, as measured by nest building and nursing behavior, declines as the litter approaches weaning (Figs. 1 and 2). After the sixth day the control mothers begin to reduce the time spent on nursing, as well as on the care expended on nest building.

Mothers of hypothyroid litters prolonged the care provided to their young considerably. Mothers whose litters were given replacement thyroid therapy are in between the control and hypothyroid group with respect to extent of maternal care provided.

These results are somewhat surprising. They refute the assumption that hypothyroid litters receive less maternal care than control litters; the opposite seems to be the case. The neuropathology that emerges in the cretinoid brain does not seem to result from any deficiency in maternal care.

The fact that maternal care was not prolonged in PTU-treated mothers whose litters received thyroid-replacement therapy argues against the

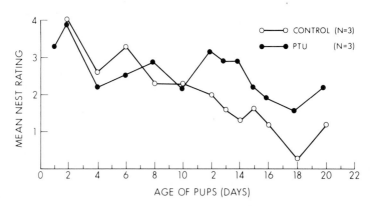

FIG. 1. Nest rating test. Control and hypothyroid mothers with hypothyroid litters scored for nestbuilding on a scale from 0 to 4: 0, no nest; 1, shavings trampled down in one corner; 2, shavings pushed aside to make bare spot in corner; 3, low ring of shavings around bare spot in corner; 4, all shavings in cage piled into high ring around bare spot in corner.

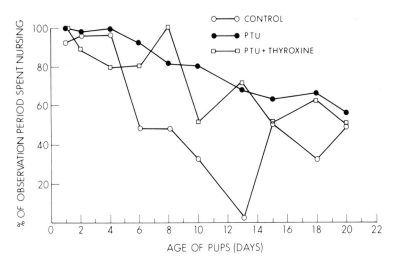

FIG. 2. Nursing test. Control, hypothyroid mothers with hypothyroid litters, and hypothyroid mothers whose litters were receiving thyroxine-replacement therapy were scored over a 10-min interval for percent of time spent nursing their young.

assumption that the thyroid state of the mother determines the quality of maternal care. The failure of our replacement therapy to return maternal behavior to control levels is probably related to the fact that our replacement therapy was insufficient. Spot checks on thyroid weights of litters receiving such replacement confirmed this interpretation, because thyroid weights of "replacement" litters were greater than controls, but less than hypothyroid young. It would seem, therefore, that some subtle signal reaches the mother from the litter, causing her to modify maternal behavior. The need of hypothyroid litters for prolonged maternal care is obvious. In its absence, the unavailability of thyroid hormone to the developing young animal may be fatal. Turkewitz (1974) has shown a similar relationship between maternal behavior and a starved litter.

INFLUENCE OF T$_4$ ON MATURATION OF PERIPHERAL INPUT SYSTEMS

Behavorial Tests

The similarity of the changes described by Cragg (1970) on the visual cortex of neonatally thyroidectomized rats with those raised in darkness (Gyllensten, Malenfors, and Norlin, 1967) suggested that some of the cortical changes obtained in thyroid-deprived rats may be mediated by hormonal influences exerted on the optic input system and that the abnormal histogenesis of the visual cortex may be a consequence of deficiency induced in the sensory system by lack of hormone during critical phases of development. This hypothesis is strengthened by the observation that neonatally induced hyperthyroidism accelerates eye opening in newborn rodents, whereas in hypothyroid young rats eye opening is delayed by 4 or 5 days. To test this proposition two experiments were devised.

Experiment 1 measured the emergence of home orientation behavior, which in normal young rats presumably reflects the switch from olefactory to visual orientation.

The home orientation test devised by Rosenblatt, Turkewitz, and Schneria (1969) was started 4 days after birth, and continued every other day until the pups were 20 days old. Pups were tested in three corners of the home cage between noon and 4 P.M. The home quadrant was determined by observing the location of the nest. The nearest neighboring corner was designated the adjacent corner (its quadrant was the adjacent quadrant). The corner diagonally opposite the home corner was designated the diagonal corner and its quadrant the diagonal quadrant. The fourth corner of the home cage was designated the neutral corner and its quadrant as the neutral quadrant.

Pups were tested in each corner of the home cage, except the neutral corner, in random order, every other day. The pup was placed on the cage floor with its head facing away from the test corner, toward the center of the cage, and released. The distance between the pup's head and the border of the home quadrant in tests of the adjacent corner was about 10 cm; in tests of the diagonal corner it was about 17 cm.

The mother and the remaining litter were removed from the home cage before testing was started. Food dishes were removed and nest shavings were brushed into the home corner. Each pup was then taken individually to be tested. Before a test the pup was placed on a flat surface for approximately 15 sec, then gently placed in the test corner and released. Tests lasted for 2 min. The pup's movements during a test were traced on a facsimile of the cage floor.

In order to subtract random movements from movements that were "nest-oriented," the percentage of pups terminating in the neutral corner when tested in the diagonal corner was compared to the percentage terminating in the home corner when tested in the adjacent corner. Because the distance between corners in both cases was identical, any difference between the two was attributed to nest orientation. Likewise, the percentage of pups terminating in the neutral corner when tested in the adjacent corner was compared with the percentage of pups terminating in the home corner when tested in the diagonal corner.

After making allowance and subtracting random movement, by the 14th postnatal day 85% of the young rats exhibit definite preference for the home nest and return there within 2 min after they have been displaced (Fig. 3). Hypothyroid rats reach comparable behavior on day 18, and even as late

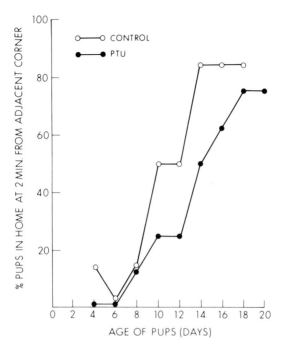

FIG. 3. Home orientation test. Observations on movement of control and hypothyroid young rats and their preference to land in the home corner in apposition to the neutral or adjacent corner, scored over a 10-min interval.

as day 20 the percentage of animals orienting toward "home" within the 2-min test period is lower than controls (75%).

If the emergence of home orientation behavior in rats is indeed indicative of a switch from olefactory to visual discrimination, the retardation of this behavior in hypothyroid rats may be a reflection of delayed maturation of the visual input system. The delayed eye opening of hypothyroid rats may be operative in delaying the organization of the visual cortex and leading to permanent reduction of the synaptic profile in this area (Cragg, 1970).

EFFECT OF T_4 ON MYELIN SYNTHESIS

We studied the rate of myelin synthesis in the visual cortex of control, hypothyroid, hyperthyroid young rats, and hypothyroid rats that were treated with epithelial growth factor (EGF), a substance that promotes, among other things, premature eye opening (Cohen, 1971). We did this in order to test the hypothesis that lack of T_4 may not only delay eye opening but may delay the maturation of the whole visual input system and thus secondarily suppress the organization of the visual cortex.

Hypothyroidism was induced with PTU, as described. Lyophilized EGF (obtained from the laboratory of Dr. Stanley Cohen, Vanderbilt University School of Medicine) was dissolved in 0.9% physiological saline (3,000 μg/10 ml of fluid). Injections of EGF were administered with a microsyringe subcutaneously into newborn rats, whose average weight was 5 to 5.5 g, starting on day 2 and continuing until day 21. The following dosages were administered: 15 μg in 0.05 ml of fluid to rats 2 to 4 days old; 30 μg in 0.10 ml of fluid to rats 5 to 7 days old; and 45 μg in 0.15 ml fluid to rats 8 to 21 days old.

Because variations in weight among controls, hypothyroid, and hyperthyroid animals did not emerge until after the 10th day of age, dosages of EGF injected were not adjusted to body weight.

Four groups were prepared: group 1, controls; group 2, hypothyroid rats, thyroidectomized as indicated in Experiment 1; group 3, rats rendered hyperthyroid as indicated above; group 4, hypothyroid rats injected simultaneously with EGF. Under the influence of EGF, eye opening is considerably accelerated. Hamburgh, Burkart, and Weil (1971) have reported accelerated eye opening to times even preceding the onset of eye opening in controls.

Rats were decapitated at 25 days of age. The brain was quickly exposed and pieces of cortex from frontal and occipital lobes were immersed in cold 4% distilled glutaraldehyde (Polysciences) in 0.1 M cacodylate buffer, pH 7.2. While in the fixative, tissues were cut with a razor into blocks about 2 mm across, then transferred to fresh cold glutaraldehyde for 1 hr at 4°C, washed in cacodylate buffer (4°C) overnight, fixed in 1% osmium tetroxide in 0.1 M cacodylate buffer (pH 7.2) for 1 hr, dehydrated in alcohol and propylene oxide, embedded in Epon, sectioned with an ultramicrotome, stained with uranyl acetate and lead citrate, and examined with an electron microscope.

In randomly selected sections of frontal and occipital cortex, scanned with the electron microscope at 25 days of age, there were large numbers of myelinated axons in both frontal and occipital cortical areas in controls (Fig. 7) and in even greater number in hyperthyroid rats at this age (Figs. 6 and 9). In contrast, both the frontal and occipital cortex of 25-day-old hypothyroid rats seems to be almost devoid of myelinated axons. Few or no myelinated axons were found in areas of comparable size in hypothyroid rats (Figs. 4 and 8).

In hypothyroid rats simultaneously treated with EGF the deficiency of myelinated fibers in the visual cortex was somewhat alleviated (Fig. 5), but in no case did EGF-treated animals ever equal controls with respect to extent of myelinated fibers. EGF seemed to alleviate the suppression of myelin synthesis in the visual cortex of hypothyroid animals, but never succeeded in repairing it to control levels.

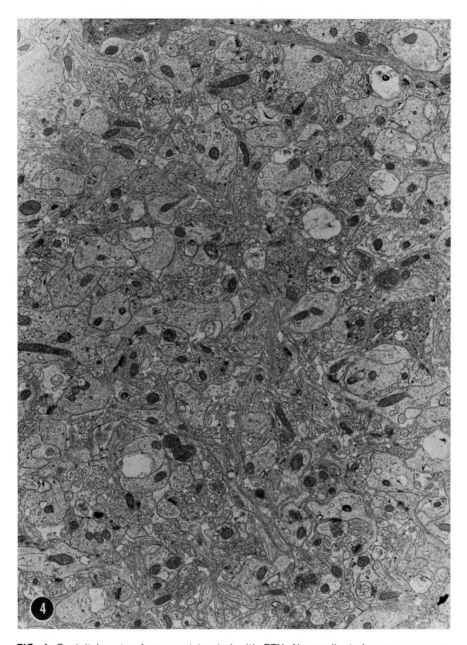

FIG. 4. Occipital cortex from a rat treated with PTU. No myelinated axons are seen. ×3,400.

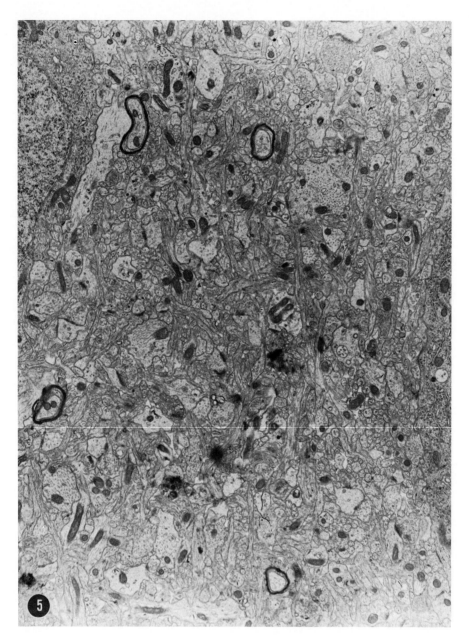

FIG. 5. Occipital cortex from a rat treated with PTU and EGF. Note four profiles of myelinated axons. ×3,400.

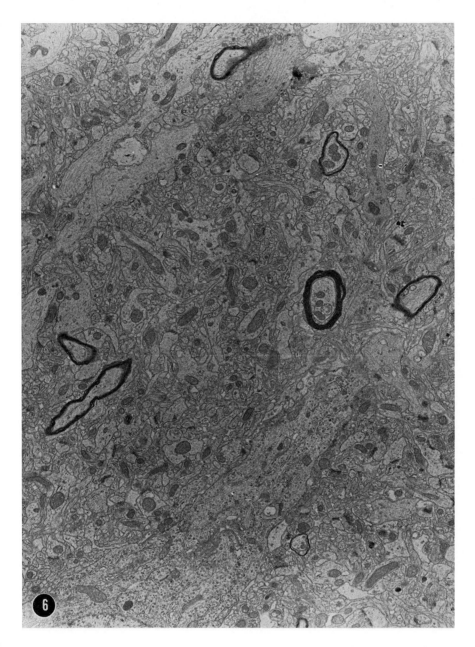

FIG. 6. Occipital cortex from a rat treated with PTU and T$_4$. Note at least seven profiles of myelinated axons. ×3,400.

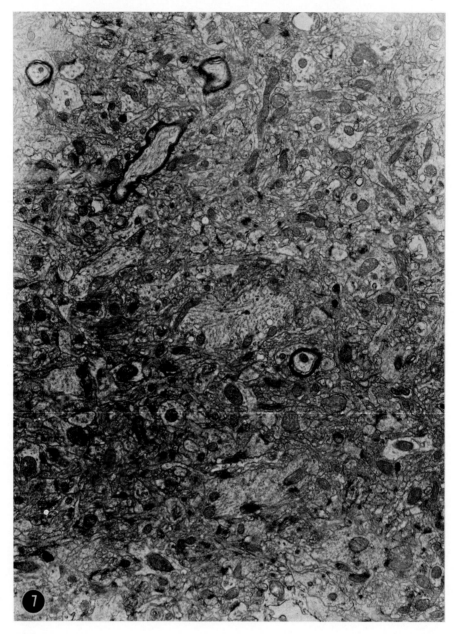

FIG. 7. Frontal cortex from an untreated control rat. Note four profiles of myelinated axons. ×2,975.

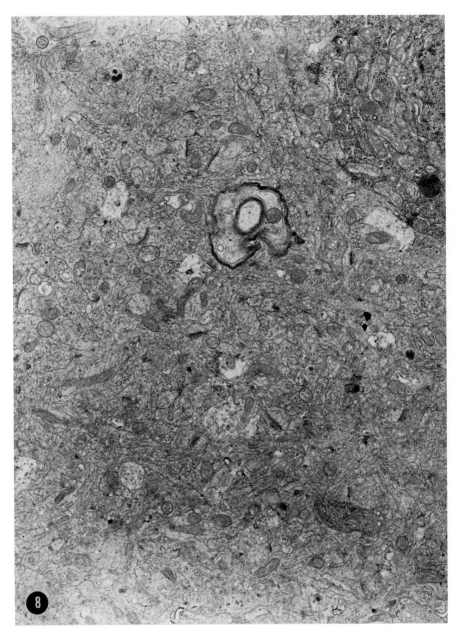

FIG. 8. Frontal cortex from a rat treated with PTU. A myelinated axon is seen near the center of the micrograph. ×3,400.

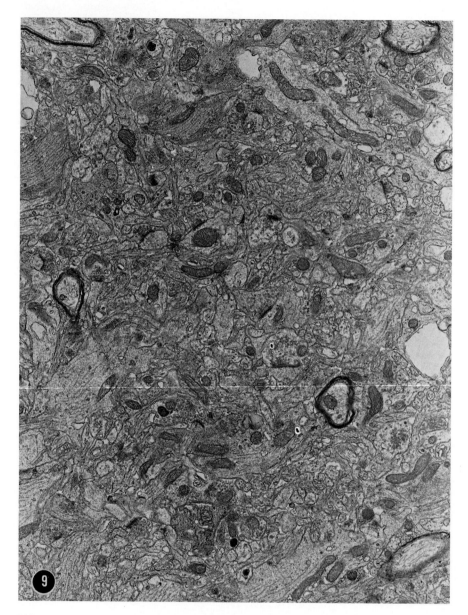

FIG. 9. Frontal cortex from a rat treated with PTU and thyroxine. Six profiles of myeli-nated axons are seen near the periphery of the micrograph. ×3,400.

CONCLUSIONS

Considerable evidence, mostly from biochemical studies, has been amassed to demonstrate the influence of thyroid hormone on myelin synthesis within the cortex and peripheral nervous system. Only a few morphological studies are available on this aspect, except for a study by Barnett (1948) and some recent reports by Reier and Hughes (1972*a,b*), Rosman (1972), and Matthieu, Reier, and Sawchak (1975). The data presented here provide additional morphological evidence for thyroid influence on myelin synthesis in cerebral cortex.

The choice of myelin as an indicator to test whether some central effects are mediated via peripheral factors is probably a poor one, because there is some evidence from tissue culture studies by Hamburgh (1966) that thyroid hormone probably accelerates myelin formation by direct action on the myelin-synthesizing components of the brain. The observation that the defect in myelin synthesis in the occipital cortex of hypothyroid young rats could be ameliorated by EGF, though not reversed, may be interpreted to mean that some of the thyroid effects on central maturation are mediated by hormonal action on the sensory periphery.

Failure of the hypothyroid rats to form myelin in the visual cortex may be due in major part to unavailability of thyroid hormone to act directly on the developing brain, and, in part, to the delayed arrival of visual signals in the developing cortex (possibly because of the delayed eye opening). Substantiation of this hypothesis would depend on demonstrating by electrophysiological studies that onset of eye opening and transmission of impulses over the visual systems are causally and/or temporally related.

Schapiro's studies (Schapiro, 1968; Schapiro, Salas, and Vukovich, 1970) in cortisone-treated young rats show that eye opening is accelerated, emergence of swimming behavior is delayed, and maturation of some other components of the CNS is probably retarded. This throws doubt on the automatic assumption that advancing the onset of eye opening must necessarily accompany accelerated maturation of all components of the CNS.

These observations should not be construed as indicating that the effect of thyroid hormone is essentially indirect. Cortical organization during ontogeny of the brain is undoubtedly influenced by many extraneous (nongenetic) factors, among them availability of such hormones as corticosteroid, sex hormones, and T_4; connection of afferent fibers with the center; access to sensory information; supply of nutrients, etc. The precise role and mechanism of hormone action is difficult to assess *in vivo* because manipulation with one hormone invariably affects the availability and concentration of many others. Removal or addition of any hormone during ontogeny not only disturbs the remaining endocrine balance but also initiates diverse metabolic changes in the mother, the embryo, or both; it is therefore difficult to determine whether the developmental changes that follow hormone manipulation are not mediated through effects on blood supply, nutritional state, or metabolic rate, rather than through direct intervention of the hormone with differentiation of the target cell.

Tissue culture has provided a tool to resolve some of these doubts, and in those cases where the *in vivo* effect of a hormone on developing tissue can be continued *in vitro*, a direct action is indicated.

Unfortunately, available tissue culture methods do not always lend themselves well to the study of the effects of hormones on neurogenesis. Successful culturing of nervous tissue usually requires the presence in the culture medium of plasma, serum, or chick embryo extract and cannot be carried out successfully in any known synthetic medium. It is therefore not possible to control or exclude hormones from the medium in which embryonic nervous tissue is to be grown. Tests for the effects of hormones on neurogenesis *in vitro* therefore, rely heavily on experiments in which excess of hormone is made available to the developing neuroblasts. Studies in this direction have been started (Hamburgh, 1966), but the information to be obtained in this manner is limited. Our own tissue culture experiments (Hamburgh, 1966) have at least shown that the onset of myelin synthesis of cerebellum is accelerated by excess T_4 supplied to the culture, and that the hormonal effect must therefore be a direct one.

We have reinvestigated these earlier findings and confirmed the original impression that in cultures maintained under less than optimal conditions (e.g., low temperatures), myelin synthesis can be improved by the addition of T_4. These observations would tend to reinforce the impression that T_4 influences myelin synthesis in the developing brain, in part at least, by direct action of the hormone on the myelin-synthesizing components of the central nervous system. The extent of myelin formation may be improved additionally by afferent connections or informational input to the center, the rate of development of both of which may also be under the control of T_4.

EXPERIMENT II

The question has never been resolved as to whether the T_4 molecule itself controls maturation of developing tissues directly or whether there is an intermediate molecule produced in the target cells after exposure to thyroid hormone which is the physiologically active agent.

Our interest was aroused by observations on a system different from the brain-thyroid model, namely the metamorphosing tissue of amphibians.

The investigation of hormone physiology has emphasized the search for mechanisms of hormone action at the cellular and subcellular level. The prevailing framework is that those cells sensitive to a particular hormone probably have specialized receptor molecules which recognize the hormone and which bind to it. The complex so formed then initiates a series of biochemical events including gene activation. Etkin worked on the problem of the action of thyroid hormones as controlling factors in the metamorphosis of the frog (see summary in Etkin, 1970). Etkin and Kim (1970) became concerned with the problems of thyroid action at the cellular and tissue levels and developed a system *in vitro* for the study of this phenomenon that promises a novel approach to the analysis of early biochemical actions of the hormone in tadpole tissues. (For a review on thyroid hormone in metamorphosis see also Kollros, 1961; Frieden, 1967, 1968; and Frieden and Just, 1970.)

We have been studying *in vitro* the response of tail tissue of *Xenopus laevis* larvae to thyroid hormone. This system was developed by Shaffer (1963) and has since been used by a number of other investigators (Weber, 1962, 1969*a;* Flickinger, 1963; Tata, 1966; Ryffel and Weber, 1973). This system has been refined in our laboratory (Derby, 1968; Derby and Etkin, 1968) so that we can now quantify the shrinkage which constitutes the tissue response. Pieces of tail fin tissue with no components of the tail axis are cut and allowed to heal, closed over by epidermal migration, in sterile saline solution. Such disks consist of connective tissue bags enclosed by a thin integument. The disks remain stable for 2 to 4 weeks in sterile medium and can be measured readily by projecting their image, outlining it, and determining the area with a planimeter. If T_4 is added to the culture medium at appropriate concentration, the tissues show the characteristic tail response, culminating after 3 days in tissue shrinkage.

Pieces of agar soaked in T_4 solution and implanted into a tail fin disk induce a local area of shrinkage similar to that reported in intact tadpoles by Derby (1968), Derby and Etkin (1968), and Weber (1969*a*). Agar soaked in control substances has no such effect. Fragments of tail tissue from tadpoles previously injected with T_4 also induce such local shrinkage. This reaction to T_4 suggests a technique for analyzing the sequence of events preceding the response of this and/or other tissues in an animal exposed to T_4 during a critical stage of development.

If tail fin disks from previously injected animals are allowed to fuse with pieces from noninjected animals (fusion is readily achieved by maintaining contact between freshly cut pieces), both tissues show initiation of shrinkage at the same time. When pieces from uninjected animals are fused with pieces from animals injected 0, 1, 2, or 3 days previously, the uninjected pieces of recipients tend to show shrinkage synchronously with the T_4 injected pieces of donors. Because the shrinkage takes less than 3 days in disks joined to donor pieces exposed to T_4 hormone for 3 to 4 days, the material transferred from the donor pieces is probably not residual T_4 but must be a subsequent derivative which diffused from the injected donor to its mate.

Methods and Materials

Experiments were undertaken to test more systematically the hypothesis that a diffusable substance is formed under the influence of T_4 in cells preparing for metamorphosis, which can subsequently initiate metamorphic changes in tissues that have not yet been exposed to T_4.

Eggs of *Rana pipiens* were fertilized and raised until they had grown to 25 to 30 mm. They were then immersed in a solution of T_4 at concentration 1.2×10^{-5} M in 1/10 Ringer (10,000 ppb) and kept in a constant-temperature box at 25°C. Three days after immersion, the tadpoles were removed, washed thoroughly with several changes of dilute Ringer's solution to eliminate contamination by T_4, and placed in culture. The culture medium consisted of Hank's balanced salt solution and distilled water (70:30 proportion). To 500 ml of this solution was added penicillin and streptomycin (500,000 units), and sulfadiazine sodium into 500 ml of medium. The 1:1 Hank's solution served as a medium in which all operations were carried out, and freshly operated disks were allowed to heal there for a period of 4 to 5 hr.

One disk from the recipient and two donor disks were introduced into a small sterile dish oriented in a manner so that the short edge of the recipient disk was in contact with the edge of the donor disk. Contact was maintained by pressure from glass pellets. A series of fused disks obtained from tadpoles which had not received T_4 but had been roused in 1/10 Ringer throughout were prepared in the identical manner to serve as controls. The second group of controls consisted of single disks placed into culture medium supplemented with T_4 at 2.4×10^{-7} M.

After fusion was achieved, all specimens were outlined by projection

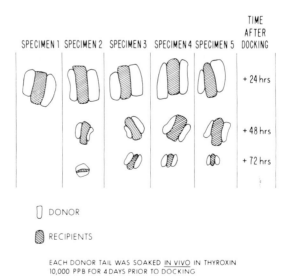

FIG. 10. Shrinkage of amphibian tail disks during metamorphosis. Two donor disks obtained from 25-mm tadpoles raised in T_4 solution of 10,000 ppb were docked to tail disks obtained from control tadpoles and maintained in culture for 72 hr.

to establish initial size relations. All specimens were observed continuously from days 4, 5, 6, and 7 after coupling. On day 7 all specimens were fixed in Bouin's fluid and prepared for histological analysis. The best cultures were selected for drawing and photography.

Results and Conclusions

Our results confirm the initial observation that under these conditions, docking of a recipient tail disk with one or two donor disks that had been exposed to T_4 previously, but before they had actually initiated regressive changes, can induce resorption in a recipient disk that has never been exposed to T_4. Particular attention was paid to the duration of the intervening latent period. The latent period between onset of shrinkage after exposure to thyroid hormone by immersion of *Rana pipiens* tadpoles containing T_4 is usually 4 days. In 60% of recipient disks coupled in culture to disks obtained from T_4-exposed donors, shrinkage was already well under way 48 hr after docking (Fig. 10.) None of the control recipients docked to tail disks obtained from tadpoles not exposed to hormones showed any shrinkage at all.

Conclusions

Exposure to massive doses of T_4 is always followed by a latent period of 72 to 96 hr at 24°C before any physiological or morphological changes are noted prior to metamorphosis. Tail disks are no exception to this generalization. During the latent period, physiological and biochemical events take place which prepare the changes that are subsequently revealed in morphology.

The results of the docking experiments lead us to postulate a diffusible substance the synthesis of which is induced by T_4 in hormone-sensitive cells. This hypothetical substance, in turn, may induce the various changes associated with metamorphosis. It may be argued that the material diffusing from the shrinking tail disk may contain massive quantities of lytic enzymes which are produced in premetamorphic resorbing tail disks under the influence of T_4. Evidence for stimulation of various lytic enzymes that operate in tail resorption has been presented by the work of Gross and Lapiere (1962); Weber (1969a,b); Frieden (1968); Frieden and Just (1970); and Greenfield and Derby (1972).

Weber (1969, 1969a) has also proposed that tail regression may be due to activation of macrophages under the influence of thyroid hormone. Both of these mechanisms can plausibly account for our observations.

The important point we wish to emphasize in this preliminary report is that the tail disk may provide a useful model to test the action of the various components that have been suggested as operative in activating tissue resorption under hormone influence.

The usefulness of the tail disk model to study the physiologically active agent mobilized by T_4 hormone would be much enhanced if it could be applied to a variety of different CNS targets that are normally thyroid-sensitive. If the hypothetical T_4-induced intermediate agent, so effective in tail shrinkage, is ineffective on other thyroid-sensitive targets of the metamorphosing animal, then it might be argued that, under the influence of T_4, each sensitive target produces its own physiologically active intermediate. If, on the other hand, the environment of the docked tail disk brings on metamorphic changes with the same accelerated speed normally associated with T_4 in other tissues implanted in the tail disk, it might then be argued that a hypothetical generally acting intermediate is produced. Experiments are now in progress to test these alternatives.

ACKNOWLEDGMENTS

This investigation was supported by a Faculty Research Grant from the City University of New York to Dr. Max Hamburgh; a research grant from the National Institute of Neurological and Communicative Disorders and Stroke NIH B1716 and NIH Grant AI 102070, Biomedical Sciences Support Grant PHS 5 SO RR7132–05, and the City University of New York Faculty Research Program (P. L. Krupa).

We gratefully acknowledge Miss Cassandra Kirk for technical assistance; Smith, Kline and French for supplying the T_4 used in this investigation; Dr. Stanley Cohen of the Department of Biochemistry, Vanderbilt University, School of Medicine, for supplying epithelial growth factor; and Mr. M. Kurtz, medical photographer, for his assistance with the photographic work.

The experiments on amphibian tail disk shrinkage and evidence for an intermediate substance, other than T_3 or T_4, active on metamorphosis were carried out by Mr. Young Kim in partial fulfillment for the requirements of the Ph.D. degree. We also gratefully acknowledge Professor William Etkin for his critical evaluation of the experimental procedures used in the amphibian experiments. The behavior tests were proposed, formulated, and carried out by I. Bennett in partial fulfillment for the Ph.D. degree at the City University.

REFERENCES

Balázs, R. (1972): Effects of hormones and nutrition. In: *Human Development and the Thyroid Gland*, edited by J. B. Stanbury and R. L. Kroc. Plenum Press, New York.
Balázs, R., Brooksbank, B. W. L., Davison, A. N., Eayrs, J. T., and Wilson, D. A. (1969*a*): The effect of neonatal thyroidectomy on myelination in the rat brain. *Brain Res.*, 15:219–232.

Balázs, R., Kovacs, P., Cocks, W. A., Johnson, A. L., and Eayrs, J. T. (1971*a*): Effect of thyroid hormone on the biochemical maturation of rat brain: Postnatal cell formation. *Brain Res.*, 25:555–570.

Balázs, R., Kovacs, P., Teichgraber, P., Cocks, W. A., and Eayrs, J. T. (1969*b*): Biochemical effect of thyroid deficiency on the developing brain. *J. Neurochem.*, 15:1335–1349.

Balázs, R., Kovacs, P., Teichgraber, P., Cocks, W. A., and Eayrs, J. T. (1971*b*): Biochemical effect of thyroid hormones on the developing brain. In: *Proceedings of an International Symposium on Hormones in Development,* edited by M. Hamburgh and E. J. W. Barrington. Appleton-Century-Crofts, New York.

Barnett, R. J. (1948): Some aspect of the experimental cretinlike animal. Thesis, Yale University School of Medicine.

Clos, J., and Legrand, J. (1972): Influence de l'hypothyroidisme sur l'incorporation de leucine tritiee dans les proteines des cellules de Purkinje et des motoneurones chez le jeune rat. Etude radioautographique. *Gen. Comp. Endocrinol.,* 18:583, abstract.

Clos, J., and Legrand, J. (1973): Effects of thyroid deficiency on the different cell populations of the cerebellum in the young rat. *Brain Res.,* 63:450–455.

Clos, J., Rebière, A., and Legrand, J. (1973): Differential effects of hypothyroidism on the development of glia in the rat cerebellum. *Brain Res.,* 63:445–449.

Cohen, S. (1971): Studies on the mechanism of action of epidermal growth promoting factor EGF. In: *Hormones in Development,* edited by Max Hamburgh and E. J. W. Barrington. Appleton-Century-Crofts, New York.

Cragg, B. G. (1970): Synapses and membranous bodies in experimental hypothyroidism. *Brain Res.,* 18:297–307.

Dainat, J., and Legrand, J. (1971): Influence de l'hyperthyroidisme neonatal sur l'incorporation *in vivo* de la L-³H-leucine dans les proteines du cervelet chez le jeune rat. *C. R. Soc. Biol. (Paris),* 169:1377.

Davenport, J. W., and Dorcey, T. P. (1972): Hypothyroidism: Learning deficit induced in rats by early exposure to thiouracil. *Horm. Behav.,* 3:97–112.

DeRaveglia, I. F., Gomez, C. J., and Ghittoni, N. E. (1972): Effect of neonatal thyroidectomy on lipid change in cerebral cortex and cerebellum of developing rats. *Brain Res.,* 43:181–187.

Derby, A. (1968): An *in vitro* quantitative analysis of the response of tadpole tissues to thyroxine. *J. Exp. Zool.,* 168:147–156.

Derby, A., and Etkin, W. (1968): Thyroxine induced tail resorption *in vitro* as affected by anterior pituitary hormones. *J. Exp. Zool.,* 169:1–8.

Eayrs, J. T. (1954): The vascularity of the cerebral cortex in normal and cretinous rats. *J. Anat.,* 88:164–173.

Eayrs, J. T. (1971): Thyroid and developing brain. Anatomical and behavioral effect. In: *Hormones in Development, Proceedings of an International Conference on Hormones in Development,* edited by M. Hamburgh and E. J. W. Barrington. Appleton-Century-Crofts, New York.

Eayrs, J. T., and G. Horn. (1955): The development of the cerebral cortex in hypothyroid and starved rats. *Anat. Rec.,* 121:53–61.

Eayrs, J. T., and Lishman, W. A. (1955): The maturation of behavior in hypothyroidism and starvation. *Br. J. Anim. Behav.,* 3:17–24.

Etkin, W. (1970): The endocrine mechanism of amphibian metamorphosis, an evolutionary achievement. In: *Hormones and the Environment,* edited by G. K. Benson and J. G. Phillips, pp. 137–156. Cambridge University Press, Cambridge.

Etkin, W., and Kim, Y. S. (1970): Development of thyroxin sensitivity in tadpole tail tissue (Abst.) *Am. Zool.,* 10:321.

Flickinger, R. A. (1963): Iodine metabolism in thyroidectomized frog larvae. *Gen. Comp. Endocrinol.,* 3:606–615.

Frieden, E. (1967): Thyroid hormones and the biochemistry of amphibian metamorphosis. *Recent Prog. Horm. Res.,* 23:139, 194.

Frieden, E. (1968): Biochemistry of amphibian metamorphosis. In: *Metamorphosis,* edited by W. Etkin and L. Gilbert, pp. 349–399. Appleton-Century-Crofts, New York.

Frieden, E., and Just, J. J. (1970): Hormonal responses in amphibian metamorphosis. In: *Biochemical Action of Hormones,* Vol. 2, edited by G. Litwack, pp. 2–52. Academic Press, New York.

Geel, S., and Timiras, P. (1967): The influence of neonatal hypothyroidism and of thyroxine on the ribonucleic acid and deoxyribonucleic acid concentration of rat cerebral cortex. *Brain Res.*, 4:135–142.

Geel, S. E., and Timiras, P. S. (1970a): Influence of growth hormone on cerebral cortical RNA metabolism in immature hypothyroid rat. *Brain Res.*, 22:63–72.

Geel, S. E., and Timiras, P. S. (1970b): The role of hormones in cerebral protein metabolism. In: *Protein Synthesis of the Nervous System*, edited by A. Lajtha. Plenum Press, New York.

Geel, S. E., and Timiras, P. S. (1971): The role of thyroid and growth hormones on RNA synthesis in the developing brain. In: *Proceedings of an International Symposium on Hormones in Development*, edited by M. Hamburgh and E. J. W. Barrington. Appleton-Century-Crofts, New York.

Gomez, C. (1971): Hormonal influences of the biochemical differentiation of the rat cerebral cortex. In: *Hormones in Development*, edited by M. Hamburgh and E. J. W. Barrington. Appleton-Century-Crofts, New York.

Gomez, C. J., Ghittoni, N. E., and Delacha, J. M. (1966): Effects of L-thyroxine or somatotrophin on body growth and cerebral development in neonatally thyroidectomized rats. *Life Sci.*, 5:243–246.

Gourdon, J., Clos, J., Coste, C., Dainat, J., and Legrand, J. (1973): Comparative effects of hypothyroidism, hyperthyroidism and undernutrition on the protein and nucleic acid contents in the young rat. *J. Neurochem.*, 21:861–871.

Greenfield, P., and Derby, A. (1972): Activity and localization of acid hydrolases in the dorsal tail fin of *Rana pipiens* during metamorphosis. *J. Exp. Zool.*, 179:129–140.

Gross, J., and Lapiere, E. M. (1962): Collagenolytic activity in amphibian tissues: A tissue culture assay. *Proc. Nat. Acad. Sci. (USA)*, 48:1014.

Gyllensten, L., Malenfors, T., and Norlin, M. L. (1967): Effect of visual deprivation on the optic centers of growing and adult mice. *J. Comp. Neurol.*, 124:149–160.

Hamburgh, M. (1966): Evidence for a direct effect of temperature and thyroid hormone myelinogenesis *in vitro. Dev. Biol.*, 18:15–30.

Hamburgh, M. (1968): An analysis of the action of thyroid hormone on development based on *in vivo* and *in vitro* studies. *Gen. Comp. Endocrinol.*, 10:198–213.

Hamburgh, M. (1969): Role of thyroid and growth hormone in neurogenesis. In: *Current Topics in Developmental Biology*, Vol. 4, edited by A. Moscona and A. Monroy, pp. 109–148. Academic Press, New York.

Hamburgh, M., Burkart, J., and Weil, F. (1971): Thyroid-sensitive processes in the developing nervous system in the rat. *Nottingham Conference on Hormones in Development*, edited by M. Hamburgh and E. J. W. Barrington. Appleton-Century-Crofts, New York.

Hamburgh, M., and Flexner, L. B. (1957): Biochemical and physiological differentiation during morphogenesis. XXI. Effect of hypothyroidism and hormone therapy on enzyme activities of the developing cerebral cortex of the rat. *J. Neurochem.*, 1:279–288.

Holt, A. B., and Cheek, D. B. (1961): Prenatal hypothyroidism and brain composition in a primate. *Nature*, 243:413–414.

Holt, A. B., Cheek, D. B., and Kerr, G. R. (1973): Prenatal hypothyroidism and brain composition in a primate. *Nature*, 243:413–414.

Klee, C. B., and Sokoloff, L. (1964): Mitochondrial differences in mature and immature brain. Influence on rate of amino acid incorporation into protein in response to thyroxine. *J. Neurochem.*, 11:709–716.

Kollros, J. J. (1961): Mechanism of amphibian metamorphosis. *Am. Zool.*, 1:107–114.

Matthieu, J. M., Reier, P., and Sawchak, J. (1975): Proteins of rat brain myelin in neonatal hypothyroidism. *Brain Res.*, 84:443–451.

Nicholson, J. L., and Altman, J. (1972a): Synaptogenesis in the rat cerebellum: Effects of early hypo- and hyperthyroidism. *Science*, 176:530–531.

Nicholson, J. L., and Altman, J. (1972b): The effects of early hypo- and hyperthyroidism on the development of rat cerebellar cortex I. cell proliferation and differentiation. *Brain Res.*, 44:13–23.

Pesetsky, I. (1973): The development of abnormal cerebellar astrocytes in young hypothyroid rats. *Brain Res.*, 63:456–460.

Pesetsky, I., and Model, P. G. (1969): Thyroxin-stimulated ultrastructural changes in ependymoglia of thyroprivid amphibian larvae. *Exp. Neurol.*, 25 (2):238–245.

Rabié, A., and Legrand, J. (1973): Effects of thyroid hormone and undernourishment on the amount of synaptosomal fraction in the cerebellum of the young rat. *Brain Res.*, 61:267–278.

Rastogi, R. B., and Singhal, R. L. (1974): Alterations in brain norepinephrine and tyrosine hydroxylase activity during experimental hypothyroidism in rats. *Brain Res.*, 81:253–266.

Rebière, A., Bout, M. C., and Legrand, J. (1972): Influence de la sousalimentation et de la deficience thyroidienne sur l'ontogenese des epines dendritiques de cellules de Purkinje. *Gen. Comp. Endocrinol.*, 18:619, abstract.

Reier, P. J., and Hughes, A. F. (1972a): An effect of neonatal radiothyroidectomy upon non-myelinated axons and associated Schwann cells during maturation of the mouse sciatic nerve. *Brain Res.*, 41:263–282.

Reier, P. J., and Hughes, A. F. (1972b): An effect of neonatal radiothyroidectomy upon non-myelinated axons and associated Schwann cells during maturation of the mouse sciatic nerve. *Brain Res.*, 41:263–282.

Rosenblatt, J. S., Turkewitz, G., and Schneria, T. C. (1969): Development of home orientation in newly born kittens. *Trans. N.Y. Acad. Sci.*, Series II, 31 3): 231–250.

Rosman, N. P. (1972): The neuropathology of congenital hypothyroidism. In: *Human Development and the Thyroid Gland*, edited by J. B. Stanbury and R. L. Kroc. Plenum Press, New York.

Ryffel, G., and Weber, R. (1973): Changes in the pattern of RNA synthesis in different tissues of *Xenopus* larvae during induced metamorphosis. *Exp. Cell Res.*, 77:79–88.

Schapiro, S. (1968): Some physiological, biochemical and behavioral consequences of neonatal hormone administration: Cortisone and thyroxine. *Gen. Comp. Endocrinol.*, 10:214–228.

Schapiro, S., Salas, M., and Vukovich, K. (1970): Hormonal effects on ontogeny of swimming ability in the rat: Assessment of central nervous system development. *Science*, 161:147–150.

Seitz, P. F. D. (1958): The maternal instinct in animal subjects. I. *Psychosom. Med.*, 20:214–226.

Shaffer, B. M. (1963): The isolated *Xenopus laevis* tail: A preparation for studying the central nervous system and metamorphosis in culture. *J. Embryol. Exp. Morphol.*, 11:77–90.

Szigan, I., Chepelinsky, A. B., and Piras, M. M. (1970): Effect of neonatal thyroidectomy on enzymes in subcellular fraction of rat brain. *Brain Res.*, 20:313–318.

Szigan, I., Kalbermann, W. E., and Gomez, C. J. (1971): Hormonal regulation of brain development IV. Effect of neonatal thyroidectomy upon incorporation *in vivo* of L phenylalanine into proteins of developing rat cerebral tissues and pituitary glands. *Brain Res.*, 27:309–317.

Tata, J. R. (1966): Requirement for RNA and protein synthesis for induced regression of the tadpole tail in organ culture. *Dev. Biol.*, 11:352–370.

Turkewitz, G. (1974): *Private communication.*

Walravens, P., and Chase, H. P. (1969): Influence of thyroid on formation of myelin lipid. *J. Neurochem.*, 16:1477–1488.

Weber, R. (1962): Induced metamorphosis in isolated tails of *Xenopus* larvae. *Experientia*, 18:84–85.

Weber, R. (1969a): The isolated tadpole tail as a model system for studies on the mechanism of hormone dependent tissue involution. *Gen. Comp. Endocrinol.*, Suppl. 2:408–416.

Weber, R. (1969b): Tissue involution and lysosomal enzymes during anuran metamorphosis. In: *Lysosomes*, edited by J. T. Dingle and H. B. Fell, pp. 437–461. North Holland, Amsterdam.

DISCUSSION

Ford: Did you consider retrieval as a test for behavior?

Hamburgh: That is one of the tests planned. The retrieval data are less uniform than those of the other test we reported.

Sokoloff: In our work on protein synthesis in liver. we found a 5-min lag that precedes the stimulation of protein synthesis. These experiments were done at 37°C. We wanted to know what was happening during those 5 min, so we lowered the temperature to 27°C, thinking we might extend the lag to 10 min. To our surprise, we found no effects of T_4 at all at that low temperature. In these docking experiments. have you looked to see whether there are any lytic enzymes in the medium?

Hamburgh: We assume that a large quantity of lytic enzymes must be liberated eventually, because the tail literally dissolves. It literally eats itself up. This is not, however, the initial event, because when we transplant pituitaries into the disk, the pituitary is not destroyed immediately.

Sokoloff: But the lytic enzymes would not work until they got into the cell. Perhaps they are initially excluded by the pituitary cells.

Hamburgh: If it turns out that the docking effect can be produced in tail tissue only and mimics no effect of T_4 on other tissues that have been transplanted into docked tails, I would assume that, as far as the tail is concerned, we were dealing with a lytic effect only.

Timiras: One of the points that Dr. Hamburgh brought out should be underscored. In interpreting the mechanism of action of thyroid hormones postnatally, we are concerned with factors such as nutrition, but we often disregard other factors such as the influence of sensory input on normal development. Normal sensory development is very much delayed in the hypothyroid animal. When we quantified the difference in time required for complete eye opening in the offspring of hypothyroid animals and controls, we found a differential of 3 days. During these 3 days (days 15 to 18) many synapses develop, and the lack of visual input at the proper time would be critical.

Kollros: I presume that collagenase is the operative enzyme, since the disks (as well as the whole tail fin) are largely acellular internally. The tail fin is comprised primarily of cell products rather than cells.

Hamburgh: Do you think that a large enzyme like collagenase can cross from cell to cell?

Kollros: Why not? There are no cellular barriers.

Hamburgh: But the disks fuse and heal. We disregard the disks that do not heal.

Geller: Is it possible to interpose a semipermeable membrane between them? That would eliminate the problem and would be an interesting experiment. I also wanted to ask about whether T_3 and T_4 compete for uptake into the cell.

Hamburgh: In our tail disk system?

Geller: In any system. In the brain you said that T_3 was more effectively accumulated.

Ford: It appears to be more effective because it is less tightly bound. Were the degree of binding equal, it would be interesting to see if one hormone were more potent than the other.

Geller: Do they compete with one other in a single transport system, or are they taken up independently?

Ford: I think they are taken up independently.

Thyroid Hormones and Brain Development,
edited by Gilman D. Grave. Raven Press,
New York, 1977.

Biochemical Mechanisms of the Action of Thyroid Hormones: Relationship to Their Role in Brain

Louis Sokoloff*

It is almost 50 years since the chemical structure of thyroxine (T_4) was first established by Harington and Barger (1927). This active principle of the thyroid gland was found to have a relatively simple chemical structure (Fig. 1). With the exception, perhaps, of epinephrine, this was the first hormone to have its chemical structure fully defined. The simplicity of its structure led biochemists to believe that it would prove equally simple to determine its mechanism of action. In fact, this simple molecule has proved to be a source of frustration for the last 50 years and continues to be so.

An elaborate system has evolved in animals to synthesize this specialized molecule, as well as its analogue, 3,3',5-triiodo-L-thyronine (T_3), a related hormone with similar actions, also synthesized in the thyroid gland (Fig. 1). For present purposes we will assume that these two thyroid hormones have qualitatively similar modes of action. It would seem unlikely that so highly specialized a hormonal structure would have many different biochemical actions. The molecule, however, has a number of special chemical properties, and all the structural requirements for its biological actions have not yet been unequivocally established. To a large extent this has been because the hormone has many diverse biological and biochemical effects which are affected to different degrees by modification of specific aspects of its structure. The major problem in defining the biochemical mechanism of its action is that it has too many actions.

One of the most intriguing biological actions of the thyroid hormones is their role in anuran metamorphosis. The metamorphosis of a tadpole into a frog represents a progressive, orderly sequence of structural and anatomical changes which lead ultimately to the complete transformation of one phenotype into another. This process is completely dependent on the presence of thyroid hormones; it does not occur if the hormones are absent from the animal or the medium. If the morphological changes in the transformation from tadpole to frog are so profound, imagine the complexity of the associated biochemical changes. These biochemical changes are not all simultaneous but are ordered and sequential, just like the morphological changes. It is almost certain that not all the biochemical changes are the

---

* Laboratory of Cerebral Metabolism, National Institute of Mental Health, U.S. Department of Health, Education, and Welfare, Public Health Service, Bethesda, Maryland 20014.

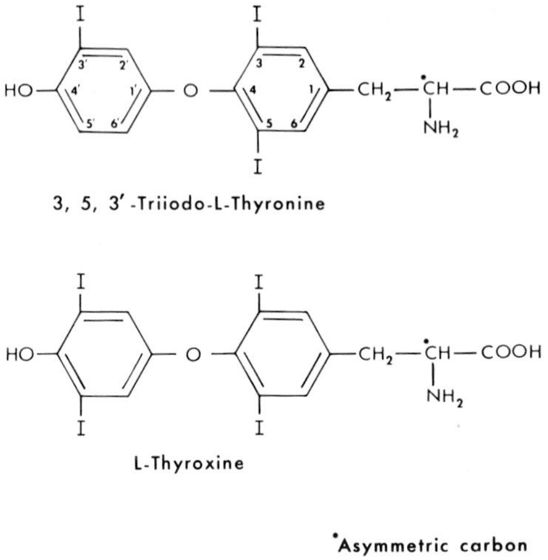

3, 5, 3'-Triiodo-L-Thyronine

FIG. 1. Chemical structure of the thyroid hormones.

L-Thyroxine

*Asymmetric carbon

result of direct action or participation by the thyroid hormones. Many, probably most, are the consequences of changes in the intracellular chemical environment that resulted from earlier actions of the hormones. One bias in our studies of the action of thyroid hormones has been to assume the most parsimonious hypothesis, namely, that there is a single biochemical mechanism of action of thyroid hormones and that most of the biochemical and morphological effects seen *in vivo* are secondary, tertiary, quaternary, etc., consequences of that initial action.

Chemists deal with molecular interactions and transformations which they describe by chemical equations. To a biochemist, the delineation of the mechanism of action of a chemical substance, such as a hormone, implies at the very least the ability to formulate a balanced chemical reaction in which the hormonal molecule participates. The eventual goal is to define the chemical mechanisms of that reaction. In organized biological systems hormones have numerous biochemical effects, but most are secondary consequences of the initial action or represent adaptative and compensatory changes in the cells to the consequences of earlier effects. These secondary effects do not directly involve the hormonal molecule. The goal of our research on thyroid hormones has been and remains the determination of their biochemical mechanism of action. To achieve that we have been attempting to tease out from their myriad chemical effects the initial biochemical reaction in which the hormonal molecule directly participates. Our strategy has been to work backwards from their most prominent and characteristic effects through the series of antecedent reactions that lead eventually to them.

The thyroid hormones have a number of characteristic effects, depending on the species and age or degree of maturity of the animal and the specific tissue. For example, in the frog the most prominent effects of thyroid hormones are the morphogenetic and biochemical changes characteristic of metamorphosis, but once the mature stage is achieved, the hormones appear to be without further effect. In mammals, however, thyroid hormones have developmental and growth-promoting effects in the immature, but stimulation of energy metabolism and metabolic rate is historically their most prominent effect and persists throughout the life span.

EFFECTS OF THYROID HORMONES ON CEREBRAL ENERGY METABOLISM

The actions of thyroid hormones in mammalian brain resemble in several ways their effects in tadpole metamorphosis. The brain of many mammalian species, including man, is relatively immature at birth, and undergoes a major part of its morphological, physiological, and biochemical maturation after birth. These changes are so extensive as to be nearly analogous to the transformation of the tadpole into frog. Also, as in anuran metamorphosis, the maturation of the brain is largely dependent on the thyroid hormones, and once complete, the thyroid hormones appear to have no further direct effects.

Figure 2 illustrates the effects of thyroid state on the cerebral cortical O_2 consumption of the rat during the postnatal maturation of the brain (Fazekas, Graves, and Alman, 1951). Cerebral cortical O_2 consumption is normally low at birth and remains so for approximately the first 10 days. It then rises in a sigmoid fashion until it reaches the adult level at approximately 45 days.

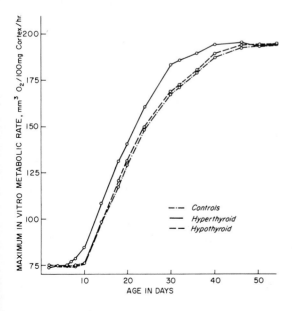

FIG. 2. Effects of thyroid state on cerebral cortical O_2 consumption of the rat from birth to maturity. (Redrawn from Fazekas et al., 1951.)

Administration of T_4 daily from birth shifts this curve to the left, increases O_2 consumption during the period of growth and development, and causes a more rapid rise of the cerebral metabolic rate to the normal adult level. Once that level is reached, however, further administration of T_4 is without apparent effect. In the studies of Fazekas et al. (1951) summarized in Fig. 2, hypothyroidism appears to have no effects on cerebral O_2 consumption. The reason for this is probably that the animals were not truly hypothyroid because of inappropriate dosage and timing of the antithyroid drugs administered. There is ample evidence in the literature that infantile hypothyroidism in the rat leads to impaired and retarded postnatal development of cerebral oxidative enzymes and capacity (Sokoloff and Kennedy, 1973). We were able to confirm that thyroid hormones also have no effects on the cerebral O_2 metabolism of the mature human brain. Patients with clinical thyrotoxicosis with a mean total body basal metabolic rate (BMR) of $+52\%$ had normal rates of cerebral O_2 consumption, and in those patients in whom effective treatment for the hyperthyroidism lowered the BMR from a mean of $+57\%$ to $+7\%$, there was no significant change in cerebral O_2 consumption (Table 1) (Sokoloff, Wechsler, Mangold, Balls, and Kety, 1953). The stimulation of energy metabolism, a characteristic effect of thyroid hormones in most tissues, is manifested in brain only during the period of its growth and development.

TABLE 1. *Cerebral metabolic rate in human adult thyrotoxicosis*

Subjects	Total body BMR (%)[a]	Cerebral O_2 consumption (ml/100 g brain/min)[a]
Normal (9 subjects)	—	3.5 ± 0.1
Hyperthyroid (11 subjects)	$+52 \pm 6$	3.5 ± 0.2
Treated hyperthyroid: (7 patients)		
Before treatment	$+57 \pm 7$	3.3 ± 0.2
After treatment	$+7 \pm 9$[b]	3.1 ± 0.3

From Sokoloff et al. (1953).
[a] Means $\pm$ standard errors.
[b] Statistically significantly changed by treatment ($p < 0.05$).

These studies on human hyperthyroidism first aroused our interest in the actions of thyroid hormones. Our initial goal was to explain the biochemical difference between mature and immature brain (or between mature brain and most other body tissues) that was responsible for the varying responses of their energy metabolism to thyroid hormones. It soon became clear that no such explanation was possible without more understanding of the mechanism of the hormonal stimulation of metabolic rate.

The lack of T_4 effects in mature brain appeared to offer a possible lead to the mechanism of its action. The mature brain shares with only two other tissues, the testis and reticuloendothelial tissue (e.g., spleen), the property of having a T_4-insensitive metabolic rate (Gordon and Heming, 1944). Of these refractory tissues, two (the mature brain and the testis) have a respiratory quotient (RQ) of approximately unity. No T_4-sensitive tissue is known to have a RQ of unity. Although this correlation might be fortuitous, it seemed that a RQ of 1 indicated some unique metabolic properties that were related to the lack of T_4 sensitivity. As summarized in Table 2, the metabolism of mature brain does exhibit some unique features. They all indicate that carbohydrate is normally an essential and almost exclusive substrate for cerebral energy metabolism and that protein and lipid turnover are almost negligible when compared with that of carbohydrate. These considerations, and a number of others beyond the scope of this report, led us to the work-

TABLE 2. *Some special characteristics of the metabolism of the normal mature brain in vivo*

Respiratory quotient of almost unity.
Utilization of O_2 and glucose in almost exact stoichiometric relationship for complete oxidation of glucose to CO_2 and water.
Lack of uptake by brain of any oxidizable substrate other than glucose in more than trace amounts under normal circumstances.
Inability of any other naturally present substrate to substitute adequately for glucose as the oxidizable substrate in hypoglycemia.

Interpretations:
Carbohydrate is almost the exclusive and essential ultimate substrate for the energy metabolism of the brain.
The quantities of protein and lipid turned over per unit time in brain are almost too negligible compared to that of carbohydrate to have an impact on the overall oxidative and energy metabolism.

From Sokoloff (1960).

ing hypothesis that the thyroid hormones act first to stimulate the energy-consuming process of protein synthesis and that the effects on metabolic rate are secondary (Sokoloff et al., 1953). In such tissues as mature brain, in which protein turnover and, therefore, also protein synthesis, are negligible compared with that of carbohydrate, effects of the hormone on energy metabolism would not be expected to be readily apparent. On the other hand, in developing brain in which protein synthesis is considerably more active and represents a major energy-dependent metabolic activity, the stimulation of protein synthesis by thyroid hormone would be expected to be reflected measurably in increased consumption of O_2. An action on protein synthesis appeared to be a reasonable possibility because protein synthesis is fundamental to many other biochemical processes in the cell; an effect on it could lead to the many diverse and disparate metabolic and biological effects of thyroid hormones.

EFFECTS OF THYROID HORMONES ON PROTEIN
BIOSYNTHESIS

The design of our studies on the action of thyroid hormones on protein biosynthesis was conditioned by a number of strategic considerations. Although hypothyroid animals are more sensitive to thyroid hormones, we decided to use euthyroid animals as much as possible, because hypothyroid animals are basically sick animals in which numerous processes are disturbed indirectly as a result of a deficiency disease and its consequences. When a disturbed process is restored to normal by replacement therapy, it may be a consequence of the amelioration of the disease rather than of a specific action of the hormone. On the other hand, euthyroid animals are normal, so that a change in a process as a result of hormone administration might then be more closely related to the specific action.

We also had the choice of *in vitro* or *in vivo* experiments. *In vitro* the conditions can be more rigorously controlled so that it is easier to isolate and identify specific actions. There is the danger, however, that an effect observed *in vitro* might be physiologically irrelevant. It was, therefore, decided to utilize both types of experiments, *in vitro* to identify effects and *in vivo* to test the physiological relevance of the findings *in vitro*.

The experimental studies confirmed the hypothesis that thyroid hormones stimulate protein synthesis. This effect was observed both *in vivo* and *in vitro*. Michels, Cason, and Sokoloff (1963) studied the effects of hyperthyroidism on the rates of protein synthesis in a variety of organs in the in-

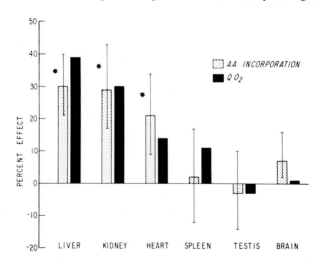

FIG. 3. Organ distribution of the effects of hyperthyroidism on amino acid incorporation into protein *in vivo* (AA) and tissue oxygen consumption (Q_{O_2}) in the rat. The asterisk indicates statistically significant effect ($p < 0.05$). The means ± standard errors are indicated. (Data on protein synthesis from Michels et al., 1963; on oxygen consumption from Gordon and Heming, 1944.)

tact adult rat. They found the rates of protein synthesis to be significantly increased in the liver, heart, and kidney when compared with the rates observed in euthyroid rats; there were no significant changes in the brain, testis, and spleen (Fig. 3). The organ distribution of the effects on protein synthesis was, therefore, identical to that of the effects on O_2 consumption previously observed by Gordon and Heming (1944). In contrast to the lack of effect in mature brain, protein synthesis in the developing brain of immature rats is stimulated by thyroid hormone treatment (Schneck, Ford, and Rhines, 1965) as is cerebral O_2 consumption (Fazekas et al., 1951).

The increased rate of protein synthesis is not secondary to the increased rate of energy metabolism; it appears to be quite the contrary. The stimulation of O_2 consumption lags behind the effect on protein synthesis (Tata, Ernster, Lindberg, Arrhenius, Pederson, and Hedman, 1963) and can be prevented or even reversed by inhibitors of protein synthesis which also, therefore, block the effects of thyroid hormones on protein synthesis (Tata, 1963; Weiss and Sokoloff, 1963).

STUDIES OF MECHANISM OF EFFECT OF T_4 ON PROTEIN SYNTHESIS

The stimulation of protein synthesis by thyroid hormones administered *in vivo* persists in cell-free preparations from T_4-sensitive tissues. In Table 3 we summarize the result of studies on the effects of experimental hyper- and hypothyroidism on the rate of amino acid incorporation into protein [assayed *in vitro* in cell-free preparations from rat liver (Sokoloff and Kaufman, 1961)]. Hyperthyroidism increased the rate of protein synthesis to approximately 42% above the level observed in similar preparations from matched normal control animals. Thyroidectomy was followed by a significant decrease in the rate of protein synthesis, suggesting that the effect on protein synthesis represents a true tonic physiological action of the hormone.

The subcellular fractions contained in the cell-free system used *in vitro* consisted of mitochondria, microsomes, and cell sap. In order to ascertain which of these fractions was responsible for the increased protein synthetic activity of hyperthyroid liver, the three subcellular components were isolated from both euthyroid and hyperthyroid livers, and all combinations of mitochondria, microsomes, and cell sap derived from the two sources were assayed for protein synthesis. The results demonstrated some increased activity associated with the hyperthyroid microsomes, but most of the increased activity in the preparations was attributable to their mitochondrial component (Sokoloff and Kaufman, 1959, 1961). Euthyroid preparations in which the mitochondria were replaced by hyperthyroid mitochondria exhibited hyperthyroid rates of protein synthesis; hyperthyroid preparations in which the mitochondria were replaced by euthyroid mitochondria exhibited euthyroid rates of protein synthesis (Fig. 4). Al-

TABLE 3. *Effects of altered thyroid state on* [^{14}C]*leucine incorporation into protein in cell-free rat liver preparations*

Thyroid state	Protein specific activity		Effect of altered state	
	Control	Experimental		
	(cpm/mg protein)		(Δ cpm/mg)	(%)
Hyperthyroid (8)	30 ± 3	41 ± 4	+11.0 ± 4[a]	+42
Hypothyroid (8)	29 ± 3	20 ± 3	− 9 ± 4[a]	−28

From Sokoloff and Kaufman (1961).

[a] Statistically significant difference; $p < 0.05$ as determined by method of paired comparison.

Adult male albino rats were paired according to age and weight. In the studies on hyperthyroidism one of each pair received almost daily intraperitoneal injections of 100 μg of sodium L-thyroxine dissolved in 1 ml of 0.01 N NaOH for 6 to 16 days (mean = 10 days); the other received equivalent amounts of the NaOH solution only. On the day after the last dose, liver homogenates were prepared simultaneously from both animals, and DL[1-^{14}C]leucine incorporation activity was assayed in a single combined experiment. In the studies on hypothyroidism one rat of each matched pair was surgically thyroidectomized, and the other subjected to sham operation. Liver homogenates were prepared simultaneously from both animals 28 to 41 days (mean = 32 days) after operation, and DL[1-^{14}C]leucine incorporation activity into protein was assayed in paired flasks. The incubation mixture contained the following components in micromoles: sucrose, 150; AMP, 5; potassium phosphate buffer, pH 7.4, 20; MgCl$_2$, 5; potassium α-ketoglutarate, 50; DL[1-^{14}C]leucine (specific activity = 5.33 or 5.47 mCi/mmole), 0.8. In addition, 0.45 ml of liver homogenate containing mitochondria and microsomes equivalent to the yield from 200 mg and cell sap equivalent to the yield from 30 mg of fresh liver were added. The reaction mixture was brought to a final volume of 1.7 ml with water. Incubation time at 37°C was 60 min. The preparation of the homogenates, incubation procedures, and assay of specific activity were as described by Sokoloff and Kaufman (1961). Radioactivity was measured with an end-window tube-type Geiger-Mueller counter with an overall efficiency of less than 5%, but sufficient counts were collected to achieve a coefficient of variation of less than 2%. The values represent the means ± standard errors; % represents the mean of the individual percent effects. The numbers in parentheses represent the numbers of paired experiments in each series.

though the presence of hyperthyroid mitochondria was required for the full expression of the stimulation of protein synthesis, it was microsomal protein synthesis that was stimulated (Sokoloff and Kaufman, 1961). These results suggest that the mitochondrial fraction of the cell was implicated in the mechanism of the stimulation of microsomal protein synthesis by thyroid hormones *in vivo*.

Studies of the mechanism of the effect were greatly facilitated by the finding that the same cell-free preparations that exhibited the effects of thyroid hormones administered *in vivo* responded similarly to the direct addition of the hormones *in vitro* (Sokoloff and Kaufman, 1961). With cell-free preparations from euthyroid rat liver, small but statistically significant effects were observed in the presence of added T$_4$ at concentrations as low as 1.3×10^{-7} M. The magnitude of the effect was concentration-dependent; graded increases in the percent stimulation occurred with progressively increasing concentrations of T$_4$ until a maximum stimulation of +77% was achieved

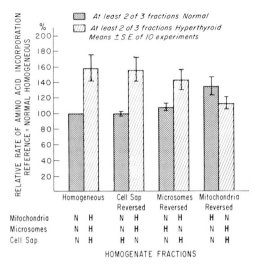

FIG. 4. Substitution experiments to determine the contributions of each of the various subcellular components of the liver homogenates to the stimulation of protein synthesis following T_4 administration *in vivo*. Paired euthyroid and hyperthyroid rats prepared as described in Table 3, and mitochondria, microsomes, and cell sap prepared separately from their livers as described by Sokoloff and Kaufman (1961). Amino acid incorporation into protein was assayed in the presence of all combinations of these three cell fractions derived from the paired animals, a total of 8 possible combinations. Assay conditions were the same as those described in Table 3. N, normal (euthyroid); H, hyperthyroid. (From Sokoloff, 1968.)

at about 4×10^{-4} M (Fig. 5). Above this concentration the effect of T_4 reversed abruptly from stimulation to inhibition, probably because of the superseding effects of uncoupling of oxidative phosphorylation and/or Mg^{2+} binding by T_4 (Sokoloff and Kaufman, 1961).

The existence of an effect of thyroid hormones in a cell-free protein synthesizing system *in vitro* opened up the possibility of a range of studies on the mechanism of the effect. It is beyond the scope of this chapter to describe the numerous and extensive studies of the mechanism of the stimulation of protein synthesis by T_4 *in vitro*. In essence they showed that the stimulation is a translational one at the level of the transfer of the tRNA-bound amino acid into the protein being synthesized on the ribosomes (Sokoloff, Kaufman, Campbell, Francis, and Gelboin, 1963). The effect is to

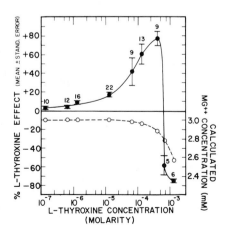

FIG. 5. Effects of T_4 added *in vitro* on [^{14}C]leucine incorporation into protein in cell-free preparations from normal rat liver. Assay conditions are the same as those described in Table 3, except that the preparations were always from normal, euthyroid rat liver, and T_4 was pipetted directly into the incubation mixtures in amounts sufficient to achieve the final concentrations indicated. Incubation time at 37°C was 25 min. The dashed line represents the estimated Mg^{2+} remaining free in the solution after binding and precipitation of Mg^{2+} by complex formation with T_4. (From Sokoloff and Kaufman, 1961.)

enhance the rate of growth of the nascent polypeptide chain and, perhaps, also the release of the completed chains from their ribosomal attachment (Krause and Sokoloff, 1967).

There is, however, one aspect of the mechanism that is of special relevance to the disparity of the effects of thyroid hormones in developing and mature brain. The results in Fig. 4 implicate mitochondria in the mechanism of the stimulation of protein synthesis by thyroid hormones *in vivo*. The role of mitochondria was even more dramatically apparent *in vitro* when T_4 was added directly to the cell-free preparations. Mitochondria are not essential for microsomal protein synthesis and can be replaced in the reaction system by some alternative ATP-generating system, such as a creatine kinase system. Then, the control rates of protein synthesis are essentially unchanged, but the stimulation by T_4 *in vitro* is lost (Table 4) (Sokoloff, 1968). In other words, the stimulation of microsomal protein synthesis by T_4 *in vitro* is characterized by an absolute dependency on the presence of mitochondria in the reaction system.

Table 4 also provides evidence about the nature of the mitochondrial involvement in the mechanism of the effect. In early studies of the stimulation of protein synthesis by T_4 *in vitro* it was noted that a 5-min lag precedes the stimulation of protein synthesis (Sokoloff and Kaufman, 1961). This lag can be eliminated by preincubation of the entire system, less the labeled amino acid, for 5 min or by preincubation only of the mitochondria, oxidizable substitute, AMP or ADP, and phosphate with the hormone for 5 min, before the addition of the complete protein-synthesizing system (Sokoloff and Kaufman, 1961; Sokoloff, 1968). If the mitochondria are removed by centrifugation from the preincubated mixtures, and the supernatant solutions are added to a mitochondria-free protein synthesizing system, in which T_4 alone has no effect, then the stimulation by T_4 is still observed. The effect is even more apparent with supernatant solutions from which the protein has been precipitated by boiling and removed by centrifugation before addition to the protein-synthesizing reaction system (Table 4). Thus, the role of the mitochondria appears to consist of participation in an energy-dependent interaction with the hormone, leading to a soluble heat-stable product which mediates the stimulation of protein synthesis. The active product has not yet been identified, but appears to be a small, dialyzable, heat-stable, organic molecule (Sokoloff, 1968).

In vivo, the mechanism of the stimulation of protein synthesis is more complicated. The overall effect consists of two distinct mechanisms. First, there is the mitochondria-dependent, cytoplasmic stimulation of translational activity at the ribosomal level, followed several hours later by an increase in cellular and microsomal RNA, leading to an increased rate of protein synthesis which is no longer mitochondria-dependent (Sokoloff, Roberts, Januska, and Kline, 1968). The two effects *in vivo* are illustrated in Fig. 6. Following a single small dose of T_3 to rats, protein synthesis, assayed

TABLE 4. Role of mitochondria in the stimulation of microsomal protein synthesis by L-thyroxine in vitro in cell-free liver systems

Protein synthesis assay system and additions	Type of incubated mitochondrial supernatant fraction added to protein synthesis assay system	Protein specific activity (cpm/mg protein)	Thyroxine effect	
			(Δ cpm/mg)	(%)
Complete (+ mitochondria, + β-hydroxybutyrate):				
Control	None	59	–	–
+ thyroxine	None	100	+41	+69
Minus mitochondria, minus β-hydroxybutyrate, + creatine phosphate, + creatine kinase:				
Control	None	49	–	–
+ thyroxine	None	42	–7	–14
+ Crude mitochondrial preincubation supernatant	Control	26	–	–
	+ thyroxine	29	+ 3	+12
+ Boiled extract of mitochondrial preincubation supernatant	Control	43	–	–
	+ thyroxine	61	+18	+42

From Sokoloff (1968).

Assay conditions for the complete system were the same as described in Fig. 5, except that 0.25 μmoles GTP were included in the reaction mixture, and Na$^+$ DL-β-hydroxybutyrate was used as the oxidizable substrate in place of potassium α-ketoglutarate. In the assay lacking mitochondria, the mitochondria and β-hydroxybutyrate were replaced by 40 μmoles of creatine phosphate and 0.25 mg of creatine kinase in an equivalent volume. When added directly to the assay system, the T$_4$ concentration was 6.5×10^{-5} M. Incubation time at 37°C was 25 min. At the end of the incubation the reaction was terminated by the addition of 5 ml of ice-cold 0.25 M sucrose solution containing 1 mg/ml of nonradioactive DL-leucine. The mitochondria were then removed by centrifugation at 12,800 $\times$ g for 15 min, and the microsomal and cell sap protein in the supernatant fraction was precipitated by the addition of an equal volume of 12% trichloroacetic acid. The precipitated protein was purified and assayed for specific activity as described by Sokoloff and Kaufman (1961). Radioactivity was measured by means of an end-window gas-flow Geiger-Mueller counter with an overall efficiency of approximately 17%. Sufficient counts were collected to achieve a coefficient of variation of less than 2%.

The mitochondrial supernatant solution added to the protein synthesis assay system was prepared as follows: mitochondria were incubated for 5 min at 37°C in the identical reaction mixture used for the complete protein synthesis system, except that the GTP was absent, and the microsomes and cell sap were replaced by equivalent volumes of 0.25 M sucrose. The T$_4$ concentration, when present, was 2.6×10^{-4} M. The incubation was terminated by chilling to 0°C in ice, and the mitochondria then removed by centrifugation at 12,800 $\times$ g for 15 min. The volumes of the supernatant fraction added to the protein synthesis assay system were such that their T$_4$ content was diluted to 6.5×10^{-5} M. Boiled extracts of the mitochondrial supernatant fraction were prepared by quick-boiling small volumes of the crude fraction for 10 min, then removing precipitated material by centrifugation at 100,000 $\times$ g for 1 hr.

FIG. 6. Time course of the initial mitochondria-dependent cytoplasmic stimulation of microsomal protein synthesis and the delayed increases in cytoplasmic RNA, and associated secondary changes in microsomal protein synthesis following a single small dose of T_3 to euthyroid animals. Normal adult male albino rats were paired for age and weight. One of each pair was given a single intraperitoneal injection of sodium triiodo-L-thyronine (60 μg/100 g of body weight) contained in 0.01 N NaOH at a concentration of 75 μg/ml; the paired control animal received an equivalent volume of the NaOH solution alone. The animals were killed at the indicated times, and mitochondria, microsomes, and cell sap were prepared from their livers as described (Sokoloff et al., 1968). In each experiment, microsomal protein synthesis was assayed simultaneously in cell-free liver systems from both types of animals in the presence and absence of mitochondria under assay conditions as described in Table 4. RNA contents were measured by the method of Fleck and

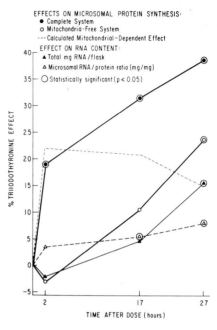

EFFECTS ON MICROSOMAL PROTEIN SYNTHESIS:
● Complete System
○ Mitochondria-Free System
--- Calculated Mitochondrial-Dependent Effect
EFFECT ON RNA CONTENT:
▲ Total mg RNA/flask
△ Microsomal RNA/protein ratio (mg/mg)
○ Statistically significant (p < 0.05)

% TRIIODOTHYRONINE EFFECT

TIME AFTER DOSE (hours)

Begg (1965). Each point in the figure represents the mean of 9 to 12 experiments. The dashed line (mitochondria-dependent stimulation of microsomal protein synthesis) was calculated by subtracting the percent effect on protein synthesis in the absence of mitochondria from the percent effect in their presence; it is assumed that in the presence of mitochondria, the total effect represents the sum of mitochondria-dependent and mitochondria-independent effects. The circled points represent statistically significant changes ($p < 0.05$). (From Sokoloff et al., 1968.)

in cell-free liver systems, is increased with essentially no lag and prior to any change in RNA content of the microsomes or the system as a whole, but only if the mitochondria are included in the assay system. In the absence of mitochondria, there is no early effect on protein synthesis, but an increased rate appears about one day later associated with a rise in the RNA content of the microsomes. The increased microsomal RNA content probably reflects increased synthesis and accumulation of ribosomes (Tata and Widnell, 1966). The initial mitochondria-dependent effect is analogous to the effect of T_4 *in vitro;* the mitochondria-independent effects, both on protein and on RNA synthesis, appear later, never occur *in vitro,* and can be prevented by an overnight fast. It appears that the early mitochondria-dependent effect is closer to the true biochemical action of the hormone molecule itself, whereas the later effects on RNA and protein synthesis may represent secondary cellular adjustments to the intracellular alterations produced by the earlier effects. The overall response appears to represent the integration of a primary response and a functional cellular adaptation. An initial, mitochondria-dependent, cytoplasmic stimulation of the activity of the existing protein-synthesizing machinery is followed by a nuclear-mediated increase in the amount of protein-synthesizing machinery. The secondary effect serves to amplify and prolong the consequences of the initial effect. Also, inasmuch as the nucleus is involved in the secondary response, it may also offer the means for regulation of gene expression. However, the initial biochemical event which precedes the entire sequence is a cytoplasmic action of the hormone, and present evidence points to the mitochondrion as the locus of that action (Sokoloff, 1968).

The mechanism responsible for the delayed or second phase of the increased rate of protein synthesis following thyroid hormone administration *in vivo* is still uncertain. Certainly it is due to the increased synthesis of ribosomal RNA and accumulation of functional ribosomes (Tata and Widnell, 1966). These changes are the result of alterations of nuclear functions and increased RNA polymerase activities (Tata and Widnell, 1966). It is still uncertain, however, whether the increased nuclear RNA polymerase activity is the result of direct actions of the hormones in the nucleus or a secondary change initiated by altered intracellular conditions arising from earlier cytoplasmic actions of the hormone. Nuclear RNA polymerase activity and, specifically, nucleolar synthesis of ribosomal RNA are extremely sensitive to the chemical environment of the nuclei, e.g., the monovalent and divalent ionic composition (Johnson, Jant, Kaufman, and Sokoloff, 1971) and the amino acid concentration (Franze-Fernandez and Pogo, 1971) of the medium. These components of the intracellular fluid, the medium for the nucleus, could be altered by earlier cytoplasmic actions of the hormone. On the other hand, recent evidence of specific, high-affinity binding sites for thyroid hormones in the nucleus (Oppenheimer, Koerner, Schwartz, and Surks, 1972) raises the possibility of direct actions of the hormones in the nucleus. These issues remain to be resolved.

EFFECTS OF THYROID HORMONES ON PROTEIN SYNTHESIS IN BRAIN

The studies of the mechanism of action of thyroid hormones in liver and other tissues have led to better understanding of the unique features of their actions in the central nervous system. The thyroid hormones stimulate the metabolic rate and induce maturation in the developing mammalian brain but have no apparent effects once the brain has matured; the effects on protein synthesis show a similar age differentiation both *in vivo* (Fig. 3) and *in vitro* (Gelber, Campbell, Deibler, and Sokoloff, 1964). The effects on protein synthesis *in vitro* are illustrated in Table 5. The rates of protein synthesis in cell-free liver preparations from infant and adult rats are almost the same, and both are equally stimulated by T_4. The rate of protein synthesis in cell-free preparations from immature brain is almost the same as

TABLE 5. *Effects of L-thyroxine in vitro on [¹⁴C]leucine incorporation into protein in cell-free preparations from adult and infant rat liver and brain*

Tissue	Animal age		Protein specific activity		Thyroxine effect	
			Control	Thyroxine		
			(cpm/mg protein)		(Δ cpm/mg)	(%)
Liver	Adult	(3)	39	61	+ 22	+ 57
	Infant	(2)	32	45	+ 13	+ 42
Brain	Adult	(7)	12	9	− 3^a	− 21
	Infant	(6)	44	50	+ 6^a	+ 14

From data of Gelber et al. (1964).

^{a} Statistically significant effects; $p < 0.05$ by method of paired comparison. The values presented are the means of the results of the number of experiments indicated in the parentheses. % represents the mean of the percent effects obtained in the individual experiments.

The assay conditions were the same as those described for the complete protein synthesis assay system in Table 4. The liver and brain homogenates were prepared as described by Gelber et al. (1964). Adult rats were 40 to 50 days old; infant rats were 15 to 16 days old. Thyroxine concentration was 6.5×10^{-5} M. Incubation time at 37°C was 25 min.

that in liver and, like it, is stimulated by T_4. In similar preparations from mature brain, however, protein synthesis proceeds at only one-fourth to one-third the rate of that in the immature brain preparations, and the responsiveness to T_4 has disappeared. The inhibition by T_4 observed with the mature brain preparation in Table 5 is of doubtful physiological significance. It is not observed *in vivo* (Fig. 3) and probably reflects the lack of stimulation sufficiently great to overcome the effects of otherwise inhibitory conditions, such as Mg^{2+} binding by the hormone in the *in vitro* assay (Sokoloff and Kaufman, 1961).

The difference in the responses of the immature and mature brain preparations to the hormone is related to the fundamental role which mitochondria play in the mechanism of its action. Figure 7A illustrates the results of mixing experiments in which mitochondria, microsomes, and cell sap were isolated from both mature and immature brain; the effect of T_4 on protein synthesis was assayed in the presence of all combinations of these three cell fractions from both types of brain. The results indicate that the source of the mitochondria determines the presence or absence of stimulation by T_4. The hormone stimulates protein synthesis in the presence of mitochondria from immature brain and fails to stimulate in the presence of adult brain mitochondria, regardless of the source of the microsomes and cell sap. The role of the mitochondria is even more clearly demonstrated in Fig. 7B, in which similar mixing experiments with cell fractions from mature brain and liver are presented. The protein-synthesizing system (consisting of the microsomes and crude cell sap) of mature brain is apparently fully capable of responding to T_4 with increased activity, but only if mitochondria from a

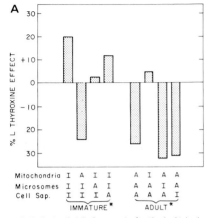

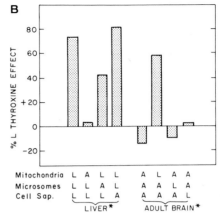

A

I – Indicates that the homogenate fraction is obtained from immature brain.

A – Indicates that the homogenate fraction is obtained from adult brain.

* – At least two components derived from sources as indicated.

B

L – Indicates that the homogenate fraction is obtained from liver.

A – Indicates that the homogenate fraction is obtained from adult brain.

* – At least two components derived from sources as indicated.

FIG. 7. Role of mitochondria in the difference in effects of T_4 on protein synthesis in mature brain compared with immature brain and liver. Protein synthesis and the effects of T_4 on the rate were assayed *in vitro* in cell-free preparations as summarized in Table 5. The final T_4 concentration was 6.5×10^{-5} M. The cell-free system contained mitochondria, microsomes, and cell sap derived from immature brain (I), mature brain (A), or mature liver (L). Immature rats were 15 to 16, and mature rats were 40 to 50 days of age. The effects of T_4 on protein synthesis were examined in all possible combinations of these three cell fractions. Note that stimulations by T_4 are observed when the mitochondria are either from immature brain (**Fig. 7A**) or from liver (**Fig. 7B**) and never with mature brain mitochondria, regardless of the source of the cell sap and microsomes. (From Klee and Sokoloff, 1964.)

T_4-sensitive tissue are present. This is further confirmed by experiments in which the addition of a boiled extract of the supernatant solution from an incubated liver mitochondrial-T_4 reaction mixture has been found to stimulate the rate of protein synthesis by a mitochondria-free adult brain protein-synthesizing system (Sokoloff and Roberts, *unpublished data*).

The mitochondria of immature brain, like those of liver and other T_4-sensitive tissues, appear to contain a functional site which is the locus of the primary action of the thyroid hormone. The mitochondria of fully mature brain have apparently lost this site and with it the ability to participate in the initial reaction with the hormone which triggers the chain of events comprising its overall physiological action. A change in mitochondria appears to be the basis for the change in T_4 sensitivity of brain during its maturation. Further understanding of the mechanisms by which thyroid hormones promote brain maturation, however, must await more precise definition of their biochemical mechanisms of action in general.

REFERENCES

Fazekas, J. F., Graves, F. B., and Alman, R. W. (1951): The influence of the thyroid on cerebral metabolism. *Endocrinology,* 48:169–174.

Fleck, A., and Begg, D. J. (1965): The estimation of ribonucleic acid using ultraviolet absorption measurements. *Biochim. Biophys. Acta,* 108:335.

Franze-Fernandez, M. T., and Pogo, A. O. (1971): Regulation of the nucleolar DNA-dependent RNA polymerase by amino acids in Ehrlich ascites tumor cells. *Proc. Natl. Acad. Sci. (USA),* 68:3040–3044.

Gelber, S., Campbell, P. L., Deibler, G. E., and Sokoloff, L. (1964): Effects of L-thyroxine on amino acid incorporation into protein in mature and immature rat brain. *J. Neurochem.,* 11:221–229.

Gordon, E. S., and Heming, A. E. (1944): The effect of thyroid treatment on the respiration of various rat tissues. *Endocrinology,* 34:353–360.

Harington, C. R., and Barger, G. (1927): (XXIII) Chemistry of thyroxine. III. Constitution and synthesis of thyroxine. *Biochem. J.,* 21:169–183.

Johnson, J. D., Jant, B. A., Kaufman, S., and Sokoloff, L. (1971): Effects of ionic strength on the RNA polymerase activities of isolated nuclei and nucleoli of rat liver. *Arch. Biochem. Biophys.,* 142:489–500.

Klee. C. B., and Sokoloff, L. (1964): Mitochondrial differences in mature and immature brain. Influence on rate of amino acid incorporation into protein and responses to thyroxine. *J. Neurochem.,* 11:709–716.

Krause, R. L., and Sokoloff, L. (1967): Effects of thyroxine on initiation and completion of protein chains of hemoglobin *in vitro. J. Biol. Chem.,* 242:1431–1438.

Michels, R., Cason, J., and Sokoloff, L. (1963): Thyroxine: Effects on amino acid incorporation into protein *in vivo. Science,* 140:1417–1418.

Oppenheimer, J. H., Koerner, D., Schwartz, H. L., and Surks, M. I. (1972): Specific nuclear triiodothyronine binding sites in rat liver and kidney. *J. Clin. Endocrinol. Metab.,* 35:330–333.

Schneck, L., Ford, D. H., and Rhines, R. (1965): The uptake of S^{35}-L-methionine into the brain of euthyroid and hyperthyroid neonatal rats. *Acta Neurol. Scand.,* 40:285–290.

Sokoloff, L. (1960): Metabolism of the central nervous system *in vivo.* In: *Handbook of Physiology-Neurophysiology,* edited by J. Field, H. W. Magoun, and V. E. Hall, Vol. III, pp. 1843–1864. American Physiological Society, Washington, D.C.

Sokoloff, L. (1968): Role of mitochondria in the stimulation of protein synthesis by thyroid hormones. In: *Regulatory Mechanisms for Protein Synthesis in Mammalian Cells,* edited by A. Pietro, M. R. Lamborg, and F. T. Kenney, pp. 345–367. Academic Press, New York.

Sokoloff, L., and Kaufman, S. (1959): Effects of thyroxin on amino acid incorporation into protein. *Science,* 129:569–570.

Sokoloff, L., and Kaufman, S. (1961): Thyroxine stimulation of amino acid incorporation into protein. *J. Biol. Chem.,* 236:795–803.

Sokoloff, L., Kaufman, S., Campbell, P. L., Francis, C. M., and Gelboin, H. (1963): Thyroxine stimulation of amino acid incorporation into protein. Localization of stimulated step. *J. Biol. Chem.,* 238:1432–1437.

Sokoloff, L., and Kennedy, C. (1973): The action of thyroid hormones and their influence on brain development and function. In: *Biology of Brain Dysfunction,* edited by G. E. Gaull, Vol. 2, pp. 295–332. Plenum Publishing Corporation, New York.

Sokoloff, L., Roberts, P. A., Januska, M. M., and Kline, J. E. (1968): Mechanisms of stimulation of protein synthesis by thyroid hormones *in vivo. Proc. Natl. Acad. Sci. (USA),* 60:652–659.

Sokoloff, L., Wechsler, R. L., Mangold, R., Balls, K., and Kety, S. S. (1953): Cerebral blood flow and oxygen consumption in hyperthyroidism before and after treatment. *J. Clin. Invest.,* 32:202–208.

Tata, J. R. (1963): Inhibition of the biological action of thyroid hormones by actinomycin D and puromycin. *Nature,* 197:1167–1168.

Tata, J. R., Ernster, L., Lindberg, O., Arrhenius, E., Pedersen, S., and Hedman, R. (1963): The action of thyroid hormones at the cell level. *Biochem. J.,* 86:408–428.

Tata, J. R., and Widnell, C. C. (1966): Ribonucleic acid synthesis during the early action of thyroid hormones. *Biochem. J.,* 98:604–620.

Weiss, W. P., and Sokoloff, L. (1963): Reversal of thyroxine-induced hypermetabolism by puromycin. *Science*, 140:1324–1326.

DISCUSSION

Valcana: Dr. Sokoloff, in seeking a fundamental cellular effect of T_4 you started with protein synthesis, but something may even precede that. For example, have you studied permeability properties of mitochondrial membranes from hypo- and hyperthyroid animals in terms of amino acid uptake? If so, was there any influence on amino acid uptake? All the studies show incorporation of amino acid into protein, but what precedes that is amino acid uptake. In the mitochondrial system, protein synthesis is very much dependent on adequate amino acid uptake.

Sokoloff: This is an example of the reasons why we adhered to the strategy that any effects we saw *in vivo* should be paralleled by results *in vitro* before drawing any conclusions about mechanisms. Our *in vitro* system is cell-free, and therefore has no amino acid permeability limitations.

Valcana: But the mitochondrial membrane is there.

Sokoloff: But the amino acids, being incorporated into protein, do not get into the mitochondria. This is microsomal protein synthesis that we are studying.

Valcana: It may be preceded by an effect on mitochondrial protein synthesis. You synthesize something within the mitochondria that can, in turn, be dependent on the permeability of that membrane to amino acids.

Sokoloff: We doubt that a protein is being made which then stimulates microsomal protein synthesis, because the mitochondrial factor is dialyzable and heat-stable. If it is, it is a very small one. It could be a small peptide. If it is, then it is possible that it exists normally in the mitochondria, and that the T_4 releases it as it does NAD^+ and other substances.

Valcana: Or that it is synthesized as a response of the T_4 interaction with the mitochondrion and then, because of changes in the membrane barrier, it is diffused into the medium where it might stimulate microsomal protein synthesis. Although not demonstrated, it is thought that ribosomes do exist within the mitochondria, and the ribosomal effect may follow a mitochondrial protein stimulation.

Sokoloff: It is quite possible that there might have been a stimulation of mitochondrial protein synthesis, but what is released is not protein, at least as far as dialyzability and heat stability indicate. It could be a fragment of a protein.

Valcana: A small peptide.

Sokoloff: We have not excluded that; it is one of the possibilities we must consider.

Ford: There is a recent review by Turakulov (1972) which summarizes much of the Russian literature, as well as that of Western investigators, but it has not appeared in English yet. While he did not speak of thyroid hormone's effect in brain, he did discuss its effect on almost every other organ. He concluded that the basic effect of thyroid hormone is at the level of electron transport.

Sokoloff: That is an old theory that has never been proved. Thyroid hormones have many effects, most of them secondary to earlier effects, such as protein and enzyme synthesis. We have been studying some effects which may have broad consequences in cellular metabolism. Thyroid hormones *in vivo* stimulate the Ca^{2+}- and Mg^{2+}-ATPases of liver microsomes and liver plasma membranes. They do not have such effects in mature brain, but there have been reports of stimulations of Na^+, K^+-ATPase in developing brain. Such effects would probably result in changes in the intracellular ionic composition. Johnson, Jant, Kaufman, and Sokoloff (1971) have shown that nucleolar ribosomal RNA synthesis is very sensitive to the ionic strength of the medium. It may be that ionic effects are responsible for some of the changes in RNA and protein synthesis associated with the action of thyroid hormones. These can result in increased levels of a number of enzymes.

Bass: The comparison between infant and adult brain in terms of the actual crude mitochondrial fraction is interesting. Rather than creating a new process, is it possible that your actual mitochondrial fraction contains a higher concentration of something that might be present in the adult, because of the nature of the fractionation procedure?

Sokoloff: Yes, and one might ask another question. Are the mitochondria really changing during development, or are we just sampling a different population of mitochondria? We do not know.

Gona: Dr. Sokoloff, you made a comment that in the adult amphibian, the thyroid hormone has no effect at all on energy metabolism.

Sokoloff: That has been reported in the literature. It does not stem from my personal experience.

Salas: Until now we have been talking about changes produced by thyroid deficiency on a subcellular level, like mitochondrial fraction, enzymes, protein synthesis, etc. I would like to ask Dr. Ford if the increase in number of microglia might explain the impaired behavioral capabilities, as demonstrated by Eayrs (1964); Schapiro (1968); and Davenport et al. (1973). Do you think that the increased amount of glial cells, by reducing the space available, interfered with the growth of neuronal processes and thereby caused behavioral changes at later ages?

Ford: There were about the same number of microglia, but the microglia of the hypothyroid animals contained increased amounts of lysosomal material, so that any difference in the amount of space occupied by these microglia would be insignificant.

Salas: Yes, but according to studies of Diamond et al. (1966); Kuhlenkampf (1952), and Murray (1968), many such stress conditions such as dehydration and increased sensory and locomotor activity in both adult and infant may result in an increase in the rate of glial multiplication at different levels of the brain.

Ford: A point in relation to glia which we have not really explored is to what degree does the hypothyroid state influence the postnatal gliogenesis at about day 5 or 6? This could be very important for the subsequent function of the nerve cells. If this is influenced in any significant way almost any place in the brain, I would expect to find many biochemical and behavioral abnormalities.

Bass: There is considerable debate about the existence of microglia in developing brain. James Vaughn has described a third neuroglial cell type. What we have been calling microglia may be not the same type of scavenger cells that really are undifferentiated glial cells. Could you comment on that?

Ford: There are a number of theories about the source of microglia, one of which is that they might be derived from pericytes. To what degree the cells we are examining are microglia in the classical sense or to what degree are they a modified, perhaps even a third category of glia, is an unresolved question. Our criteria are those described by LeBlond for microglia, which are not quite the same as those used by other investigators.

Initially, we thought that we might have been looking at oligodendroglia, except that the nuclei contained material which was much more electrondense than would be found in normal oligodendroglia. The oligodendroglia which we expected to see at this age were relatively scarce. We have not tried to quantitate this glial population, but if oligodendroglia are scarcer in the hypothyroid brain than in the normal brain, cerebral function might be impaired.

Pesetsky: Dr. Nicholson also has reported on increases in the number of Bergmann glial cells in the hypothyroid state, and LeGrand recently reported observations by electron microscopy that profiles of Bergmann glial cytoplasm around the Purkinje dendrites are increased. There is growing evidence that the glia do respond to changes in thyroid state.

Timiras: As a physiologist, speaking of glia and neurons separately is not very appealing; I prefer to speak in terms of neuroglial units. If, for example, normal function of the neuron is impaired, you would expect, even in the hypothyroid, an increase in glial population, a normal reaction to any malfunction in the neurons. In other words, it is difficult to separate one from the other physiologically.

Pesetsky: Perhaps the glia will also respond to whatever goes right with the neuron.

Timiras: Both circumstances must be considered, as well as the implications of regional differences.

DISCUSSION REFERENCES

Davenport, J. W., and González, L. M. (1973): Neonatal thyroxine stimulation in rats: Accelerated behavioral maturation and subsequent learning deficit. *J. Comp. Physiol. Psychol.,* 85:397–408.

Eayrs, J. T. (1964): Effect of neonatal hyperthyroidism on maturation and learning in the rat. *Anim. Behav.,* 12:195–199.

Johnson, J., Jant, B., Kaufman, S., and Sokoloff, L. (1971): Effects of ionic strength on the RNA polymerase activities of isolated nuclei and nucleoli of rat liver. *Arch. Biochem, Biophys.,* 142:489–500.

Schapiro, S. (1968): Some physiological, biochemical and behavioral consequences of neonatal hormone administration: Cortisol and thyroxine. *Gen. Comp. Endrinol.,* 10:214–228.

Turakulov, Y. K. (1972): *The Thyroid Hormones.* Fan. Tashkent.

Thyroid Hormones and Brain Development,
edited by Gilman D. Grave. Raven Press,
New York, 1977.

Role of Thyroid Hormones in Development of GABA-Metabolic Enzymes in Cerebellar Neurons and Glia: Loss of Enzymatic Activity in Bergmann Cells of Hypothyroid Rats

Irwin Pesetsky* and John F. Burkart**

A variety of functional, morphological, and biochemical deficits have been described in the brains of animals rendered hypothyroid at birth or earlier in development (reviewed by Kollros, 1968; Hamburgh, 1969). The development of Purkinje cell dendrites in the cerebellum of hypothyroid neonatal rats is severely curtailed (Legrand, 1967), synaptogenesis is reduced, there is a decrease in the number of basket cells, and an increase in the number of granule cells and astrocytes (Bergmann glia) (Nicholson and Altman, 1972*a,b*). The work of Ramírez De Guglielmone and Gomez (1966) indicated that such morphological changes are accompanied by changes in levels of a number of amino acids in the brain, among them γ-aminobutyric acid (GABA), which has been implicated as an inhibitory neurotransmitter in the central nervous system. Hypothyroidism apparently also results in permanent reduction in cerebellar levels of γ-aminobutyric acid transaminase (GABA-T), the enzyme which catalyzes the oxidation of GABA to succinic semialdehyde (SSA) (García Argiz, Pasquini, Kaplún, and Gómez, 1967). A subsequent investigation by Krawiec, García Argiz, Gómez, and Pasquini (1969) demonstrated that GABA-T concentration could be restored to normal by administering thyroid hormone to hypothyroid rats prior to 15 days of age but not thereafter. In neither of the latter studies was it possible to determine whether these changes occurred in all cells or whether the various kinds of neurons and glial cells in the cerebellar cortex might differ chemically in their response to thyroid hormone deprivation.

We will summarize the results of our recent histochemical studies on GABA-degradative enzymes in cerebellar cortical cells of animals rendered chronically hypothyroid and in normal controls. In addition to GABA-T activity, we have also studied the activity of succinic semialdehyde dehydrogenase (SSADH), which mediates the oxidation of SSA to succinate. Our observations indicate that, in hypothyroid animals, activity of these enzymes is depressed, and that this depression is of a transient nature in

* Department of Anatomy, Albert Einstein College of Medicine, Bronx, New York 10461.
** Department of Biology, State University of New York at Farmingdale, Farmingdale, New York 11735.

neuronal elements but long-term or permanent in certain glial cells (Pesetsky, Burkart, and Hamburgh, 1973; Pesetsky, 1975).

METHODS

Pregnant Charles River CD-strain rats were fed a diet of powdered Rockland Mouse Diet containing 0.2% propylthiouracil (PTU) during the last week of gestation. This regimen was maintained in the young after birth until they were weaned. Thereafter, these hypothyroid young were fed the same goitrogenic diet. Pregnant controls and their young were fed unsupplemented food. Hypothyroid rats and controls of the same sex were killed at 3- to 4-day intervals between 1 and 60 days of age and at 10- to 12-day intervals up to the age of 100 days. At least 3 pairs of animals were studied in each age group. The cerebellum of each animal was rapidly removed and frozen in powdered Dry Ice. These tissues were then transferred to the cryostat, and parasaggital sections were cut through the vermis at 14 μm. The sectioning of control and experimental tissues was alternated, cutting the brain of a control animal prior to that of a hypothyroid rat in one experiment and reversing this order for the next run. Both animals of a pair intended for comparison were always sectioned within the same 1-hr period. Sections were mounted on warm coverslips and air dried in the cryostat at $-15°C$ for 12 to 24 hr prior to incubation.

Intracellular GABA-T activity in these sections was visualized by the method of Van Gelder (1965), but modified by substituting Ficoll (35%) for the agar originally recommended (Pesetsky, 1975). This change in the procedure significantly increases the viscosity of the incubation medium, diminishes diffusion of intrinsic cellular enzyme, and provides more precise localization of enzyme activity. The medium is entirely homogeneous when Ficoll is used in place of agar; therefore, the resulting histochemical

---

FIG. 1. GABA-T activity in cerebellar cortex of a 6-day-old control. Purkinje cells are large and heavily "stained."

Abbreviations for Figs. 1 through 8: P, Purkinje cells; a, axon; d, dendrite; B, Bergmann glia; M, molecular layer; G, internal granule layer; g, glomeruli; e, external granule layer. ×240.

FIG. 2. GABA-T activity in cerebellar cortex of 6-day-old, hypothyroid rat. This section was incubated "back to back" with the section in Fig. 1, and displays considerably less GABA-T activity in Purkinje cells. ×240.

FIG. 3. SSADH activity in cerebellar cortex of a control, 15 days of age. High levels of activity are seen in Purkinje cells and Bergmann glia. Moderate levels are visualized around internal granule layer cells and in molecular layer neuropil. ×400.

FIG. 4. SSADH activity in a section of cerebellar cortex of a 15-day-old hypothyroid rat incubated "back to back" with preparation in Fig. 3. Enzyme activity is lower in Purkinje cells of this animal, with moderate to high levels in Bergmann cells, molecular layer neuropil, and around internal granule layer cells. ×400.

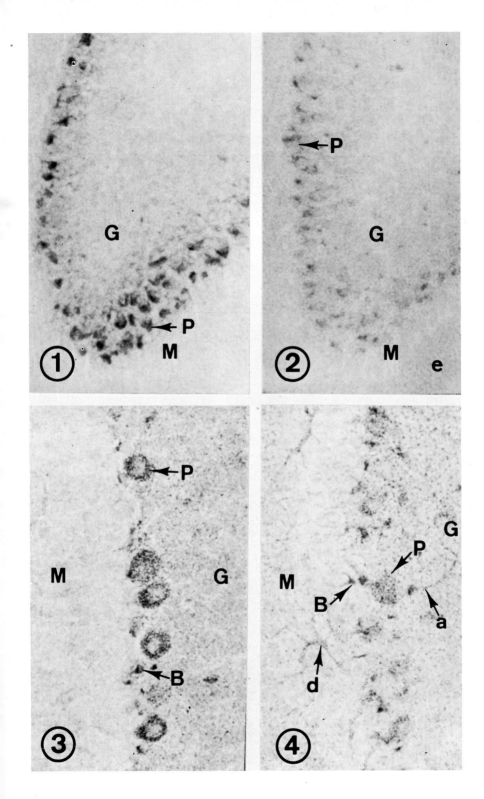

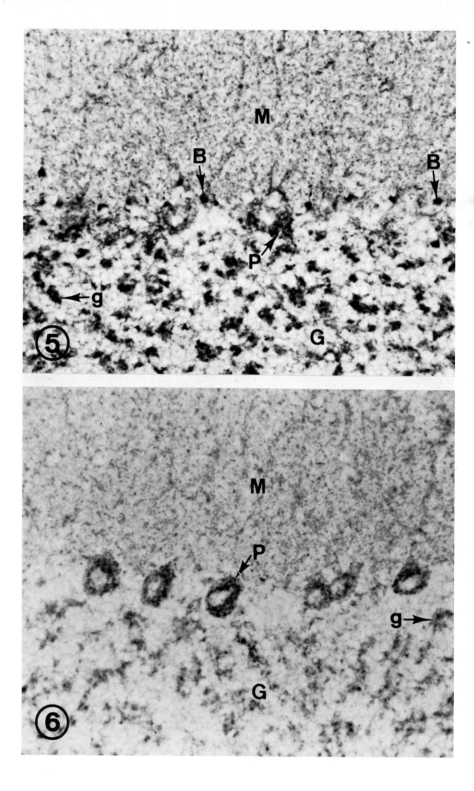

reaction is invariably uniform. In addition, the sections are more easily washed clean at the end of the incubation period.

SSADH activity was studied using the method of Sims, Weitsen, and Bloom (1971), modified, as above, with 35% Ficoll in place of agar. Initial samples of SSA, the substrate, were generously supplied by Dr. K. L. Sims. In later experiments we used SSA synthesized in our laboratory by the method of Bruce, Sims, and Pitts (1971). Results were the same with either substrate.

For each experiment, 10 ml of the appropriate incubation medium were prepared to fill a Columbia dish. Control and experimental sections intended for histochemical comparison were incubated "back to back," simultaneously, in the same dish of medium for 60 or 90 min at 38 °C. In each dish, as many as 14 sections from each member of each pair of animals could be incubated at the same time.

RESULTS

In the cerebellum of normal, adult animals, we found GABA-T and SSADH in the same cells (Figs. 5 and 7). Moderately high levels of these GABA-degradative enzymes were demonstrable in Purkinje cell bodies and their processes, in the neuropil of the molecular layer, and in glomeruli of the granule cell layer. Considerable "staining" was apparent around or between granule cells, but it could not be determined with any certainty whether activity was in granule cell cytoplasm or in glial processes between these cells. High levels of enzyme activity were also found in Bergmann glial fibers, in perikarya of their cells of origin, as well as in astrocytes dispersed throughout the white matter. We could detect no GABA-T or SSADH activity in newborn animals. By 3 days of age, low levels of activity were seen in Purkinje cell perikarya, by 6 days these enzymes were demonstrable in Purkinje cell dendrites, in molecular layer neuropil, and in synaptic glomeruli of the granule layer (Fig. 1). Until day 6, comparison of control and hypothyroid animals revealed no differences between the two groups. On day 6, and more obviously on days 8 and 10, activity in controls was clearly more intense than in the hypothyroid young (Figs. 1 and 2). These differences were confined on days 6 to 10 to Purkinje cells perikarya, but thereafter were seen in Purkinje dendrites, in molecular layer neuropil,

FIG. 5. GABA-T activity in a control 62 days of age. High levels of activity are seen in Purkinje cells, Bergmann glia, molecular layer neuropil, and synaptic glomeruli in the internal granule layer. ×440.

FIG. 6. GABA-T in hypothyroid rat 62 days of age incubated "back to back" with section seen in Fig. 5. Although "staining" intensity in this animal is somewhat less than that in the control, most animals older than 26 days show no such differences. Note, however, that Bergmann glia in this animal contain little GABA-T and thus cannot be readily visualized. ×470.

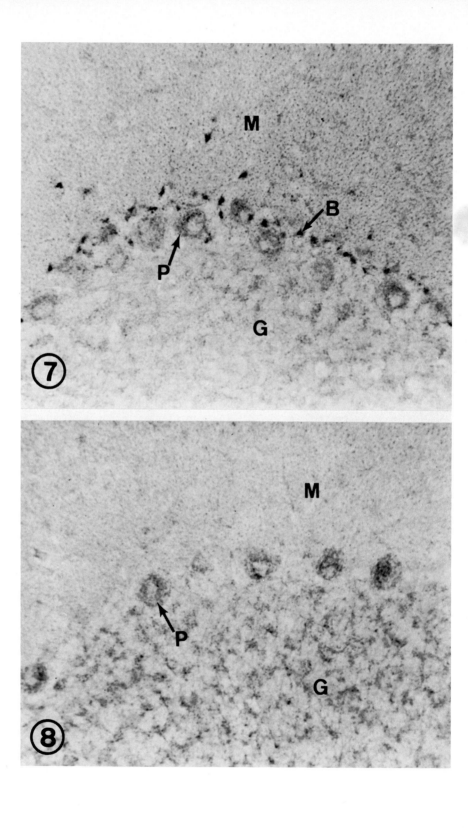

glomeruli, and glia (Figs. 3 and 4). From day 6 through 23, activity of GABA-T and of SSADH in these elements was consistently more intense in controls (Figs. 1 and 3) than in PTU-treated rats (Figs. 2 and 4); these "staining" differences were generally apparent even to the naked eye. After the 26th postnatal day, such differences were no longer apparent in most cells nor in the neuropil of the molecular layer. In animals as old as 100 days, tissues from either group were approximately equal in staining intensity or varied individually with no relation to the thyroidal states of the animals from which they were taken.

With respect to the Bergmann glia, the situation was quite different. In PTU-treated rats, as in controls, Bergmann fibers and cells displayed considerable GABA-T and SSADH activity between days 10 and 23. Enzyme activity was high in the patch of cytoplasm just distal to the nucleus as well as in the radial processes which course through the molecular layer to reach the pia. In normal controls 40 days of age or older, a considerable amount of activity was demonstrable in Bergmann cells and fibers (Figs. 5 and 7). However, in preparations from hypothyroid animals processed "back to back" with those controls, Bergmann cells were difficult, indeed often almost impossible, to identify; most displayed little or no GABA-T or SSADH activity and were therefore nearly invisible (Figs. 6 and 8).

DISCUSSION

The biochemical study of García Argiz et al. (1967) on cerebellar homogenates shows that normal levels of GABA-T in the rat increase sixfold between postnatal days 5 and 40. In hypothyroid animals, these levels are depressed as much as 55% between days 5 and 50. The authors indicate that these differences between control and hypothyroid animals are transient (beginning on day 5 and diminishing after 40 days) if the data are analyzed on a wet-weight basis, but permanent if calculated on the basis of cerebellar DNA.

Our histochemical studies indicate the onset of GABA-T activity in the cerebellum as early as postnatal day 3, and confirm the findings of García Argiz et al. (1967) that GABA-T activity at day 5 is approximately equal in control and hypothyroid rats and that depression of GABA-T activity below normal levels first becomes apparent between 5 and 10 days of age. Our

FIG. 7. SSADH in a 72-day-old control. Bergmann cells display high levels of activity. Moderate activity is seen in Purkinje cells, molecular level neuropil, and glomeruli in the internal granule layer. ×400.

FIG. 8. SSADH activity in hypothyroid rat 72 days old, incubated "back to back" with section illustrated in Fig. 7. Note the virtual absence of activity in Bergmann glia. In this section moderate activity is seen in Purkinje cells and molecular layer neuropil, and higher levels are present in glomeruli of the internal granule layer. ×400.

histochemical observations indicate that the decrease in GABA-T activity in Purkinje cells, glomeruli, and neuropil persists until no later than 26 days of age, and not 50 or more days as suggested by García Argiz and his co-workers. Our histochemical methods may not be sufficiently sensitive to detect the more persistent differences reported by the latter investigators. However, it may be significant that Sims, Witztum, Quick, and Pitts (1968) report that GABA-T activity in whole rat brain rises rapidly until day 26, then plateaus at a level approximating that of adults. In hypothyroid animals, the rate of GABA-T synthesis in neurons may be temporarily retarded, catching up with adult levels on or about 26 days of age. On the other hand, the methods employed in the biochemical assays of brain homogenates do not permit analysis of the contributions made by neurons as opposed to those of glia. In hypothyroid rats, neuronal GABA-T activity (in Purkinje cells, in synaptic glomeruli, and in molecular layer neuropil) may be transiently suppressed, and long-term or permanent depression in GABA-T activity may be attributable largely to loss of enzymatic activity in Bergmann glial elements.

Our findings with regard to localization and activity of SSADH in normal and hypothyroid rats parallel those for GABA-T. Our failure to observe SSADH activity in the cerebellum prior to day 3 is at variance with the results of biochemical assays of Pitts and Quick (1966), who showed high levels of SSADH activity in all layers of the rat cerebellum at birth. Again, histochemical methods may not be sufficiently sensitive to detect the level of SSADH activity prior to day 3. However, Pitts and Quick (1967) also speculate on the possibility that the enzyme synthesized until the second day of life may be a fetal protein species, different from the adult enzyme synthesized later. Their study on SSADH in whole brain shows a sharp increase in synthesis on postnatal day 6, the age at which we first observed activity of this enzyme in Purkinje cell dendrites, in molecular layer neuropil, and in synaptic glomeruli of the internal granule layer. In our study, day 6 also marks the onset of consistent differences in SSADH and GABA-T activity between control and hypothyroid rats.

Growing evidence suggests that GABA functions as an inhibitory neurotransmitter in the central nervous system of vertebrates (Krnjević, 1974). There is also considerable concern regarding the manner in which extracellular GABA is removed from the synaptic environment and inactivated following performance of its inhibitory function. It is known that free GABA is taken up by a variety of nerve endings and presynaptic inhibitory interneurons (review by Krnjević, 1974), but the capacity of glial cells to accumulate GABA is considerably greater (Hamberger and Sellström, 1974). Exogenous [³H]GABA is taken up by glioma cells (Schrier and Thompson, 1972), by satellite cells in sensory ganglia (Gottesfeld, Kelly, and Schon, 1973), by Müller cells in retina (Neal and Iverson, 1972), and by glial cells in cerebral cortex (Henn and Hamberger, 1971).

Hökfelt and Ljungdahl (1972) have reported uptake of [³H]GABA by Bergmann glia in rat cerebellum. The presence in Bergmann glia of GABA-T and SSADH (Pesetsky et al., 1973; Pesetsky, 1975) indicates that these cells not only take up GABA, but are also capable of breaking down the GABA they accumulate. The entire dendritic arborization of each Purkinje cell is enveloped in sheaths of Bergmann cell cytoplasm. Since GABA is an important neurotransmitter in the brain, the loss of GABA- degradative enzyme activity by Bergmann glia could have significant effects on synaptic function in the cerebellar cortex.

Hypothyroidism in children and in adults may result in a variety of neurological complications. Among these, ataxic symptoms attributable to cerebellar dysfunction are frequent, and, in adults, often severe (reviewed by Sokoloff and Kennedy, 1973; Mancall, 1975). There is a high incidence of cerebellar ataxia in patients hypothyroid during their first 3 months of life, but such symptoms occur less often in those treated with thyroid hormones sufficiently early in life (Wiebel, 1976). Smith, Blizzard, and Wilkins (1957) report abnormal neurological findings (including incoordination, intention tremors, and disturbances of gait attributable to cerebellar dysfunction) in 18% of severe congenital cretins whose thyroid hormone therapy had been initiated within the first 6 months of life, but in 37% of those whose treatment was delayed until after 6 months of age. These neurological signs showed little evidence of improvement with hormone administration. In contrast, most older children and adults with cerebellar dysfunction arising from hypothyroidism acquired later in life show relatively prompt and often complete clearing of ataxic symptoms after replacement therapy with thyroid hormones (Jellinek and Kelly, 1960; Cremer, Goldstein, and Paris, 1969).

Animal experiments indicate that cerebellar structures are particularly dependent on an adequate supply of thyroid hormones during prenatal, perinatal, and early postnatal life. In rats rendered hypothyroid during these periods, cerebellar morphogenesis is delayed, and the histological characteristics of the maturing cerebellar cortex are considerably altered (Legrand, Kriegel, and Jost, 1961; Legrand, 1965, 1967a; Geloso, Hemon, Legrand, Legrand, and Jost, 1968; Nicholson and Altman, 1972b). Administration of thyroxine during the first 2 weeks of postnatal life reverses these effects of the hypothyroid state, but when treatment is initiated later than the second week, cerebellar development remains abnormal (Legrand, 1967b). Similarly, the striking decrease in cerebral and cerebellar levels of GABA-T produced by the absence of thyroid function can be restored to normal only by thyroid treatment before 15 days of age (Krawiec et al., 1969). Legrand (1967b) has suggested that in the rat the first 2 weeks of life constitute a "critical period" for the development of the cerebellum, and that adequate levels of thyroid hormone must be available then for normal cerebellar development. Clinical experience suggests the existence of a similar, thyroid-dependent critical period for cerebellar morphogenesis in man (Hagberg and Westphal, 1970; Wiebel, 1976). The ataxic syndromes of patients with congenital hypothyroidism may be attributable, at least in part, to abnormal cerebellar histogenesis during this critical period. Ataxias in such patients are nonprogressive (Hagberg and Westphal, 1970) and not reversed by hormone therapy. However, cerebellar ataxia is also found in individuals who become hypothyroid long after cerebellar morphogenesis has been completed. The rapid, often complete loss of ataxic symptoms following appropriate hormonal therapy suggests a metabolic or other neurochemical etiology for these cerebellar dysfunctions.

Elevated levels of GABA in the cerebellum are associated with ataxia in experimental animals (Grimm, Gottesfeld, Wassermann, and Samuel, 1974; Anlezark, Horton, Meldrum, and Sawaya, 1976). In these studies, GABA levels were markedly increased by agents that depress the activity of GABA-T and/or SSADH. Ataxias also occur in humans given high doses of antiepileptic drugs that inhibit these catabolic enzymes (Sawaya, Horton, and Meldrum, 1975). GABA-T and SSADH are intracellular, mitochondrially bound enzymes. Since synaptically released GABA is probably inactivated largely by glial reuptake, (Henn and Hamberger, 1971; Hamberger and Sellström, 1974), inhibition of these enzymes may cause an accumulation of GABA in glia. Increased levels of intracellular GABA could interfere with reuptake, thus raising GABA levels in synaptic clefts and prolonging inhibitory activity. The results of Bowery and Brown (1972), showing that GABA accumulated by glial cells can be released by depolarization, suggest also that glia may play a direct role in modulating neuronal excitation.

Purkinje cells comprise the only output from the cerebellar cortex. Basket and stellate cells make inhibitory, GABA-ergic synapses on Purkinje cell somata and dendrites (Roberts, 1974), and the sheaths of Bergmann glial cell cytoplasm that enclose Purkinje cells are intimately associated with these synaptic sites. Our demonstration that Bergmann cells of hypothyroid rats lose capacity to degrade GABA suggests the possibility that in such animals, GABA levels in inhibitory synapses on Purkinje cells may be altered, thus contributing to abnormal cerebellar function.

ACKNOWLEDGMENTS

The work reported here was supported by grant NS 04555 from the National Institutes of Health, U.S. Public Health Service.

REFERENCES

Anlezark, G., Horton, R. W., Meldrum, B. S., and Sawaya, M. C. B. (1976): Anticonvulsant action of ethanolamine-0-sulphate and DL-n-propylacetate and the metabolism of γ-aminobutyric acid (GABA) in mice with audiogenic seizures. *Biochem. Pharmacol.*, 25:413–417.

Bowery, N. G., and Brown, D. A. (1972): γ-Aminobutyric acid uptake by sympathetic ganglia. *Nature (New Biol.)*, 238:89–91.

Bruce, R. A., Sims, K. L., and Pitts, F. N., Jr. (1971): Synthesis and purification of succinic semialdehyde. *Anal. Biochem.*, 41:271–273.

Cremer, G. M., Goldstein, N. P., and Paris, J. (1969): Myxedema and ataxia. *Neurology*, 19:37–46.

García Argiz, C. A., Pasquini, J. M., Kaplún, B., and Gómez, C. J. (1967): Hormonal regulation of brain development. II. Effect of neonatal thyroidectomy on succinate dehydrogenase and other enzymes in developing cerebral cortex and cerebellum of the rat. *Brain Res.*, 6:635–646.

Geloso, J. P., Hemon, P., Legrand, J., Legrand, C., and Jost, A. (1968): Some aspects of thyroid physiology during the perinatal period. *Gen. Comp. Endocrinol.*, 10:191–197.

Gottesfeld, Z., Kelly, J. S., and Schon, F. (1973): Uptake of γ-aminobutyric acid (GABA) by sensory root ganglia. *Br. J. Pharmacol.*, 47:640P.

Grimm, V., Gottesfeld, Z., Wassermann, I., and Samuel, D. (1975): The level of GABA in the brain and locomotor behavior. *Pharmacol. Biochem. Behav.*, 3:573–578.

Hagberg, B., and Westphal, O. (1970): Ataxic syndrome in congenital hypothyroidism. *Acta Paediat. Scand.*, 59:323–327.

Hamburgh, M. (1969): The role of thyroid and growth hormones in neurogenesis. In: *Current Topics in Developmental Biology*, edited by A. A. Moscona and A. Monroy, Vol. 4, pp. 109–148. Academic Press, New York.

Hamberger, A., and Sellström, A. (1974): Techniques for separation of neurons and glia and their application to metabolic studies. In: *Metabolic Compartmentation and Neurotransmission, NATO Advanced Study Institute on Metabolic Compartmentation in Relation to Structure and Function of the Brain, Oxford, 1974*, edited by S. Berl, D. D. Clarke, and D. Schneider, pp. 145–166. Plenum Press, New York.

Henn, F. A., and Hamberger, A. (1971): Glial cell function: Uptake of transmitter substances. *Proc. Natl. Acad. Sci. USA*, 68:2686–2690.

Hökfelt, T., and Ljungdahl, Å. (1972): Histochemical determination of neurotransmitter distribution. In: *Neurotransmitters*, edited by I. J. Kopin, *Ass. Res. Nerv. Dis. Proc.*, Vol. 50, pp. 1–24. Williams & Wilkins, Baltimore.

Jellinek, E. H., and Kelly, R. E. (1960): Cerebellar syndrome in myxedema. *Lancet*, 2:225–227.

Kollros, J. J. (1968): Endocrine influences in neural development. In: *Ciba Foundation Symposium on Growth of the Nervous System*, edited by G. Wolstenholme and M. O'Connor, pp. 179–192. J. and A. Churchill, London.

Krawiec, L., García Argiz, C. A., Gómez, C. J., and Pasquini, J. M. (1969): Hormonal regulation of brain development. III. Effects of triiodothyronine and growth hormone on the biochemical changes in the cerebral cortex and cerebellum of neonatally thyroidectomized rats. *Brain Res.*, 15:209–218.

Krnjević, K. (1974): Chemical nature of synaptic transmission in vertebrates. *Physiol. Rev.*, 54:418–540.

Legrand, J. (1965): Influence de l'hypothyroïdisme sur la maturation du cortex cérébelleux. *C.R. Acad. Sci.*, 261:544–547.

Legrand, J. (1967a): Analyse de l'action morphogénétique des hormones thyroidiennes sur le cervelet du jeune rat. *Arch. Anat. Micr. Morphol. Exp.*, 56:205–241.

Legrand, J. (1967b): Variations en fonction de l'age de la response du cervelet à l'action morphogénétique de la thyroide chez le rat. *Arch. Anat. Micr. Morphol. Exp.*, 56:291–308.

Legrand, J., Kriegel, A., and Jost, A. (1961): Déficience thyroidienne et maturation du cervelet chez le rat blanc. *Arch. Anat. Micr. Morphol. Exp.*, 50:507–519.

Mancall, E. L. (1975): Late (acquired) cortical cerebellar atrophy. In: *Handbook of Clinical Neurology*, edited by P. J. Vinken and G. W. Bruyn, Vol. 21, Part 1, p. 496. North Holland, Amsterdam.

Neal, M. J., and Iverson, L. L. (1972): Autoradiographic localization of ^{3}H-GABA in rat retina. *Nature (New Biol.)*, 235:217–218.

Nicholson, J. L., and Altman, J. (1972a): Synaptogenesis in the rat cerebellum: Effects of early hypo- and hyperthyroidism. *Science*, 176:530–531.

Nicholson, J. L., and Altman, J. (1972b): The effects of early hypo- and hyperthyroidism on the development of rat cerebellar cortex. I. Cell proliferation and differentiation. *Brain Res.*, 44:13–23.

Pesetsky, I. (1975): Glial GABA degradative enzyme activity in cerebellar cortex of the rat: Effect of altered thyroidal state. *J. Cell Biol.,* 67:331.

Pesetsky, I., Burkart, J., and Hamburgh, M. (1973): Cerebellar development: Histochemical studies of succinic semialdehyde dehydrogenase and γ-aminobutyric acid transaminase activities in euthyroid, hypothyroid, and hyperthyroid rats. *Anat. Rec.,* 175:411.

Pitts, F. N., Jr., and Quick, C. (1967): Brain succinate semialdehyde dehydrogenase—II. Changes in the developing rat brain. *J. Neurochem.,* 14:561–570.

Ramírez De Guglielmone, A. E., and Gómez, C. J. (1966): Influence of neonatal hypothyroidism on amino acids in developing rat brain. *J. Neurochem.,* 13:1017–1025.

Roberts, E. (1974): γ-Aminobutyric acid and nervous system function. A perspective. *Biochem. Pharmacol.,* 23:2637–2649.

Sawaya, M. C. B., Horton, R. W., and Meldrum, B. S. (1975): Effects of anticonvulsant drugs on the cerebral enzymes metabolizing GABA. *Epilepsia,* 16:649–655.

Schrier, B. K., and Thompson, E. J. (1972): Glutamate and gamma-aminobutyrate metabolism in cultured glial cells. *Fed. Proc.,* 31:490.

Sims, K. L., Weitsen, H. A., and Bloom, F. E. (1971): Histochemical localization of brain succinic semialdehyde dehydrogenase—A γ-aminobutyric acid degradative enzyme. *J. Histochem. Cytochem.,* 19:405–415.

Sims, K. L., Witztum, J., Quick, C., and Pitts, F. N., Jr. (1968): Brain 4-aminobutyrate:2-oxoglutarate aminotransferase. Changes in the developing rat brain. *J. Neurochem.,* 15:667–672.

Smith, D. W., Blizzard, R. M., and Wilkins, L. (1957): The mental prognosis in hypothyroidism of infancy and childhood. *Pediatrics,* 19:1011–1022.

Sokoloff, L., and Kennedy, C. (1973): The action of thyroid hormones and their influence on brain development and function. In: *Biology of Brain Dysfunction,* edited by G. E. Gaull, Vol. 2, pp. 295–332. Plenum Press, New York.

Van Gelder, N. M. (1965): The histochemical demonstration of γ-aminobutyric acid metabolism by reduction of a tetrazolium salt. *J. Neurochem.,* 12:231–237.

Wiebel, J. (1976): Cerebellar-ataxic syndrome in children and adolescents with hypothyroidism under treatment. *Acta Paediatr. Scand.,* 65:201–205.

DISCUSSION

Hamburgh: Do these animals, particularly the older ones that you assayed, look like animals that have a neuromuscular defect, or do they behave normally, like animals with intact cerebella?

Pesetsky: Many of these animals have an abnormal gait, but we have not yet done a proper behavioral study.

Ford: Some years ago we were studying the effect of irradiation on developing brain, and some of the rats were allowed to attain maturity. Their behavior seemed perfectly normal until picked up by the tail. Then they showed a prompt scissoring of the hind limbs and problems in subsequent locomotion. Had you tested your hypothyroid rats, you might have found a similar disorder of posture, in turn reflecting a possible defect in neuroglial interrelationships.

Have you studied the spinal cord? GABA seems to be effective in that part of the neuroaxis.

Pesetsky: We have not yet studied the cord.

Balázs: Eayrs has investigated the behavioral effects of neonatal thyroid deficiency; he noted that the motor coordination of the animals was impaired when they grew up. When rats were exposed to insults of various kinds, e.g., undernutrition, during the early postnatal period, the effects on motor coordination were similar, i.e., the result was a clumsy animal, indicating that cerebellar functions are not as good as in the normal rat.

In regard to GABA-T activity in thyroid deficiency, histochemical methods are useful in demonstrating the pattern of localization of chemical constituents, but they are of limited help in quantification. The potential GABA-T activity exceeds the overall GABA flux in the cerebellum. Thus, it is possible that even a fraction of the normal enzyme activity in the Bergmann glia may be sufficient to cope with the small amounts of GABA that are released as a result of synaptic function adjacent to those cells. Therefore, the observation that the histochemically discernible GABA-T activity is depressed in the Bergmann glia in thyroid deficiency does not necessarily imply a functional impairment of the inactivation of GABA in the cerebellar cortex.

It must also be remembered that the neurophysiological action of GABA is exerted only when this substance reaches the proper receptors on the outside of neurons. Functional problems involving GABA in thyroid deficiency would arise by a failure of the Bergmann glia to take up GABA released into the synapse, rather than from a decrease in the activity of GABA-T which is exclusively an intracellular, mitochondrial enzyme. Indeed, it seems that Bergmann glia can accumulate GABA. Although this has not yet been studied in thyroid deficiency, your gold-impregnated sections indicate that the Bergmann glia is normal, so certain functions other than GABA-T activity, including GABA uptake, may not be impaired in the hypothyroid animals.

It seems that this applies not only to the molecular layer, but also to the internal granular layer. In comparison with controls, there are more glial profiles in thyroid deficiency.

Rosman: I would like to underscore the occurrence of motor deficits as a complication of malnutrition. It is difficult to attribute such deficits to an abnormality of cerebellum. Several years ago, when feeding pregnant rats a commercially available iodine-deficient diet (to induce hypothyroidism in their offspring), we noted that the mother rats developed ataxia, which we initially thought to be of cerebellar origin. While they ate this diet, the ataxia progressed to paresis, and then to total paralysis of the hind limbs. We investigated the animals in detail, and found that we had produced a myopathy, as evidenced by electrophysiological and morphological criteria. We then ascertained that this myopathy was not caused by a deficiency of iodine, but rather by more generalized malnutrition. These observations illustrate that malnutrition can cause motor abnormalities which may mimic those of cerebellar origin.

Pesetsky: The abnormal gait I see in PTU-treated rats also occurs in some rats thyroidectomized at birth with [131]I. These thyroidectomized animals are maintained on normal laboratory chow. Although their growth is retarded, there is no evidence that they are malnourished.

Bass: In humans, hypothyroidism has been reported to produce morphologically aberrant Purkinje cells containing odd cytoplasmic bodies. However, Dr. King-Engel has indicated that these bodies may be artifacts associated with tetrazolium salt staining.

Balázs: But in Dr. Pesetsky's experiments, the activity of GABA-T in the hypothyroid animals was compared with GABA-T activity in controls, thus all the variables except the thyroid state were comparable.

Bass: But, are we really staining the GABA enzyme system?

Sokoloff: The tetrazolium reaction depends on NADH generation. But suppose that the enzyme is not affected at all, but for some reason there is a loss of NAD^+ from the mitochondria. Would that not give the same result?

Pesetsky: No, I do not believe it would. We are dealing with NAD^+-dependent reactions, and exogenous NAD^+ is an ingredient of the histochemical incubation medium. I think Dr. Bass's question has to do with the possibility that our reactions might actually be demonstrating nonspecific diaphorase activity rather than SSADH or GABA-T. In histochemical tests for NAD^+-dependent dehydrogenases using nitro-blue tetrazolium (NBT), the substrate is oxidized by the cellular dehydrogenase, and NAD^+ becomes reduced to NADH. Reduction of the tetrazolium salt (NBT) to an insoluble blue precipitate within the cell is effected by oxidation of the NADH back to NAD^+ through mediation of a NADH-diaphorase. It is assumed that the primary dehydrogenase will be close to a diaphorase system within the same cellular locale, but one cannot be certain that the observed reduction of the tetrazole has not been caused by NADH diffusing from some other site.

To deal with this possibility, we employed a number of controls. If tissues were incubated in histochemical media which were complete except for the omission of substrate (GABA or SSA), there was little or no formazan production, and sections were either very pale or blank. When sections were tested for NADH-diaphorase activity using exogenous NADH as substrate, staining was similar in some respects to that with GABA or SSA, but no differences were seen between control and hypothyroid animals. Sims, Weitsen, and Bloom (1971) have shown that a 1 mM concentration of nordihydroguaiaretic acid (NDGA) in the incubation medium will inhibit NADH-diaphorase activity, but not SSADH. We have employed this test with similar results. In addition, the reaction for SSADH is buffered at pH 9. Sims et al. (1971) demonstrated that at pH 9, NBT is reduced directly by NADH and that the reaction is not mediated by diaphorase. We are therefore confident that the methods employed are reliable.

Sokoloff: But when you replace GABA in your reaction, you may not get the maximal amount of product, either, especially if only a small fraction of the GABA pool functions as a transmitter pool.

Balázs: I do not think that, in this particular case, the difference between the experimental and the hypothyroid animal could be accounted for by an artifact.

Sokoloff: We, too, had problems with the low-iodine diet supplied by Nutritional Biochemical Corporation. We tried to do studies similar to those of LeBlond and fed the animals a normal diet of Purina Laboratory Chow after thyroidectomy. We found that the thyroidectomized animals did not grow, but the sham-operated ones did not grow well either. We then switched to the low-iodine diet, because we had learned that the regular Purina Chow contains thyroactive substances. The thyroidectomized animals did not grow, and again neither did the controls. We found that by supplementing the low-iodine diet with brewer's yeast, as LeBlond had suggested, normal growth of the sham-operated animals could be achieved. You must be careful with low-iodine diets, because they may also be nutritionally deficient.

Rosman: There is now available a vitamin-fortified low-iodine diet that is more expensive than the nonsupplemented one. Actually, the diet that we had used was vitamin-fortified, but it clearly was in need of more fortification!

DISCUSSION REFERENCE

Sims, K. L., Weitsen, H. A., and Bloom, F. E. (1971): Histochemical localization of brain succinic semialdehyde dehydrogenase – A γ-aminobutyric acid degradative enzyme. *J. Histochem. Cytochem.*, 19:405–415.

Thyroid Hormones and Brain Development,
edited by Gilman D. Grave. Raven Press,
New York, 1977.

Thyroid-Induced Maturation of the Cerebellar Cortex in the Frog

Amos G. Gona*

At the time of metamorphosis, the frog tadpole undergoes dramatic morphological and biochemical changes (Etkin, 1968; Frieden, 1968). Since Gudernatsch (1912, 1914) discovered that metamorphosis of the frog tadpole is controlled by the thyroid, many of the different aspects of the metamorphic phenomenon have been analyzed. The question of whether these various metamorphic changes are under direct or indirect control of thyroid hormone has been the subject of numerous studies.

By implanting T_4-impregnated agar, Hartwig (1940) demonstrated that metamorphic changes could be induced in small, localized regions of the skin. Kaltenbach (1953a–c; 1959) and Kollros and Kaltenbach (1952) applied this ingenious method extensively for testing the action of T_4 on metamorphic changes. They implanted T_4-containing cholesterol pellets at selected sites and produced local resorption of the tail fin (Kaltenbach, 1959) or perforation of the opercular integument to form the skin window (Kaltenbach, 1953c) in *Rana pipiens* tadpoles. More recently, tadpole tail has been shown to undergo resorption *in vitro* in media containing T_4 (Derby, 1968; Gona, 1969) in a manner identical to the resorption *in vivo* described by Usuku and Gross (1965). These experiments indicate that thyroid hormone induces metamorphic changes by a direct action on the target tissues. However, other work has shown that not all metamorphic events are induced by a direct action of thyroid hormone. Helff (1928, 1931, 1937), for example, demonstrated that the immediate causative factor in the formation of tympanic membrane is the influence of the annular cartilage and columella, and that the latter structures are under thyroid control. It is thus important to study every metamorphic event to determine whether the effect of the thyroid is direct or indirect.

Development of the amphibian brain is dependent on thyroid hormone. Allen (1918) reported that development of the brain in thyroidectomized *Rana pipiens* tadpoles was retarded. Similar observations were made by Hoskins and Hoskins (1919) in thyroidectomized *Rana sylvatica* larvae. More recently, several studies have demonstrated the dependence of neuronal and neuroglial elements of the amphibian brain on the maturational

* Department of Anatomy, College of Medicine and Dentistry of New Jersey, Newark, New Jersey 07103.

effects of thyroid hormone (Tusques, 1949a,b,c; Weiss and Rosetti, 1951; Kollros and McMurray, 1956; Pesetsky and Kollros, 1956; Pesetsky, 1962, 1965; Pesetsky and Model, 1969). In general, these studies indicate that thyroid hormone induces precocious growth and differentiation of the cells of the tadpole brain. For example, Kollros and McMurray (1956) demonstrated that the neurons of the mesencephalic V nucleus not only respond to T_4 by growth, but also show a dramatic regression when the hormone action ceases.

Our interest in the metamorphic changes in the cerebellum was generated by the paucity of information on this particular aspect of metamorphosis. Although Larsell (1925) had studied the developmental changes in the frog cerebellum long ago, the rapid metamorphic changes in this part of the brain were barely appreciated. For example, Larsell made no mention of the formation of an external granular layer in the tadpole cerebellum. We found that a conspicuous external granular layer, similar to that seen in mammals, is established during metamorphosis and that the cells from this layer migrate into the internal granular layer primarily just before and during metamorphic climax (the period following the emergence of the fore limbs (Figs. 1 through 3).

Our first concern, then, was to determine whether treatment with thyroid hormone would induce precocious cerebellar maturation in the premetamorphic tadpole. This was of particular interest to us in view of the evidence that the mammalian cerebellum is very sensitive to the maturational effects of the thyroid hormone (see Legrand, 1967a,b; Hamburgh, Mendoza, Burkart, and Weil, 1971). In one series of experiments we injected premetamorphic bullfrog tadpoles intraperitoneally with either thyroid-stimulating hormone (TSH) or T_4. We found that the maturational changes seen in

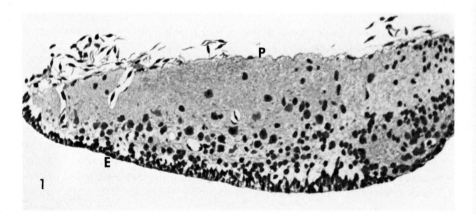

FIG. 1. Cerebellum of a premetamorphic bullfrog tadpole. Sagittal section. P, pia; E, ependyma. ×200 (From Gona, 1972.)

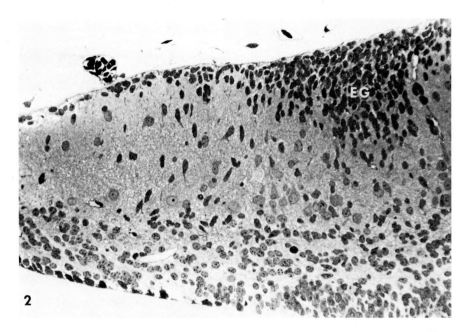

FIG. 2. Cerebellum of a bullfrog tadpole on the day of emergence of the fore legs. Note the cone of external granular layer cells (EG) migrating down toward the ependymal region. ×250. (From Gona, 1972.)

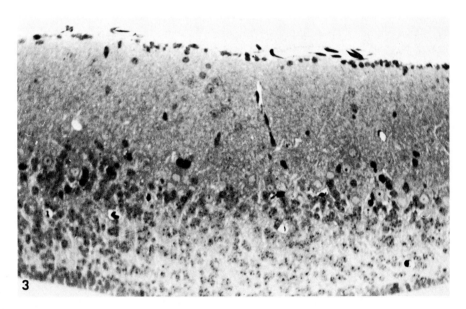

FIG. 3. Cerebellum of *R. pipiens* froglet 4 weeks after fore leg emergence. Note the disappearance of the external granular layer except for a few scattered cells. ×200.

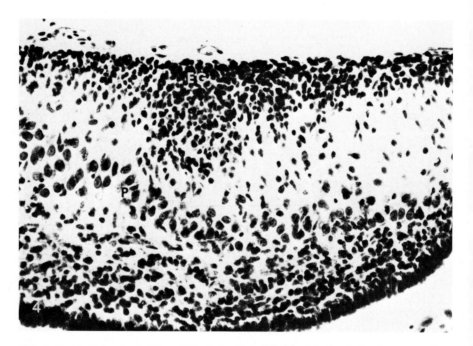

FIG. 4. Cerebellum of a bullfrog tadpole treated with thyroid-stimulating hormone. Note the massive migration of the external granule cells (EG) in the form an inverted cone and also the conspicuous Purkinje cell stratum (P). ×200. (From Gona, 1973.)

the cerebellum of spontaneously metamorphosing tadpoles could be duplicated by such hormone therapy (Fig. 4). However, we also found that growth hormone (GH), at a dose of 0.1 unit per animal, was effective in inducing cerebellar maturation (Gona, 1973).

MATERIALS AND METHODS

We explored the role of GH in the maturation of the frog cerebellum to determine if GH is capable of inducing cerebellar maturation as well as thyroid hormone. Premetamorphic bullfrog (*Rana catesbeiana*) tadpoles (8 to 12 g body weight) were obtained either through commercial suppliers or collected in the field. They were maintained in tap water at a temperature of 20 to 21°C and were fed canned spinach. Three groups of 10 tadpoles each were treated as follows:

Group 1: Ten tadpoles were thyroidectomized (method of Dent, 1959) and injected intraperitoneally, with 0.1 U of ovine GH (NIH-GH-S9) (made slightly alkaline with dilute sodium hydroxide, in 0.1 ml of 0.66% saline) on alternate days for 12 days via tail muscle with a Hamilton syringe fixed with a 30-gauge needle.

Group 2: Ten tadpoles were sham-operated and injected with GH as in group 1.

Group 3: Ten sham-operated controls were injected with saline only.

Twelve days after the first injection, all of the animals were killed and the upper jaws were fixed in Bouin's solution for 2 days. The brains were processed through paraffin. Sagittal sections were stained with hematoxylin-eosin.

A second experiment was designed to use the technique of implantation of T_4 to determine whether cerebellar maturation could be induced by a local effect of this hormone. The tadpoles were anesthetized by immersion in a solution of MS 222 (tricaine methane sulfonate), and the region of the optic tectum and cerebellum was exposed. Through an opening made in the arachnoid a few crystals of T_4 were implanted between the optic tectum and the cerebellum. Stray particles of T_4 were flushed out of the area, and the flaps of the cranium and skin were replaced. The animals were killed 12 days later, and paraffin sections were stained with cresyl violet.

RESULTS AND DISCUSSION

The cerebellum of the intact tadpoles treated with GH (group 2) showed establishment of a conspicuous external granular layer several cells thick, characteristic of normally metamorphosing tadpoles in late prometamorphic period (Fig. 5). The thyroidectomized tadpoles treated with GH (group 1) failed to show this effect and their cerebella (Fig. 6) were identical to those of the saline-injected control (group 3) animals (Fig. 8).

In our earlier study (Gona, 1973), GH (at a dose of 0.1 unit per injection given on alternate days for 12 days) induced cerebellar changes comparable with those induced by 0.1 μg of T_4 administered for 7 days. However, injections of 0.001 unit of TSH (equivalent to the impurity contained in 0.1 unit of growth hormone) also induced changes comparable to those of the preparation of GH. We surmised that this TSH impurity initiated the observed cerebellar changes in tadpoles treated with GH.

In the present work, thyroidectomized tadpoles were used to eliminate the effect of TSH impurity. Because these animals failed to develop the cerebellar changes induced by the preparation of GH in the intact animal, GH cannot be substituted for T_4 in inducing these maturational changes in the cerebellum of the frog tadpole.

Gómez, Ghittoni, and Dellacha (1966) and Hamburgh (1968) reported that GH could replace thyroid hormone in inducing maturational changes in the mammalian brain. In the frog tadpole, however, all available evidence indicates that thyroid hormones, their analogues, and TSH are the only substances that can trigger metamorphosis. The maturational changes in cerebellum seem to be equally specific in their dependence on thyroid hormones.

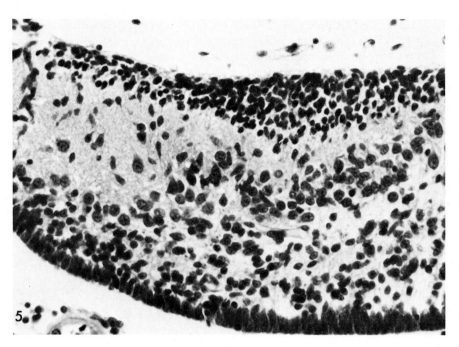

FIG. 5. Cerebellum of a growth hormone-treated, intact tadpole. Note the conspicuous bed of external granule cells (EG). ×200.

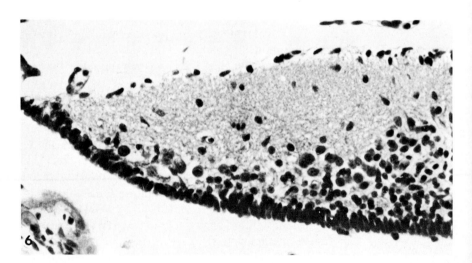

FIG. 6. Cerebellum of a thyroidectomized tadpole treated with growth hormone. ×200.

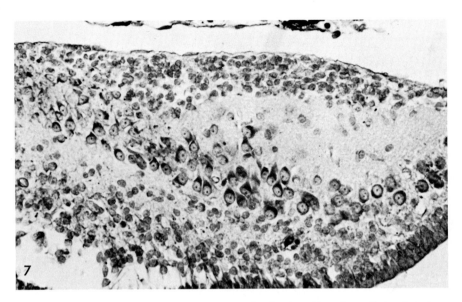

FIG. 7. Cerebellum of a tadpole carrying a thyroxine implant. Note the well-developed external granular layer and Purkinje layer. ×300.

In the second experiment involving T_4 implants, the cerebellum in the animals carrying such implants showed clear signs of cerebellar maturation. A prominent external granular layer was established, and migration of cells from this layer into the internal granular layer was observed (Fig. 7). Four animals which showed generalized metamorphic changes were discarded; the rest of the 20 animals bearing T_4 implants showed no external metamorphic changes. The control animals showed no sign of formation of a bed of external granular layer as in the first experiment (Fig. 8).

Establishment of the external granular layer as a secondary proliferative zone and the migration of cells from this layer away from the pial surface in the cerebellum are among the most remarkable developmental phenomena displayed by the CNS. The external granular layer is established early during development, and the migration of cells from this layer to their final destination is complete by the time of birth (or hatching), or soon after, in the higher vertebrates. Maturation of the human cerebellum is more protracted, and the migration of the external granule cells is not completed for several months after birth. In the bullfrog tadpole, the external granular layer is not present during the premetamorphic period, which may last for 2 or 3 years. The establishment of this layer is the first visible sign of cerebellar maturation and is seen at the onset of metamorphosis, i.e., during the prometamorphic period (Gona, 1972). For this reason, tadpole cerebellum promises to play a useful role in studies of the effects of thyroid hormone on the developing brain.

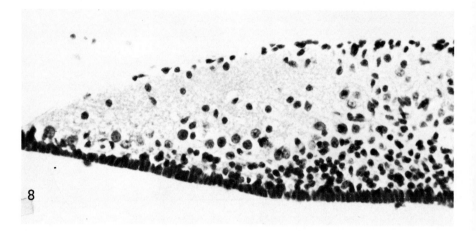

FIG. 8. Cerebellum of a saline-injected control tadpole. ×200.

Relatively large doses of mammalian TSH are needed to induce a rapid rate of metamorphosis in frog tadpoles. The fact that 0.001 unit of TSH readily induces pronounced maturational changes in the tadpole indicates that the tadpole cerebellum is highly sensitive to the maturational effect of T_4. The successful stimulation of cerebellar maturation by T_4 implants further enhances the usefulness of this experimental system for studying thyroid effects on brain development. However, more sophisticated experimental work is needed to demonstrate the direct action of thyroid hormone on the developing cerebellum. As mentioned earlier, not all metamorphic changes are directly influenced by thyroid hormone. Although maturation of many parts of the amphibian CNS depends directly on thyroid hormone (Kollros and McMurray, 1956; Kaltenbach, 1974), Beaudoin (1956) has shown that maturation of the ventral horn of the tadpole spinal cord may be stimulated by implanting T_4 pellets in the hind limb. The growth of the hind limbs appears to induce metamorphic changes in the ventral horn. In our present work, we must consider that the rapid growth of limbs during metamorphosis may stimulate cerebellar maturation. We are currently investigating this problem by other experimental approaches.

ACKNOWLEDGMENT

This work was supported by the National Institute of Child Health and Human Development, Grant HD-08157.

REFERENCES

Allen, B. M. (1918): The results of thyroid removal of *Rana pipiens*. *J. Exp. Zool.*, 24:499–519.
Beaudoin, A. R. (1956): The development of lateral motor column cells in the lumbo-sacral cord in *Rana pipiens*. *Anat. Rec.*, 125:247–259.

Dent, J. N. (1959): A technique for removing thyroid glands from anuran larvae. *Endocrinology*, 64:314–316.

Derby, A. (1968): An *in vitro* quantitative analysis of the response of tadpole tissue to thyroxine. *J. Exp. Zool.*, 168:147–156.

Etkin, W. (1968): Hormonal control of metamorphosis. In: *Metamorphosis*, edited by W. Etkin and L. I. Gilbert, pp. 313–348. Appleton-Century-Crofts, New York.

Frieden, E. (1968): Biochemistry of amphibian metamorphosis. In: *Metamorphosis*, edited by W. Etkin and L. I. Gilbert, pp. 349–398. Appleton-Century-Crofts, New York.

Gómez, C. J., Ghittoni, N. E., and Dellacha, J. M. (1966): Effect of L-thyroxine or somatotropin on body growth and cerebral development in neonatally thyroidectomized rats. *Life Sci.*, 5:243–246.

Gona, A. G. (1969): Light and electron microscope study on thyroxine-induced *in vitro* resorption of the tadpole tail fin. *Z. Zellforsch.*, 95:483–494.

Gona, A. G. (1972): Morphogenesis of the cerebellum of the frog tadpole during spontaneous metamorphosis. *J. Comp. Neurol.*, 146:133–142.

Gona, A. G. (1973): Effects of thyroxine, thyrotropin, prolactin and growth hormone on the maturation of the frog cerebellum. *Exp. Neurol.*, 38:494–501.

Gudernatsch, J. F. (1912): Feeding experiments on tadpoles. I. The influence of specific organs given as food on growth and differentiation. *Arch. Entw.-Mech. Org.*, 35:457–483.

Gudernatsch, J. F. (1914): Feeding experiments on tadpoles. II. A further contribution to the knowledge of organs with internal secretion. *Am. J. Anat.*, 15:431–481.

Hamburgh, M. (1968): An analysis of the action of thyroid hormone on development, based on *in vivo* and *in vitro* studies. *Gen. Comp. Endocrinol.*, 10:198–213.

Hamburgh, M., Mendoza, L. A., Burkart, J. F., and Weil, F. (1971): Thyroid-dependent processes in the developing nervous system. In: *Hormones in Development*, edited by M. Hamburgh and E. J. W. Barrington, pp. 403–415. Appleton-Century-Crofts, New York.

Hartwig, H. (1940): Metamorphose-Reaktionen auf einen lokalisierten Hormonreiz. *Biol. Zentralbl.*, 60:473–478.

Helff, O. M. (1928): Studies on amphibian metamorphosis. III. The influence of the annular tympanic cartilage on the formation of the tympanic membrane. *Physiol. Zool.*, 1:463–494.

Helff, O. M. (1931): Studies on amphibian metamorphosis. VII. The influence of the columella on the formation of the lamina propria of the tympanic membrane. *J. Exp. Zool.*, 59:179–197.

Helff, O. M. (1937): Studies on amphibian metamorphosis. XV. Direct tympanic membrane formation from dermal plicae integument transplanted to the ear region. *J. Exp. Biol.*, 14:1–15.

Hoskins, E. R., and Hoskins, M. M. (1919): Growth and development of amphibia as affected by thyroidectomy. *J. Exp. Zool.*, 29:1–69.

Kaltenbach, J. C. (1953a): Local action of thyroxine on amphibian metamorphosis. I. Local metamorphosis in *Rana pipiens* larvae effected by thyroxine-cholesterol implants. *J. Exp. Zool.*, (1953b): 122:21–39.

Kaltenbach, J. C. (1953b): Local action of thyroxine on amphibian metamorphosis. II. Development of the eyelids, nictitating membrane, and extrinsic ocular muscles in *Rana pipiens* larvae effected by thyroxine-cholesterol implants. *J. Exp. Zool.*, 122:41–51.

Kaltenbach, J. C. (1953c): Local action of thyroxine on amphibian metamorphosis. III. Formation and perforation of the skin window in *Rana pipiens* larvae effected by thyroxine-cholesterol implants. *J. Exp. Zool.*, 122:449–468.

Kaltenbach, J. C. (1959): Local action of thyroxine on amphibian metamorphosis. IV. Resorption of tail fin in anuran larvae effected by thyroxine-cholesterol implants. *J. Exp. Zool.*, 140:1–17.

Kaltenbach, J. C. (1974): Local action of thyroxine on amphibian metamorphosis. V. Cell division in the eye of anuran larvae effected by thyroxine-cholesterol implants. *J. Exp. Zool.*, 179:157–166.

Kollros, J. J., and Kaltenbach, J. C. (1952): Local metamorphosis of larval skin in *Rana pipiens*. *Physiol. Zool.*, 25:163–172.

Kollros, J. J., and McMurray, V. M. (1956): The mesencephalic V nucleus in anurans. II. The influence of thyroid hormone on cell size and cell number. *J. Exp. Zool.*, 131:1–26.

Larsell, O. (1925): The development of the cerebellum in the frog (*Hyla regilla*) in relation to the vestibular and lateral line systems. *J. Comp. Neurol.*, 39:249–289.

Legrand, J. (1967a): Analyse de l'action morphogénétique des hormones thyroidiennes sur le cervelet du jeune rat. *Arch. Anat. Microsc. Morphol. Exp.*, 56:205–244.

Legrand, J. (1967*b*): Variations, en fonction de l'age, de la réponse du cervelet à l'action mor-phogénétique de la thyroide chez le rat. *Arch. Anat. Microsc. Morphol. Exp.,* 56:291–307.

Pesetsky, I. (1962): The thyroxine-stimulated enlargement of Mauthner's neuron in anurans. *Gen. Comp. Endocrinol.,* 2:229–235.

Pesetsky, I. (1965): Thyroxine-stimulated oxidative enzyme activity associated with precocious brain maturation in anurans. A histochemical study. *Gen. Comp. Endocrinol.,* 5:411–417.

Pesetsky, I., and Kollros, J. J. (1956): A comparison of the influence of locally applied thyroxine upon Mauthner cell and adjacent neurons. *Exp. Cell Res.,* 11:477–482.

Pesetsky, I., and Model, P. G. (1969): Thyroxine-stimulated ultrastructural changes in epen-dymoglia of thyroprivic amphibian larvae. *Exp. Neurol.,* 25:238–245.

Rakic, P. (1971): Neuron-glia relationship during granule cell migration in developing cere-bellar cortex. A Golgi and electron microscopic study in *Macacus rhesus. J. Comp. Neurol.,* 141:283–312.

Tusques, J. (1949*a*): Action de la thyroxine sur l'appareil olfactif des têtards de *Rana esculenta. C. R. Soc. Biol. (Paris),* 143:245–247.

Tusques, J. (1949*b*): Action de la thyroxine sur l'appareil visual des têtards de *Rana esculenta. C. R. Soc. Biol. (Paris),* 143:332–334.

Tusques, J. (1949*c*): Corrélation entre le développement des membres et le développement des structures nerveuses centrales correspondentes (axe gris médullaire, ganglions spinaux et cervelet) sous l'action de la thyroxine chez les têtards de *Rana esculenta. C. R. Soc. Biol. (Paris),* 143:380–382.

Usuku, G., and Gross, J. (1965): Morphologic studies of connective tissue resorption in the tail fin of metamorphosing bullfrog tadpole. *Dev. Biol.,* 11:352–370.

Weiss, P., and Rossetti, F. (1951): Growth responses of opposite sign among different neuron types exposed to thyroid hormone. *Proc. Natl. Acad. Sci. (USA),* 37:540–556.

DISCUSSION

Pesetsky: Rakic (1971) has reported on the possible guidance of granule cells in the cerebellum of rats and primates by Bergmann glial cells. The cerebellum of the frog has no Bergmann cells, but it does have ependymal cells, the processes of which go all the way through the brainstem. Do you have any indication that the granule cells are guided by these ependymal cells?

Gona: Some of the earliest workers have shown that the ependymal cells of the cerebellum of tadpole and frog touch the ventricular surface as well as the pia. We have done rapid Golgi studies in the tadpole and in the adult bullfrog and have con-firmed that the ependymal cells are in contact both with the roof and the floor of the brainstem. Serial electron microscopic studies show that the granule cells do seem to migrate down the ependymal glial cells in the manner described by Rakic (1971).

Timiras: In collaboration with Dr. Geel (1970) we attempted with GH to reverse the effects of neonatal thyroidectomy on cerebral cortical RNA metabolism in rat pups. We used highly purified GH which we obtained from Dr. Li. Like you, we were unable to reverse the effects of thyroidectomy with GH, although other workers have reported such a reversal in immature hypothyroid rats. In our hands pure GH was unable to effect the reversal so readily accomplished by T_4.

Gona: I am delighted, Dr. Timiras, that you have raised this point, because it is difficult to apply our observations on amphibians to mammals. I have seen the publi-cations by Zemenhof and others. They used the same kinds of NIH preparations of GH that we did. I doubt seriously the ability of pure GH to cause effects that are so characteristic of T_4, especially in the tadpole.

The tadpole is a most useful animal in which to assay the purity of GH prepara-tions. A very tiny dose of NIH bovine growth hormone (BGH) injected into these tadpoles will quickly cause the animal to turn black, because BGH contains a small amount of melanocyte-stimulating hormone (MSH). This is a dramatic bioassay for a minute impurity. The tadpole has also enabled us to detect the TSH contaminant in BGH. Purified GH is simply not capable of duplicating the effects of T_4.

Unfortunately, Dr. Gomez is not here to discuss his work. Perhaps the thyroid-like effects that he produced with GH can be explained by the response of residual thyroid tissue to the minute quantities of TSH present in his preparation of GH. Following radiothyroidectomy a certain amount of functional thyroid tissue must have remained. This TSH impurity stimulated that residual tissue enough to produce a characteristic thyroid effect. Dr. Krawiec might have something to say on this matter.

Krawiec: Histological observation does not reveal any thyroid tissue. To confirm the absence of thyroid gland we performed the test of Geel and Timiras, and the result showed that no gland remained following radiothyroidectomy. Faryna de Raveglia, Gomez, and Ghittoni (1973) reported that rats made hypothyroid from birth had significant reductions in the levels of lipids of the cerebral cortex. This defect was corrected by BGH therapy; if the residual thyroid tissue exists, it is not responsible for the correction.

Gona: Perhaps one way to clarify your observations would be to measure the plasma levels of thyroid hormone in your animals.

Kollros: We have used GH from NIH to cause growth of limbs in tadpoles. Another way to demonstrate TSH activity in GH is to use hypophysectomized tadpoles; then, if a thyroid gland develops, clearly, TSH is present.

Hamburgh: The investigators who worked with GH never insisted that it can substitute for T_4 completely. They just said that on some particular variable it might be substituted for T_4 and could reverse the hypothyroid pathology. It is still possible that GH may act on some variable to supplement or mimic the action of thyroid hormone. That is all that has ever been claimed for GH by the investigators.

Kollros: The problem with giving GH preparations to tadpoles is that the legs not only grow but that they continue to differentiate. Thus, GH is contaminated with TSH. The legs do not simply elongate without change of shape. They do change shape. Legs develop, toe after toe. Since this is precisely what thyroid hormone does to the tadpole, we assume that TSH contaminates the preparation of GH.

Hamburgh: It may be that GH has no effect on the legs. It may simply mimic the effect of T_4 on one particular target that is normally sensitive to T_4. No more has ever been claimed.

Krawiec: We measured several enzymes of the hypothyroid animal treated with GH, and we obtained an increase in activity of these enzymes as with thyroid hormone. Therefore, we suppose that the effects of thyroid hormone and BGH were alike.

DISCUSSION REFERENCES

De Raveglia, F. I., Gómez, C. J., and Ghittoni, N. E. (1973): Effects of thyroxine and growth hormone on the lipid composition of the cerebral cortex and the cerebellum of developing rats. *Neurobiology*, 3:176–184.

Geel, S. E., and Timiras, P. S. (1970): Influence of growth hormone on cerebral cortical RNA metabolism in immature hypothyroid rats. *Brain Res.*, 22:63–72.

Rakic, P. (1971): Neuron-glia relationship during granule cell migration in developing cerebellar cortex. A Golgi and electron microscopic study in *Macacus rhesus. J. Comp. Neurol.*, 141:283–312.

Thyroid Hormones and Brain Development,
edited by Gilman D. Grave. Raven Press,
New York, 1977.

Hormonal Control of the Size of Mesencephalic Fifth Nucleus in Amphibians

Jerry J. Kollros*

The mesencephalic nucleus of the trigeminal nerve appears in all classes of jawed vertebrates. The cells (M-V cells), located generally in the dorsal half of the mesencephalon, greatly resemble spinal ganglion cells and the cells of Rohon-Beard (Johnston, 1909; Coghill, 1914). They are intracentral primary sensory neurons the distribution of which appears to be to the jaw musculature (Corbin and Harrison, 1940). Although a comparative study of the numbers and distribution of the cells was published by Weinberg (1928), relatively little is known about their early growth, migration, and differentiation. Piatt (1945, 1946) established that the cells were probably derived at least in part from the neural crest in *Ambystoma* (and presumably other forms), and that the number of differentiated cells was small in young larvae and increased with larval age. A few studies dealing with changes in cell number and size during developmental phases have been published, but data on these features are still scarce. They include the partial data on *Ambystoma* by Piatt (1946), Pearson (1949*a,b*) on man, the much more complete study by Kollros and McMurray (1955) on *Rana pipiens,* more recent studies on the chicken by Rogers and Cowan (1973), and on the golden hamster by Alley (1974).

In *Ambystoma,* at the time feeding begins at Harrison stage 46, about 46 M-V cells are present (Piatt, 1945); their number increases to from 78 to 208 (average 159) shortly before metamorphosis. In animals of equal size, following extirpation of the neural crest in the embryo in an attempt to reduce M-V cell number, Piatt (1945) records as few as 15 and as many as 344 cells, well beyond both lower *and* upper limits of his 10 control animals. Numbers in intermediate stages are not provided, nor are measurements of cell or nuclear size. There is a presumption that M-V cells might be identifiable before stage 46, but no earlier stage of their identification is given. Later, Piatt (1946) records an average of 261 cells in *A. punctatum* (*maculatum*) larvae of 45 mm length. His upper value is extended to 369 in an experimental series in which levator mandibulae volume was reduced, and to a maximum of 188 for one side only after increasing the levator mandibulae mass on that side. His two studies, taken together, suggest something of

---

* Department of Zoology, University of Iowa, Iowa City, Iowa 52242.

the range of cell numbers which might be expected, and the wide divergences from any average value.

In order to provide a basis for comparisons in those amphibian species studied only slightly, it seems appropriate to summarize the information available in *Rana pipiens,* and to some extent *Xenopus laevis.* The M-V cells in *R. pipiens* (Kollros and McMurray, 1955) are absent (or at least not identifiable) in the prefeeding stages, but are evident from the start of feeding (stage I of Taylor and Kollros, 1946) onward, with 15 to 55 cells counted at that early stage. There is a gradual increase in cell number through stage X (about 440 cells). Whether or not there is a further increase, with a peak in numbers just before and at the start of metamorphic climax, is unclear. Certainly, the highest numbers are seen at stages XVI and XXI (Table 1), with a maximum of 640 cells. Postmetamorphic counts are all below those recorded at stage X.

Cell and nuclear sizes follow a different pattern from cell numbers. The average cell sizes in early larval stages vary somewhat, with maximal cell sizes growing to stage III. Nonetheless, no consistent differences in M-V cell sizes distinguish the animals in the stages between I and XIV. The same is true of average nuclear sizes. Starting with stage XVI, however, minimal, average, and maximal cell sizes increase gradually, and even more in the postmetamorphic period (Table 1). Nonetheless, great variability in individual cell sizes persists. The smallest in the adults, for example, fall within the size range of cells of stage I larvae. Size was measured from tracings of camera lucida drawings of individual cells and their nuclei, the drawings being limited to those sections in which nucleoli appeared in the cell, so that sizes are of cross-sectional area rather than of volume.

The ratio of nuclear cross section to that of the cell body (N/C ratio) is also of some interest, and is expressed as a percentage. Its value is 60% or

TABLE 1. *Cell numbers and nuclear sizes (cross-sectional areas in μm^2) in* Rana pipiens *larvae*

Stages	N	Total length (mm)	Cell sizes (μm^2)		Nuclear sizes (μm^2)		Cell number
			Range	Average	Range	Average	
I	4	14–15	68–193	106–129	50–93	68–77	15–55
III	3	19–22	64–289[a]	125–160[a]	47–112[a]	71–80	85–90
IV–VI	4	29–50	75–407[a]	128–189[a]	52–154[a]	73–99	174–376
IX–XIV	6	51–71	54–255	111–123	39–103	61–67	170–442
XVI–XXI	3	63–75	76–399	153–217	52–168	80–97	366–640
XXIV–XXV	3	22–27	100–514	189–237	42–170	87–116	290–428
Juvenile	3	28–39	95–610	233–280	55–161	93–101	270–291
Adult	4	75–83	115–650	305–369	47–232	106–140	308–417

[a] One animal of each group had cells much larger than those of others, out of the general range of the stage III to XIV measurements; cell numbers were not extraordinary.

higher at stage I, 51 to 59% in stages III to XVI, 42 to 49% during meta-morphic climax (stages XX to XXV), and generally 35% in juveniles and adults (Table 2). Even within individual animals, the N/C ratios are distributed so that the larger cells tend to have the smaller values (as if more mature), and the smaller cells tend to have the larger values (as if less mature, as in 7 of 8 cases, Table 3).

TABLE 2. *Nucleus/cell ratio × 100 (based on cross-sectional areas)*

Stage	N	Range	Average
I	4	60–69	64
III	2	56–57	56
IV–VI	3	51–58	55
IX–XIV	6	51–59	56
XVI–XXI	3	44–53	48
XXIV–XXV	3	42–49	46
Juvenile	3	36–38	37
Adult	3	32–38	35

TABLE 3. *Nuclear cell (N/C) ratios of cells with the largest and smallest nuclei[a]*

Stage	N/C ratio large	N/C ratio small	Difference[b]
V	53.85	61.59	7.74
X–	54.41	59.68	5.27
XIII	52.61	55.24	2.63
XVI	53.86	52.00	−1.86
XX	46.69	48.76	2.07
XXIV	49.09	50.50	1.41
Juvenile	30.78	44.57	13.79
Adult	31.45	35.79	4.34

[a] One animal for each stage. Sample size, large or small, 20 to 27 cells each.
[b] $p = 0.03$.

The development of the optic lobes of the frog in relation to cell addition, cell differentiation, and extension of optic tract fibers appears to proceed in an anteroposterior direction (Kollros, 1953). It is not surprising, therefore, to see M-V cell differentiation following this same pattern; i.e., cell addition (as gauged by cell counts) seems to be somewhat greater near the caudal pole of the lobe than near the cranial pole. Further, the more caudal M-V cells tend to have the larger (i.e., less mature) N/C ratios. Not until stage XIII or later are these differences abolished (Table 4). When the optic lobes first contain M-V cells, they show no significant segregation into layers of

TABLE 4. *Nuclear cell (N/C) ratios of most anterior and posterior M-V cells*

Stages	No. of cells in each group	N	N/C ratio (×100)			
			Anterior	Posterior	Difference	*p*
III	23, 24	2	55.50	58.67	3.17	0.3
IV	24, 50	2	53.26	59.30	6.04	0.01
V	50	2	56.10	62.34	6.24	0.003
XII–XIII	40, 50	2	56.00	63.47	7.47	0.005
XIII–adult	25–50	5	33–54	32–53	1 to −2.30	*p* > 0.5[a]

[a] For each case.

cells and fibers, but by stage IV or V such distinction of layers is sufficient
to permit assignment of all of the visible M-V cells to a pair of layers (Table
5). With a single exception in 23 cases (at stage XX), more than half of the
cells are found in the periventricular layers 1 and 2. In larvae, layers 5 and 6
generally contain more M-V cells than layers 3 and 4, but in juveniles and
adults this relationship is frequently reversed.

What is implied by these data, if anything, about control of cell number
and size by either hormonal or peripheral trophic influences? First, we know
from work of Just (1972) that thyroid hormone levels, as gauged by direct
determinations of protein-bound iodine, begin to increase at about stage
XV, and if the cells responded to increased hormone levels by growth, such
evidence of stimulation would be appropriate from stage XVI onward.

A possibility exists that the cell size changes might have their basis in the
change in jaw musculature, growth of which is obvious during the transformation of the small-mouthed tadpole to the adult with its very large gape.
Although careful studies of jaw musculature have not been made, there is a
presumption that significant changes are not encountered until the time of

TABLE 5. *Distribution of the M-V cells in the layers of the optic tectum*

Stage	Numbers of cells in each layer			
	1–2	3–4	5–6	Total
IV+	127	2	45	174
VI−	271	15	90	376
X−	301	50	93	444
XIII−	280	10	152	442
XVI	384	58	198	640
XX	174	58	134	366
XXI−	376	80	136	592
XXV	258	14	18	290
Juvenile	205	42	23	270
Adult	308	34	35	377

jaw widening, i.e., stages XX and XXI and later, and are thus not likely to be the basis for the M-V cell differentiation and growth which is evident as early as stage XVI.

The extent to which thyroid hormone directly is the responsible agent in the growth and differentiation of the M-V cells is explored in the work of Kollros and McMurray (1956) and of Kollros (1957). This work sought answers to the following questions:

1. Without regard to the specific mode of influence, are M-V cells equally responsive to metamorphic stimuli at all stages at which they appear?

Preliminary studies (*unpublished*) had established that at midlarval stages the M-V cells could be stimulated to grow prematurely by placing tadpoles in solutions of *dl*-thyroxine of moderate concentrations (50 μg/liter). Tadpoles in stages I and II (A), III and IV (B), and V (C) were immersed in such thyroxine solutions for 7 or 8 days. Leg growth was clearly stimulated (to stages V, VII, and X, respectively), with effects on other systems bringing about external changes to stages XVIII— and XIX (reduction of cloacal tail piece) and XX— (nearly perforate skin window), respectively. Inspection of the M-V cells revealed no apparent change in group A, some modest growth in group B, and substantially more growth in group C, with average cell and nuclear sizes significantly increased, and the N/C ratio reduced to a level almost significant statistically (Table 6). The results are consonant with the interpretation that, for the hormone levels used and the time interval employed, the M-V cells of group A animals were quite insensitive, that some sensitivity or response capacity had been gained by stages III and IV, and that by stage V (group C) a high degree of sensitivity was present.

TABLE 6. *M-V cells following immersion in* DL-*thyroxine (50 μg/liter) for 7 to 8 days*

| Group | N | Cell size (μm^2) | | Nuclear size (μm^2) | | N/C ratios | Cell number |
		Maximum	Average	Maximum	Average		
A	5	233	134	107	81	61	(damaged)
B	6	301	157	123	86	56	95
C	4	376	141	144	98	51	146
p value	A–B	0.08	0.05	0.2	0.2	0.2	—
	A–C	0.05	0.04	0.06	0.03	0.06	—
	B–C	0.05	0.03	0.2	0.04	0.06	0.001

2. If M-V cell growth is dependent on thyroid hormone, then hypophysectomized tadpoles (which do not develop, spontaneously, beyond stages VI to VIII) should have M-V cells of a small, immature sort. Do they?

They do: Hypophysectomized animals 50 to 70 mm long, usually at least 3 months of age or older, were fixed. They had attained stages III+ to VI.

The M-V cell numbers were similar to control animals of stages V to XII. Cell sizes, nuclear sizes, and N/C ratios were also appropriate for animals of such control stages (Table 7); in fact, some of the N/C ratios were at a value of 60% or higher, characteristic of stage I tadpoles. Clearly, these hypophysectomized tadpoles, siblings of controls which were metamorphosing, had M-V cells characteristic of very young larvae.

TABLE 7. *M-V cell characteristics in hypophysectomized tadpoles*

Stage	Cell number	Cell size (μm^2)		Nuclear size (μm^2)		N/C ratio
		Maximum	Average	Maximum	Average	
III+	233	222	115	82	63	54
III+	220	205	108	82	63	58
IV	156	220	120	94	72	60
IV+	245	189	98	102	56	63
V−	260	211	120	106	76	63
V+	388	202	111	82	63	57
VI−	276	260	124	109	72	58
VI−	205	327	150	106	82	55
VI	314	272	126	128	77	61
VI	289	240	123	100	69	56
VI	267	247	122	110	72	59
VI	293	287	131	102	79	60
II+	250	185	99	85	57	58
Average	261	236	119	94	69	59

3. Does thyroid hormone act directly on the M-V cells, or indirectly through influences on growth of the jaw musculature?

This question was tested by the use of implants of pellets 0.5 mm in diameter compacted from mixtures of T_4 and cholesterol in a ratio by weight of 1:4. Short pellets were placed into the cranial cavity adjacent to the diencephalon, in contact with the cranial pole of the right optic lobe of 25 tadpoles initially in stages III to VII. Nineteen tadpoles were hypophysectomized, and six were not. The hormone was expected to diffuse from the pellets fairly slowly, and hormone concentrations were expected to be greater at any point in the right optic lobe than in any corresponding point in the left optic lobe, although the differences would be less the greater the distance from the pellet. Thus, hormone concentration at the cranial pole of the right optic lobe should be considerably greater than at its caudal pole. If there is a direct growth-maturational response of the M-V cells to thyroxine, cells on the right side as an aggregate should be larger than those on the left side, and on each side cells near the cranial pole should be larger than cells near the caudal pole. If there is no direct stimulation, neither of these two expectations should be realized.

The results support the contention of a direct cellular response to the hormone stimulus. Of 10 animals fixed 2 to 4 days after pellet implantation, 8 had average and maximum cell sizes larger on the right (thyroxine) side than on the left. Another 15 animals were fixed 5 to 20 days after the implantation. They showed a somewhat greater bias for large cell and nuclear sizes on the T_4 side, and a higher level of significance of the differences between the two sides (Tables 8 and 9). The values represented were based on measurements of the most anterior 25 M-V cells, the middle 25, and the most posterior 25 on each side. Considering only the last 15 animals, differences between the most anterior 10 cells are very significant, between the middle 10 cells somewhat less significant, but of no significance between the most posterior 10 cells (Table 10).

TABLE 8. *M-V cell and nuclear sizes following unilateral pellet implantation*[a]

| | | Differences in sizes (μm^2) | | | |
| | | Cell | | Nuclear | |
Days	N	Maximum	Average	Maximum	Average
2	2	−16	1	3	1
		75	13	15	5
3	4	0	16	7	6
		28	6	4	1
		78	−6	6	3
		37	8	3	2
		30	1	−8	−2
4	4	70	22	15	9
		27	3	10	2
		−10	−8	3	−2
	p	0.02	0.1	0.03	0.05

[a] Twenty-five cells each from anterior, middle, and posterior tectum.

TABLE 9. *M-V cell and nuclear sizes following unilateral pellet implantation*[a]

| | | Average differences in size (μm^2) | | | |
| | | Cell | | Nuclear | |
Days	N	Maximum	Average	Maximum	Average
5	2	54	13	19	5
6	4	34	14	12	4
7–9	4	29	19	1	5
10–13	4	122	31	26	11
20	1	59	12	17	3
	p	0.001	0.0001	0.01	0.0001

[a] Twenty-five cells each from anterior, middle, and posterior tectum.

TABLE 10. *M-V cell and nuclear sizes following unilateral pellet implantation; anterior, middle, posterior comparisons in 15 animals 5 to 20 days after operation*

	Cells			Nuclear			N/C ratio			
		Difference	p		Difference	p		Difference	p	p
L. anterior 164		49	0.001	78	14	0.0001	48[a]	5.5	0.01	
R. anterior 213				92			42.5			0.007
L. middle 161		23	0.002	79	6	0.0003	50[a]	3	0.04	
R. middle 184				85			47			0.03
L. posterior 136		5	0.2	70	1	0.2	52[a]	1	0.05	
R. posterior 141				71			51			

[a] Differences between L. middle and L. anterior, and L. posterior are insignificant. $p = 0.03$ comparing L. anterior to L. posterior.

All the animals had advanced in stage between the time of operation and fixation. Some had advanced quite rapidly, suggesting that there had been a relatively rapid loss of hormone from the pellet to the blood as well as that blood hormone levels had been maintained high for a sufficiently long time to bring about either modestly rapid or rapid changes in stage, i.e., in stimulation of leg growth and differentiation. There is a rough correlation between time to fixation and number of stages advanced, although much of the variation must also be attributed to differences in size of pellet implanted (thus to total hormone available, and length of time available), and perhaps to some degree of individual variability in capacity to respond.

The values of the nucleocytoplasmic ratios are consistent with the data on cell and nuclear sizes. There is a fair negative correlation with time of treatment, i.e., the 2-day treatment cases having overall N/C ratios of near 60%, and those treated more than 6 days tending to be below 50%. In the 15 cases treated 5 to 20 days (Table 10), differences between the two sides are significant for the anterior groups of 10, slightly significant for the middle groups of 10, and insignificant for the posterior groups of 10 cells. On the right side, the anterior, middle, and posterior groups of cells are all significantly different from each other; on the left side the adjacent groups are not different from each other, whereas anterior and posterior groups are somewhat different ($p \leq 0.03$; the comparable difference on the right has a p value ≤ 0.0004).

4. How does the sensitivity of response of the M-V cells compare with that of other systems; i.e., are thresholds comparable to those for leg growth, lid development, or initiation of tail loss?

This question was studied by immersing hypophysectomized tadpoles in weak or very weak solutions of *dl*-thyroxine for extended periods, commonly 100 to 200 days, 502 days in one. Hormone at a dose of 0.004 μg/liter showed no effect; 0.02 μg/liter showed slight external effects, with limb growth to stage VI in this study, and to XI to XV in others (Kollros,

1961); ten times this concentration carried animals to stage XIX, whereas 0.4 μg/liter were sufficient for stage XX or beyond. Unilateral cell counts in 12 animals were in the range of 100 to 212 cells. Maximum cell sizes were in the 125 to 243 μm^2 range, (average 74 to 141 μm^2). Maximum nuclear sizes were below 100 μm^2 in 10 of 12 cases (average 57 to 80 μm^2). The N/C ratios were 57 to 80% (9 of 12 were 62% or higher).

All of these values of cell size were those expected in stages II to XIV, and the N/C ratios were those expected of only the most immature cells. Thus, although hormone levels, given a great deal of time for response, were sufficient to permit change of external characteristics to those of animals in metamorphic climax, including some tail loss and some mouth changes, none of these tadpoles showed more than a trace of M-V cell growth or maturation, and these indications were the maximum cell sizes obtained in the two animals in stages XX− and XX+ (Table 11).

TABLE 11. *M-V cells in hypophysectomized tadpoles in weak thyroxine*

Thyroxine conc. (μg/liter)	Days in thyroxine	Final stage	Cell count (left)	Cell sizes (μm^2)		Nuclear sizes (μm^2)		N/C ratio
				Max.	Ave.	Max.	Ave.	
0.02	129	VI	102	184	100	92	71	71
0.08	139	XIV	145	206	112	87	66	59
0.04	502	XV	100	123	74	66	57	77
0.4	47	XVII+	212	204	111	87	64	58
0.4	114	XIX	104	199	98	85	61	62
0.6	61	XIX+	101	125	81	87	65	80
0.4	188	XX−	146	210	92	128	62	67
0.4	203	XX+	203	243	141	137	80	57
		Nonhypox. controls						
		XVII+	363	390	172	132	93	54
		XIX	−	371	221	135	98	44
		XX+	216	354	193	160	97	50
		XXI	199	395	207	135	95	46

One can interpret these results as expressing a greater insensitivity to thyroid hormone on the part of the M-V cells than on the part of the legs, operculum, eyelids, and tail base, for example. Because growth and differentiation responses of the cells can be obtained as quickly as 5 days with much higher concentrations of thyroxine, the conclusion must be drawn that the M-V cell changes presumably have a relatively high T$_4$ threshold, i.e., above that required for the usual external changes which characterize a stage XX animal. Thus, fairly high hormone concentrations bring about M-V cell growth and external body form changes, whereas fairly low hormone concentrations elicit the external body form changes but not the M-V cell growth.

5. Is the M-V cell growth response, once elicited, permanent, as are all previously reported metamorphic changes, or can it regress?

This problem was attacked in two ways. The first was by utilization of hypophysectomized tadpoles, transitory stimulation by thyroxine, followed by a period of withdrawal from thyroxine. Would cell size, increased by the hormone treatment, be reduced as a result of hormone withdrawal? The second approach was the use of euthyroid animals. As they achieved stages characterized by M-V cell growth, we treated them with thiourea for a sufficiently long time to inhibit metamorphic progress completely. In both methods, cells are temporarily subjected to heightened hormone concentrations and then to depressed ones.

The first series (Kollros and McMurray, 1956) was composed of 39 hypophysectomized tadpoles in stages III to VI, separated into 13 sets of 3 animals each, matched as to stage and length. Two of the animals of each triplet were placed in solutions of 20 μg/liter of *dl*-thyroxine from 4.5 to 9 days; 24 hr later (at 5.5 to 10 days), one member of each pair (group I) was fixed, and 6 controls were fixed at the same time. The remaining 13 thyroxine-treated tadpoles (group II) were kept out of hormone for an additional 9 to 17 days, then fixed. The 7 remaining controls were fixed at the same times.

As can be seen from Table 12, the group I animals fixed 1 day after the end of the hormone treatment period show almost uniformly larger cell and nuclear sizes than the controls (as in Table 7), and smaller N/C ratios as well. The comparisons are all significant. In contrast, such differences for the group II animals (II vs. controls) are either less significant, or, in some cases, without significance. The differences between groups I and II are significant or very nearly so in 4 of the 5 comparisons, and lack significance in one case.

One can conclude that the relatively short stimulation with T_4 promoted rapid cell and nuclear growth (groups I and II), whereas the 9- to 17-day period thereafter, away from thyroxine influence (group II only), permitted significant reduction in both cell and nuclear sizes. In some instances size reduction was of such degree as to be nearly comparable to unstimulated control tadpoles.

Cell counts were also made of the 37 animals which had been fixed. Whereas control and group II animals had counts which were alike ($p \leq 0.3$), the cell counts of the 13 animals of group I were significantly greater than those of either the controls or group II. In fact, 8 of the 13 group I animals had cell counts greater than those of any group II or control animal, and only one animal of group I had a count below the averages of those of the other two groups.

These data raise the question as to whether or not there is a subpopulation of potential or prospective M-V cells whose expression as M-V cells requires a substantially higher hormone level than does the rest of the cell

TABLE 12. M-V cells of hypophysectomized tadpoles immersed in thyroxine (20 µg/liter)[a]

Stage fixed		Days treated	Cell numbers		Cell sizes (µm²)				Nuclear sizes (µm²)				N/C ratios	
					Maximum		Average		Maximum		Average			
I	II		I	II	I	II	I	II	I	II	I	II	I	II
VIII	IX−	7	490	238	297	304	142	122	112	102	76	66	55	54
IX	X	4.5	400	230	409	275	195	48	138	100	90	77	48	52
V	IX+	6	211	265	237	360	106	110	77	86	59	63	56	57
VII	IX+	6	360	248	316	234	144	105	110	102	76	64	56	61
VIII	−	4.5	300		293		157			108	79		50	
VIII	IX	9	371	358	288	226	127	112	103	78	66	60	52	54
X−	XII	5	406	373	317	278	162	138	92	109	84	80	52	58
IX+	X	4.5	391	282	351	316	180	145	114	106	84	78	47	54
X	XII+	5	558	283	347	243	166	142	145	111	86	83	52	58
X	XII	4.5	380	322	324	289	159	139	113	100	84	82	53	59
X	XI+	5	516	272	395	381	162	144	113	110	75	74	46	51
IX	XI	4.5	523	220	360	367	177	148	118	96	81	76	46	51
VII+	−	9	404		339		154		98		74		48	
Average			408	281	329	298	156	132	111	100	78	73	51	55
p, I vs. II			0.004		0.13		0.0002		0.04		0.006		0.001	
p, II vs. control			0.3		0.01		0.02		0.2		0.2		0.02	
p, I vs. control			0.0001		0.0001		0.0001		0.001		0.01		0.0001	

[a] Presented in same order as hypophysectomized controls in Table 7.

population, a group whose *continued* enlargement (and thus identification by the investigator) is dependent on high thyroid hormone levels. Is the reduction in numbers between groups I and II attained by cell death, or by that decrease in cell size in group II to a level characteristic of the pretreatment condition, as in the control animals?

The remaining tests of temporary vs. permanent attainment of cell size were carried out in normal tadpoles of both *Rana pipiens* and *Xenopus laevis,* and in postmetamorphic juvenile *Xenopus* (Kollros, 1957). For the tadpoles, growth was permitted to proceed normally to stages XV to XVIII (or the equivalent in *X. laevis*), at which time the animals were placed in thiourea solutions to inhibit and ultimately to stop metamorphic progress. The 0.033% thiourea was ineffective in *Rana,* although it could have been presumed to have been effective at younger stages (Gordon, Goldsmith, and Charipper, 1945). A thiourea level of 0.05 to 0.06% was successful in stopping metamorphosis in 4 of 8 larvae, and of greatly slowing metamorphic changes in the other 4 older tadpoles (Table 13). The expected differences of smaller cell sizes in the thiourea cases, and control tadpoles were observed in all 8 cases; in 6, the average nuclear sizes were also smaller. Both differences were slightly significant.

TABLE 13. *Rana pipiens tadpoles in thiourea, and untreated matched controls*

Fixed stage	Days treated	Cell size (μm^2)		Nuclear size (μm^2)	
		Exp.	Cont.	Exp.	Cont.
XVI+	32[a]	120	156	73	81
XVII+	27[a]	153	185	86	96
XVII+	26[a]	123	172	78	93
XVII+	23[a]	94	168	67	89
XXI	17	232	207	104	95
XXI	17	235	215	100	97
XXII	13	185	219	85	100
XXIII−	8	184	226	84	105
Ave. XIX+	20	166	194	85	96
p			0.05		0.04

[a] Metamorphic stasis attained.

Xenopus larvae tolerated thiourea better than those of *Rana,* and a 0.25% thiourea solution was employed for immersion. All 8 of the larvae, treated 23 to 32 days, showed slowing of metamorphic progress and then metamorphic stasis. Compared with their matched controls, all 5 indices of cell size showed changes in the expected direction (Table 14), i.e., smaller maximum and average cell and nuclear sizes, and larger N/C ratios. Cell counts were only insignificantly different.

TABLE 14. *Xenopus laevis tadpoles (above) and juveniles (below) in thiourea, and untreated matched controls*

	Ave.[a] cell size (μm^2)		Ave.[b] nuclear size (μm^2)		N/C ratio		Cell count	
	Exp.	Cont.	Exp.	Cont.	Exp.	Cont.	Exp.	Cont.
	120	203	58	68	47	33	108	118
	82	198	48	72	58	36	86	99
	140	192	64	68	45	36	89	123
	115	190	54	67	46	35	116	108
	119	187	53	71	44	38	79	127
	113	180	53	68	46	37	151	132
	124	172	63	68	51	39	86	94
	138	156	59	65	43	42	85	92
	119	185	57	68	48	37	100	112
Ave. p	0.001		0.002		0.001		.25	
	273	318	76	81	27	25	85	75
	303	310	88	87	29	28	104	105
	339	299	88	80	26	26	75	83
	263	284	68	79	26	27	94	97
	269	279	75	80	30	28	90	101
	259	260	74	80	29	30	94	77
	219	253	63	73	29	29	90	102
	213	239	64	73	30	30	105	97
	256	236	68	68	26	28	77	105
	193	208	59	66	31	32	104	83
	188	198	59	66	31	33	81	79
	163	183	54	62	33	34	106	103
	157	183	55	61	35	33	76	106
	194	174	61	60	32	34	97	102
	235	244	68	73	30	30	91	94
Ave. p	0.15		0.01		0.5		0.25	

[a] Maximum cell sizes differed (245 to 319 μm^2 larvae, $p = 0.01$; 375 to 408 μm^2 juveniles, $p = 0.05$).
[b] Maximum nuclear sizes differed (89 to 99 μm^2 larvae, $p = 0.03$; 99 to 108 μm^2 juveniles, $p = 0.01$).

Similar studies were carried out on 7 recently transformed *Xenopus* (body length 24 to 34 mm), and on 7 somewhat older juveniles (body length 43 to 68 mm). The same kind of differences were observed as in the larvae (Table 14), although of considerably diminished magnitude; differences for the small juveniles were greater than for the large ones. Overall, only 3 of the 6 comparisons showed differences; of these, one was barely significant. The N/C ratios were identical in thiourea-treated and control animals, and cell counts were nearly identical. Cell numbers were smaller than in the larvae.

The results give an impression of decreased importance of thyroid hormone in the juveniles compared with the larvae, and larger juveniles show less modification than small ones. Do the larger sizes of the cells in the juveniles imply the gradual increase in importance of the sensorial input from the periphery, i.e., the jaw musculature, in determining and maintaining cell size, and the gradual waning of an influence of thyroid hormone?

To summarize the previous paragraphs, M-V cells appear gradually during the early larval period when thyroid hormone levels in the blood are very low, and gradually acquire capacity to respond to thyroid hormone, long before hormone levels are scheduled to rise. The thresholds for their response, as gauged by cell size changes, are significantly above those for many other metamorphic changes, including leg and eyelid growth, fore limb emergence, and the earliest phase of tail resorption. At appropriate higher hormone levels, i.e., those which simulate normal metamorphosis, the cells respond rapidly by growth. If hormone levels are permitted to drop prematurely, not only will cell sizes shrink, but cell numbers will fall as well. Some capacity of the cells to respond to thyroid hormone seems to persist for a time after metamorphosis, at least as tested in *Xenopus,* but other factors, especially the sensorial input from the periphery, appear to assume a dominant role in M-V size maintenance.

What is known about other, less studied species? A brief study by Bibb (1964) on development of M-V cells in *Ambystoma* (*A. jeffersonianum* indicated, but probably *A. laterale*) reveals M-V cell appearance well before the onset of feeding. Cell size, as measured by nuclear cross-sectional area, is largest in the prefeeding larva or embryo and smallest in the oldest animals. Immersion of larvae in *dl*-thyroxine at 400 μg/liter, much stronger than used for *Rana,* resulted in premature metamorphic changes, e.g., gill resorption, but no change in cell size. Presumably the size of M-V cells of *Ambystoma,* unlike those of *Rana,* are not under hormonal control.

Although the M-V cells in *Xenopus laevis* responded by change in size to thyroid hormone level modifications, a study by Shaw (1955) confirmed that the normal development of M-V cells in *Xenopus* followed the same pattern as that in *Rana pipiens.* A similar study, with comparable results, was that of del Vecchio (1952) on the bullfrog, *Rana catesbeiana.* The bullfrog, however, in both the adult and in larval stages, has larger cells than *Rana pipiens* at comparable levels of development. The cell development pattern, however, appears to be somewhat different in the toad, *Bufo americanus* (Davis, 1951). He found very modest changes in cell and nuclear sizes between midlarval periods and animals nearly through metamorphic climax (Table 15), but a very large change from those stages to the 3-in. adult, in which average cell and nuclear sizes were larger than in any other anuran, including the much larger *R. catesbeiana.*

No experimental studies have been carried out on *Bufo,* but the post-metamorphic growth is at least suggestive of a profound influence of the periphery, rather than of thyroid hormone. Of some interest, perhaps, is the fact that, despite its very large M-V cells, *Bufo* has a relatively small number of such cells, i.e., about one-half that characteristic of *Rana pipiens*

TABLE 15. *M-V cell development in Bufo americanus*[a]

Stage	Length (mm)	Total cell no.	Cell sizes (μm^2)		Nuclear sizes (μm^2)	
			Range	Average	Range	Average
X	26	67	39–132	83	26–65	43
XVI	26	107	32–178	106	15–92	46
XIX	26	73	75–175	107	32–80	62
XXIII	9	111	51–146	95	24–81	53
Adult	75	169	300–767	517	76–187	136

[a] In all but adult the 10 most anterior cells are larger than the 10 most posterior ones (data from Davis, 1951).

TABLE 16. *M-V nucleus cells in Anurans*[a]

Species	Average length	N	Cell numbers		Tectal distribution		
			Range	Average	2	4	6
Pseudacris nigrita	30	3	113–161	132	8	62	52
Acris gryllus	33	3	126–166	149	10	78	61
Bufo americanus	76	2	164–169	166	14	71	79
Rana pipiens	76	3	289–400	338	248	64	26
Rana catesbeiana	177	3	410–746	523	205	240	87
Xenopus laevis[a]	15	3	212–227	218	40	63	115

[a] Data from Payne, 1950 and Shaw, 1955.
[b] In metamorphic climax, and juvenile.

(Table 16). This table, and the information from Shaw, are consistent with the idea that, in general, cell numbers correlate with the size of the adult animal species being observed, and that there is a rough correlation between cell size and cell number. The *Bufo americanus* material deviates from this, yet the total *volume* of M-V cell material is probably very nearly like that of *Rana pipiens*, a species somewhat larger than this toad. Do the *Bufo* M-V cells innervate substantially larger individual peripheries than the M-V cells of other anurans?

SUMMARY

The M-V cells of amphibians appear in the late embryo or early larva[1] and gradually increase in number.

---

[1] *Eleutherodactylus* embryos (provided by the late W. Gardner Lynn) show mesencephalic V nucleus cells in their optic tecta several days before hatching. The cells of the older prehatching embryos are larger than those of younger ones (Kollros, *unpublished observations*).

The M-V cells of anurans increase in size well after the midlarval period, in contrast to the one species of *Ambystoma* studied. The size increase which continues through metamorphic climax is at least partially stimulated by the higher concentrations of thyroid hormone present at that time.

The size increase which follows metamorphosis may be independent of such hormonal influences (because thyroid hormone levels fall after metamorphic climax), and may instead be dependent on the extent of the sensorial periphery innervated.[2]

Thyroid hormone stimulation of hypophysectomized *R. pipiens* brings about an increase in M-V cell numbers, sometimes seen in the early part of metamorphic climax. A drop in hormone levels demonstrates this increase to be transitory. Whether the observed cell loss is by cell death or by dedifferentiation is not known.

At the time of their first appearance, the M-V cells of *Rana pipiens* are not sensitive to thyroid hormone; application of the hormone fails to elicit cell growth. A bit later (stages III to IV), there is some sensitivity of the cells with an even higher degree of sensitivity at stage V. Because body changes characteristic of early metamorphic climax can be brought about by stimulating hypophysectomized tadpoles with 0.4 to 0.6 µg/liter of *dl*-thyroxine for a sufficiently long time without observing a concomitant growth of the M-V cells, these specialized cells may have a higher threshold for their growth response than is required by many other tadpole tissues for their metamorphic responses.

The failure of *Ambystoma* M-V cells to respond to high concentrations of thyroid hormone, and of *Bufo americanus* cells to change more than minimally at metamorphic climax, both suggest that different amphibians exhibit different levels of dependency of M-V cells on thyroid hormone during development. Such dependency is reduced after metamorphosis as demonstrated by thiourea treatment of juvenile *Xenopus laevis,* and the resulting change in cell size far smaller than seen in the larva.

REFERENCES

Alley, K. E. (1974): Morphogenesis of the trigeminal mesencephalic nucleus in the hamster: Cytogenesis and neurone death. *J. Embryol. Exp. Morphol.,* 31:99–121.

Bibb, H. D. (1964): The mesencephalic V nucleus in *Ambystoma jeffersonianum*. M. S. thesis. State University of Iowa, Iowa City, Iowa.

Coghill, G. E. (1914): Correlated anatomical and physiological studies of the growth of the nervous system in Amphibia. I. The afferent system of the trunk of *Amblystoma. J. Comp. Neurol.,* 24:161–234.

Corbin, K. B., and Harrison, F. (1940): Function of mesencephalic root of fifth cranial nerve. *J. Neurophysiol.,* 3:423–435.

---

[2] Cell size measurements (Kollros, *unpublished*) of those *A. maculatum* larvae which had undergone hyperplasia or hypoplasia as a result of additions to or subtractions from their jaw musculature (Piatt, 1946) show small changes in cell and nuclear sizes correlated with the increases and decreases in cell number recorded by Piatt.

Davis, C. E. (1951): The development of mesencephalic V nucleus cells in *Bufo americanus.* M.S. thesis. State University of Iowa, Iowa City, Iowa.

del Vecchio, M. L. (1952): A description of the sizes of the cells of the mesencephalic V nucleus in *Rana catesbeiana* and comparison with *Rana pipiens.* M.S. thesis. State University of Iowa, Iowa City, Iowa.

Gordon, A. S., Goldsmith, E. S., and Charipper, H. A. (1945): The effects of thiourea on amphibian development. *Growth*, 9:19–41.

Johnston, J. B. (1909): The radix mesencephalica trigemini. *J. Comp. Neurol.*, 19:593–644.

Just, J. (1972): Protein-bound iodine and protein concentration in plasma and pericardial fluid of metamorphosing anuran tadpoles. *Physiol. Zool.*, 45:145–152.

Kollros, J. J. (1953): The development of the optic lobes in the frog. I. The effects of unilateral enucleation in embryonic stages. *J. Exp. Zool.*, 123:153–187.

Kollros, J. J. (1957): Influence of thiourea on growth of cells of midbrain in frogs. *Proc. Soc. Exp. Biol. Med.*, 95:138–141.

Kollros, J. J. (1961): Mechanisms of amphibian metamorphosis: Hormones. *Am. Zool.*, 1:107–114.

Kollros, J. J., and McMurray, V. M. (1955): The mesencephalic V nucleus in anurans. I. Normal development in *Rana pipiens. J. Comp. Neurol.*, 102:47–63.

Kollros, J. J., and McMurray, V. M. (1956): The mesencephalic V nucleus in anurans. II. The influence of thyroid hormone on cell size and cell number. *J. Exp. Zool.*, 131:1–26.

Payne, W. F. (1950): A comparative study of mesencephalic V nucleus cells in anurans. M.S. thesis. State University of Iowa, Iowa City, Iowa.

Pearson, A. (1949a): The development and connections of the mesencephalic root of the trigeminal nerve in man. *J. Comp. Neurol.*, 90:1–46.

Pearson, A. (1949b): Further observations on the mesencephalic root of the trigeminal nerve. *J. Comp. Neurol.*, 91:147–194.

Piatt, J. (1945): Origin of the mesencephalic V root cells in *Amblystoma. J. Comp. Neurol.*, 82:35–53.

Piatt, J. (1946): The influence of the peripheral field on the development of the mesencephalic V nucleus in *Amblystoma. J. Exp. Zool.*, 102:109–141.

Rogers, L. A., and Cowan, W. M. (1973): The development of the mesencephalic nucleus of the trigeminal nerve in the chick. *J. Comp. Neurol.*, 147:291–320.

Shaw, E. D. (1955): The mesencephalic fifth nucleus of *Xenopus laevis* during development. M.S. thesis. State University of Iowa, Iowa City, Iowa.

Taylor, A. C., and Kollros, J. (1946): Stages in the normal development of *Rana pipiens* larvae. *Anat. Rec.*, 94:7–23.

Weinberg, E. (1928): The mesencephalic root of the fifth nerve. A comparative anatomical study. *J. Comp. Neurol.*, 46:249–405.

DISCUSSION

Spangenberg: Dr. Kollros, would yours be a good system in which to use electron microscopic autoradiography in order to study the uptake of labeled T_4 by M-V cells? The rate of uptake of T_4 may change as the organism metamorphoses.

Kollros: This would appear to be a perfect system for such an autoradiographic study.

Hamburgh: Does the sensorial input from the periphery determine M-V cell number more than M-V cell size?

Kollros: The best studies are partly unpublished and partly those of Piatt, who changed the area of the innervated periphery in the salamander; in some cases he noted reductions in number of cells from about 150 down to 13; but he also noted some increases. Nonetheless, there are enough data to suggest that the area of peripheral innervation has an effect on M-V cell number.

I made some measurements of the size of M-V cells in relation to areas of peripheral innervation. Those cells which innervate a reduced periphery are smaller, on the average, than those which innervate a normal or an enlarged periphery. When

Piatt enlarged the periphery threefold, he noted that the corresponding M-V cells were a little bit larger, but the increase in number in such cases was greater than the increase in size.

Alternatively, we have made grafts of extra heads to tadpoles during the embryo stage. We can graft the head without the jaw musculature. Under those circumstances, fewer M-V cells are produced. I am not sure now if they are smaller, but they are clearly fewer in number.

Pesetsky: Do the processes of these cells terminate directly in proprioceptive endings within the jaw musculature?

Kollros: I am not sure.

Pesetsky: Is there an interneurone?

Kollros: There is no interneurone. These M-V cells are primary sensory cells. They look very much like ganglion cells or Rohon-Beard cells.

Valcana: Since there appears to be such a large difference in size, have you made any attempts to separate these cells and study the two cell types individually in terms of their response to thyroxine? In view of the difference, it should be possible to isolate them; but would it be feasible, in terms of numbers, in the tadpole stage?

Kollros: I think one could. I have not tried anything like that.

Pesetsky: We have a similar situation with regard to the lateral motor column cells. Do not these respond to peripheral changes as well as to hormonal changes?

Kollros: Yes, those cells innervate the limb musculature. They have been studied in virtually the same way as the M-V cells, and they show the same kinds of responses to hormonal and sensorial changes (Reynolds, 1963; Kollros, 1968).

Hamburgh: Does not every type of neuroblast respond to peripheral loading or unloading? Or is it a specific characteristic of M-V and lateral motor column cells? If you load the periphery with a tumor or with an extra limb at the right time, you can cause changes in the developing nerve cell bodies which innervate the peripheral area affected, can you not?

Pesetsky: At least one exception may be the Mauthner neuron in amphibian larvae. Evidence from a variety of experiments indicates that this cell may not be responsive to changes in the neural periphery. Some of my studies have utilized portions of the hindbrain isolated in head grafts. The Mauthner cells in these grafts were, for the most part, normal in size, although many of the grafts lacked lateral line organs and ears, and none of these preparations contained spinal cord or tail musculature.

DISCUSSION REFERENCES

Kollros, J. (1968): Order and control of neurogenesis (as exemplified by the lateral motor column.) *Dev. Biol.,* 2:274–305.

Reynolds, W. A. (1963): The effects of thyroxine upon the initial formation of the lateral motor column and differentiation of motor neurons in *Rana pipiens. J. Exp. Zool.,* 153:237–249.

Thyroid Hormones and Brain Development,
edited by Gilman D. Grave. Raven Press,
New York, 1977.

Amphibian Metamorphosis: Studies on the Mechanisms of Action of Thyroid Hormone

Helen Robinson*

The metamorphosis of anuran tadpoles into adult frogs is a dramatic developmental event initiated and sustained by thyroid hormones. It is highly complex in that it consists of numerous tissue-specific responses occurring in orderly sequence over a relatively short period of time. Among the various changes which take place at metamorphosis are the destruction of exclusively larval features such as the gills and tail, formation of new adult structures such as limbs and lungs, and biochemical transformations in other organs which enable them to perform adult functions such as urea production in the liver. These widely differing reactions are brought about on a molecular level by the interaction of thyroid hormones with responsive target tissues.

Although many of these metamorphic reactions have been characterized biochemically, the molecular nature of the hormone-target tissue interactions responsible for their initiation is poorly understood. Thyroid hormones act directly on the various tadpole tissues in order to initiate metamorphosis. This fact has been documented in studies with implanted pellets containing thyroxine (T_4) (Kollros, 1943; Kollros and Kaltenbach, 1952; Pesetsky and Kollros, 1956; Kaltenbach, 1953*a,b,c,* 1959) and in work on isolated tadpole tissues cultured *in vitro* in the presence of thyroid hormones (Shaffer, 1957, 1963; Weber, 1962; Robinson, 1972).

The nature of the metamorphic response of a tissue is an inherent property of that particular tissue, as demonstrated in the classical experiments of Schwind (1933), where an eye grafted onto the base of a tadpole tail remained intact during metamorphosis while the tail itself underwent regression. Further, it has been shown that the sensitivity of different tadpole tissues to thyroid hormones is acquired early in development, far in advance of metamorphosis (Weber, 1967; Kaltenbach, 1968; Chou and Kollros, 1974) and by different tissues at different times (Moser, 1950; Kollros, 1961).

Although little is known about the way in which thyroid hormones interact with the various target tissues in the tadpole, there is some preliminary evidence indicating the existence of specific cellular binding sites for thyroid hormones (Tata, 1970; Griswold, Fischer, and Cohen, 1972). These

* Department of Biological Sciences, Dartmouth College, Hanover, New Hampshire 03755.

studies on tadpole liver indicate that there are temperature-sensitive binding sites for T_4 located in the nuclear chromatin fraction (Griswold et al., 1972). Additional work remains to be done to characterize these binding sites in order to determine if they are hormone receptors (limited capacity binding sites associated with hormone action), and to ascertain if separate sites exist for the different thyroid hormones, T_4, and triiodothyronine (T_3).

It is also still unclear whether there is any relationship between the action of thyroid hormones during metamorphosis and the peripheral metabolism of the hormones. The existence of a relationship has been suggested. For example, the tadpole liver, which is sensitive to thyroid hormones, has a mechanism for deiodinating T_4, whereas the adult frog liver is insensitive to thyroid hormones and lacks a deiodination system (Galton and Ingbar, 1961, 1962a). Furthermore, the neotenous amphibian *Necturus maculosa* is unresponsive to thyroid hormones and also lacks a peripheral deiodinating system (Galton and Ingbar, 1962b). These reports indicate that there may be a correlation between the sensitivity of a tissue to thyroid hormones and its ability to degrade them.

The present study was initiated to determine if a relationship exists between the action of thyroid hormone and the peripheral metabolism of T_4 and T_3 in tadpole liver and tail tissues during spontaneous metamorphosis, and in isolated tadpole tail tips induced to regress *in vitro*. These particular tadpole tissues were selected for several reasons. First, the responses of liver and tail tissues to the action of thyroid hormones has been studied extensively (see reviews by Weber, 1967, 1969; Tata, 1971). In both these tissues there are dramatic changes in the activity of specific enzymes, the appearance of urea cycle enzymes in the liver, and a sharp increase in the activity of collagenase, hyaluronidase, and lysosomal acid hydrolases in the tail. Second, both tadpole tail and liver can be cultured *in vitro,* and their respective metamorphic reactions can be induced by addition of thyroid hormones to the culture medium, allowing for considerable experimental flexibility. Thus, the metamorphic reactions of the tadpole liver and tail represent two instances where the *in vivo* effects of thyroid hormones may be demonstrated *in vitro*.

METHODS

The anuran selected for this study was *Xenopus laevis,* a species which can be bred in the laboratory throughout the year and which develops rapidly, reaching metamorphosis by approximately 3 months after hatching. Adult frogs were induced to breed by administration of human chorionic gonadotropin (HCG) (Antuitrin S, Parke-Davis), and the tadpoles were reared in well water and fed an aqueous suspension of powdered nettles. The developing and metamorphosing tadpoles were staged according to the method of Nieuwkoop and Faber (1956). According to this method, hind limb buds appear at stage 48, the hind limbs assume a paddle shape at stage 52, the fore limbs emerge at stage 59, tail regression begins at stage 60, and metamorphosis is completed by stage 64.

For studies on isolated tail tips in culture, tadpoles at stage 52 were selected as donors. Tail tips measuring 14 mm in length were amputated and prepared for culture according to methods described by Robinson (1972). The culture medium was Hank's balanced salt solution (Grand Island Biological Company) containing penicillin (100 units/ml) and streptomycin (100 μg/ml) and diluted so as to be isotonic to amphibian tissues. Tail tips were cultured individually at 21 $\pm$ 2°C in sterile disposable Petri dishes containing 10 ml of medium each. All tail tips were allowed to heal for 2 days before experiments were started. Tail regression was initiated by addition of T_4 to the culture medium in a concentration of 250 parts per billion (ppb), i.e., 2×10^{-7} M. Controls were maintained in culture in the absence of T_4. The course of regression in culture was followed by making daily measurements of the tail tips by placing the culture dishes on the stage of an inverted projector, tracing the outlines of the tail tips, and measuring the areas with a planimeter.

Assays of the rate of deiodination of T_4 and T_3 by tadpole tissues were done according to the following procedure. Tissue homogenates were prepared in amphibian Holtfreter's solution, pH 6.8. Liver homogenates were made 1% weight/volume, and tail homogenates were made 10% weight/volume. Assays on tissues from intact tadpoles were made on homogenates of individual livers and tails. Assays on tail tips cultured *in vitro* were made on pooled homogenates of 7 tail tips. Aliquots of these homogenates were incubated for 1 hr at 37°C in the presence of 10^{-9} M [^{125}I]-labeled T_4 or T_3. Both compounds were labeled in the phenolic ring only and were purchased from Industrial Nuclear Co. The reaction was stopped by addition of an equal volume of human plasma, and samples were removed for analysis to assess the percent deiodination. The organic and inorganic ^{125}I present were separated by short-term electrophoresis on paper with a glycine-acetic acid buffer, pH 8.6. After electrophoresis, the paper strips were dried and stained with palladium chloride to visualize the inorganic iodide band. The origin and iodide bands were cut out and their radioactivities measured on a Searle Automatic Gamma Counter.

In order to characterize the deiodination system, the following modifications of the assay procedure were made. The heat lability of the deiodination system was examined by boiling the homogenates for 15 min prior to their use in the reaction mixture. The effect of catalase on the rate of deiodination was studied by adding catalase (1,000 units/ml, Sigma Chemical Company) to the reaction mixture. The effect of a hydrogen peroxide-generating system on the rate of deiodination was studied by adding glucose (2 mg/ml) and glucose oxidase (5 μg/ml, Sigma Chemical Company) to the reaction mixture.

The products of deiodination were analyzed by paper chromatography using a 4:1:5 mixture of butanol:dioxane:2 N NH$_4$OH as a solvent system. Samples of the deiodinated reaction mixture were applied to paper strips and chromatographed for 17 hr. At the end of this time the paper strips were dried, streaked with palladium chloride, and then cut up in 0.5-cm sections. The radioactivity in each section was measured in a gamma counter. Identification of peaks was made by comparison with peaks on separate strips containing [^{125}I] T$_4$ or T$_3$ in equivalent amount of homogenate.

The protein concentration of tissue homogenates was determined by a microadaptation of the method of Lowry, Rosebrough, Farr, and Randall (1951).

RESULTS

The course of growth and regression of the *Xenopus* tadpole tail during development and metamorphosis is shown in Fig. 1, and for tail tip regression *in vitro* in Fig. 2. During development the tail grows progressively larger, gaining both wet weight and protein up until stage 59; then the fore limbs emerge and metamorphosis begins. Tail regression begins at stage 60 and is completed by stage 64, approximately 10 to 14 days after the onset of metamorphosis. In the *in vitro* system used for this study, there is a lag period of 3 days after the addition of T$_3$ to the culture medium before signs of regression appear. By day 4 of culture, tail regression starts, and from this time resorption proceeds at a linear rate until day 7. The first signs of regression always appear in the tail fins prior to autolysis of the central muscle core and overall tail shortening, regardless of whether the regression is occurring *in vivo* or *in vitro*.

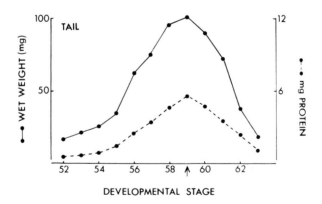

FIG. 1. The wet weight and protein content of tadpole tails at successive stages during development and metamorphosis. Each point is the mean of 20 separate measurements. The arrow indicates the onset of metamorphosis.

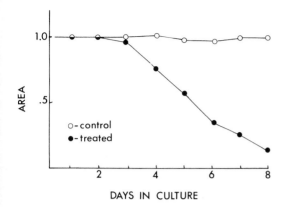

FIG. 2. The areas of tail tips on successive days in culture. Treated tail tips were cultured in the presence of 250 ppb T_4 (2×10^{-7} M); controls were cultured without T_4. Each point represents the mean of 21 separate measurements.

Changes in the wet weight and protein content of the liver during development and metamorphosis are shown in Fig. 3. The liver increases in both parameters during development and through the early stages of metamorphosis. By stage 60 the maximum size is attained. From then until the completion of metamorphosis there is a significant decrease of approximately 30% in both wet weight and protein content.

The rate of deiodination of T_4 and T_3 by tadpole tail tissues during development and metamorphosis is shown in Figs. 4 and 5. At all developmental stages, the tail tissues deiodinate T_4 several times more rapidly than T_3. However, the pattern of change in the rate of deiodination of both hormones during development and metamorphosis is essentially the same. During development, the rate of deiodination of both T_4 and T_3 remains constant when expressed as specific activity, but it rises when expressed as total activity per tail. The specific activity of deiodination of both hor-

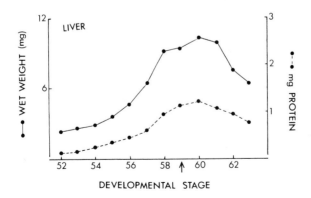

FIG. 3. The wet weight and protein content of tadpole liver at successive stages during development and metamorphosis. Each point is the mean of 10 separate measurements. The arrow indicates the onset of metamorphosis.

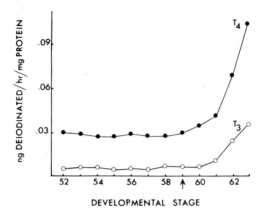

FIG. 4. The specific activity of T_4 and T_3 deiodination by tadpole tail tissues during development and metamorphosis. Rate of deiodination expressed as nanograms deiodinated per hour per milligram of protein. Each point is the mean of 10 separate determinations. The arrow indicates the onset of metamorphosis.

mones remains at a constant level up until stage 59, then starts to rise, increasing fourfold by stage 63. The total activity per tail continues to rise through the onset of metamorphosis up to stage 60, at which time it plateaus and then shows a slight decrease by stage 63. These data indicate that, during development, the system responsible for deiodinating T_4 and T_3 is increasing in amount at the same rate as the total tail protein. Furthermore, the rise in specific activity during metamorphic tail regression represents an increase in actual amount of the deiodination system, not merely a loss of total protein from the tail. There appears to be a specific accumulation of whatever is responsible for the deiodination reaction at the time when the tail is undergoing regression and its total protein content is being drastically reduced. These data indicate that there is a positive temporal correlation

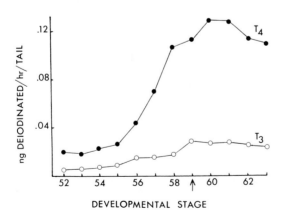

FIG. 5. The total activity of T_4 and T_3 deiodination per tadpole tail (nanograms deiodinated per hour per tail) during development and metamorphosis. Each point is the mean of 10 separate determinations. The arrow indicates the onset of metamorphosis.

between the action of thyroid hormones on tail tissues and the increase in the ability of these tissues to deiodinate the hormones.

The rate of deiodination of T_4 and T_3 by tadpole liver tissues during development and metamorphosis is shown in Figs. 6 and 7. As with tail tissues, the liver also deiodinates T_4 several times more rapidly than T_3 throughout all developmental stages. The rate of deiodination remains constant during development and metamorphosis except for a small but statistically significant rise at stage 59, the onset of metamorphosis. The total activity rises during development up until stage 59, plateaus until

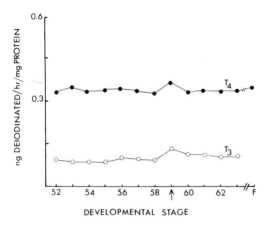

FIG. 6. The specific activity of T_4 and T_3 deiodination (nanograms per hour per milligram of protein) by tadpole liver homogenates during development and metamorphosis. Each point is the mean of 10 separate determinations. The arrow indicates the onset of meta-morphosis.

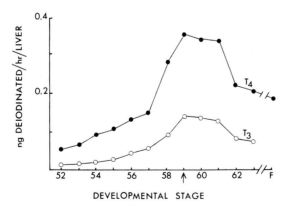

FIG. 7. The total activity of T_4 and T_3 deiodination per tadpole liver (nanograms per hour per liver) during development and metamorphosis. Each point is the mean of 10 separate determinations. The arrow indicates the onset of metamorphosis.

stage 61, then decreases by approximately 50% by stage 63. Taken together, these data indicate that during development and metamorphosis,
except at stage 59, the deiodination system increases and then decreases in
amount at the same rate as the total liver protein. The small but significant
rise in specific activity at stage 59, however, is apparently a reflection of an
actual increase in the amount of the deiodination system above the level of
increase in protein at this stage.

The rates of deiodination of T_4 and T_3 by tadpole tail tips induced to
undergo regression *in vitro* are shown in Figs. 8 and 9. The rate of deiodination expressed as specific activity by tail tips cultured in the presence of T_4
remains relatively constant throughout the entire 8-day period and does not
differ from that of the controls at any time. The specific activity remains
constant even when the treated tail tips are undergoing rapid regression
(days 4 to 8 of culture). The rate of deiodination when expressed as total
activity decreases in the T_4-treated tail tips during the course of regression,
whereas it remains relatively constant in the control tail tips. The rates of
T_4 and T_3 deiodination characteristic of control tail tips cultured *in vitro*

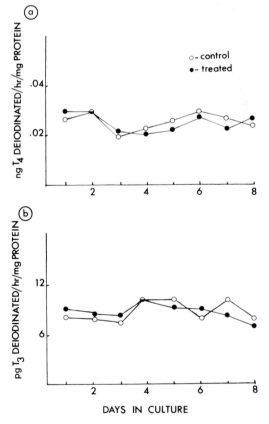

FIG. 8. The specific activity (on successive days in culture) of **(a)** T_4 deiodination and **(b)** T_3 deiodination by control and treated tail tips cultured *in vitro*. Treated tail tips were cultured in the presence of 250 ppb T_4. Each point is the mean of 3 separate determinations on homogenates of 7 tail tips.

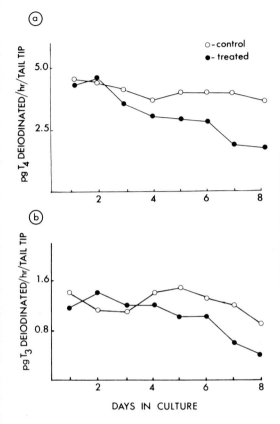

FIG. 9. The total activity/tail tip of **(a)** T_4 deiodination and **(b)** T_3 deiodination by control and treated tail tips cultured *in vitro*. Rate of deiodination = total activity per tail during 8 days in culture. Treated tail tips were cultured in the presence of 250 ppb T_4. Each point is the mean of 3 separate determinations on homogenates of 7 tail tips.

are equivalent to the rates of T_4 and T_3 deiodination by stage 52 tadpole tail homogenates (comparing Figs. 4 and 8). Further, T_4 is deiodinated several times more rapidly than T_3 by all tail tips in culture.

The deiodination system in tadpole tissues was characterized in studies to determine the effects of temperature, catalase, and a hydrogen peroxide-generating system. Temperature has the same effect on the rate of deiodination in both liver and tail tissues (Fig. 10). Boiling effectively destroys all deiodination activity, and as the temperature is increased from 0 to 37°C, the rate of deiodination also increases.

Catalase inhibits the rate of deiodination by approximately 25% and peroxide increases its rate by approximately 115% (Fig. 11). The stimulatory effect of peroxide on the rate of deiodination is completely abolished when both catalase and the peroxide-generating system are present.

Chromatographic analysis of the radioactive products of deiodination by tadpole liver and tail tissues indicates that they consist of inorganic iodide and labeled material that remained at the point of application during chromatography. When T_4 was deiodinated, there was no detectable labeled T_3;

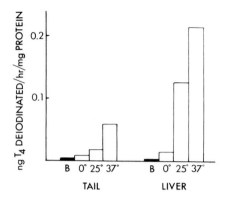

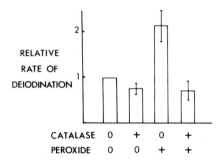

FIG. 10. The effect of temperature (0, 25, and 37°C) on the rate of T_4 deiodination by tadpole liver and tail homogenates. Also the effect of boiling (B) the homogenates prior to assay of the rate of T_4 deiodination at 37°C.

FIG. 11. The effects of catalase (1,000 units/ml) and a hydrogen peroxide-generating system (2 mg/ml glucose and 5 μg/ml glucose oxidase) on the rate of T_4 deiodination by tadpole liver homogenates. The height of each bar is the mean of 3 separate determinations and the vertical lines represent the standard deviations of the means.

only inorganic iodide and origin material were recovered. When T_3 was deiodinated, again the only labeled products recovered were inorganic iodide and origin material.

DISCUSSION

The results of this study reveal that the liver and tail tissues of *Xenopus laevis* tadpoles are capable of degrading thyroid hormones at all stages during late development and throughout metamorphosis. A system for deiodinating thyroid hormones was reported previously for *Rana pipiens* tadpole liver (Galton and Ingbar, 1961, 1962*a*). In the present work, the rate of deiodination by liver was 3 to 10 times greater than by tail tissues. Further, the rate of T_4 deiodination was 2 to 3 times greater than that of T_3 in both liver and tail homogenates. This latter finding agrees with the earlier work on *Rana* tadpole liver (Galton and Ingbar, 1962*a*). In the tadpole liver, the rate of T_4 and T_3 deiodination per milligram of protein remains constant throughout development and metamorphosis except for a small rise at stage 59. This particular stage is characterized by the emergence of the fore limbs and marks the onset of metamorphosis. This is also the stage during which the circulating level of thyroid hormones reaches a maximum (Kaye, 1961;

Gorbman, 1964; Hanaoka, Koya, Kondo, Kobayashi, and Yamomoto, 1973) and when the enzymes of the urea cycle appear (see review by Frieden and Just, 1970). Thus the onset of urea biosynthesis in the liver coincides temporally with a transient increase in the ability of the tissue to degrade thyroid hormones.

In the tadpole tail there is a completely different developmental pattern of deiodinating activity. The rate of deiodination of T_4 and T_3 per milligram of protein remains constant during development but then rises dramatically during metamorphic regression. This rise in the tail is due primarily to an actual increase in the amount of deiodinating activity rather than to a loss in protein from the tail. This conclusion is supported by the finding that the rate of deiodination per tail (total activity) shows only a slight decline during metamorphosis, a decline that is not large enough to account for the rise in rate when expressed as specific activity. Thus, it appears that there is an increase in deiodination activity in the tadpole tail at the very time when the tail is being actively resorbed.

The resorption process itself is characterized biochemically by sharp increases in numerous lytic enzymes, notably lysosomal acid hydrolases, in response to the action of thyroid hormones (Weber, 1967; Frieden and Just, 1970). The results of the present study reflect a temporal coincidence between thyroid hormone action and a rise in the rate of deiodination in tadpole tail tissues during metamorphosis.

Although there is a temporal coincidence between thyroid hormone action on tadpole tail tissues and in the deiodination activity of these tissues during metamorphosis, these two phenomena appear to be unrelated. This conclusion is supported by the results of the study on the deiodination activity in tail tips induced to undergo regression *in vitro*. Tail tips cultured in the presence of T_4 were induced to undergo typical metamorphic regression but did not exhibit any rise in deiodinating activity. Apparently the rise in deiodinating activity that characterizes tail regression during spontaneous metamorphosis is not necessary for eliciting the response to the action of thyroid hormones in that tissue.

These findings refute the suggestion that thyroid hormone action on a particular tissue depends on a high rate of deiodination by that tissue. Although the results on tails from spontaneously metamorphosing tadpoles reveal that the two phenomena occur together, the results on tail tips *in vitro* demonstrate that they are separable.

There are several possible explanations of these findings. There may be no relationship at all between thyroid hormone action in the tadpole and the peripheral metabolism of the hormones. Alternatively, there may be a requirement for only a low level of peripheral metabolism of thyroid hormones in order for the hormones to elicit metamorphosis. The peripheral deiodination of thyroid hormones in the tadpole may serve a quite different function, perhaps as a means for disposing of excess hormone. Whatever the physiological significance of the peripheral metabolism of thyroid hormones, hormone action during metamorphosis does not depend on an increase in deiodinating activity by the responding tissues.

The deiodinating system of tadpole liver and tail tissues appears to be physiological, and is probably mediated by a peroxidase. The fact that deiodinating activity was destroyed by boiling and reduced to less than 10% when assayed at 0°C indicates that the deiodination is a physiological phenomenon. The fact that the reaction rate was inhibited by catalase and stimulated by a hydrogen peroxide-generating system (glucose-glucose oxidase) indicates that the deiodinating reaction is probably mediated by a peroxidase. Peroxidases have been responsible for the deiodination of thyroid hormones in frog liver and several mammalian tissues (Galton and Ingbar, 1962*b;* Galton, Ingbar, and von der Heyde, 1965; Galton, 1970).

There was no evidence of monodeiodination of T_4 by either tadpole liver or tail tissues. That T_3 is deiodinated much more slowly than T_4 (and would be expected to accumulate if formed from T_4), coupled with the finding that no T_3 was accumulated as a product of deiodination, supports this conclusion. Further chromatographic analysis will be necessary in order to characterize completely all of the products of deiodination.

In summary, the studies presented here demonstrate the existence of a physiological mechanism for the deiodination of thyroid hormones by tadpole liver and tail tissues. This peripheral deiodination appears to be mediated by peroxidase activity. However, the physiological significance of the peripheral metabolism of thyroid hormones in the tadpole is still unclear. Further studies should serve to clarify whether or not there is any relationship between thyroid hormone action and the peripheral metabolism of these hormones, a possibility which appears unlikely in light of the results of the present investigation.

ACKNOWLEDGMENTS

This work was supported by a Brown Hazen grant from the Research Corporation and U.S. Public Health Service research grant HD-09020.

REFERENCES

Chou, H. I., and Kollros, J. J. (1974): Stage-modified responses to thyroid hormone in anurans. *Gen. Comp. Endocrinol.,* 22:255–260.
Frieden, E., and Just, J. J. (1970): Hormonal responses in amphibian metamorphosis. In: *Biochemical Actions of Hormones, I,* edited by G. Litwack, pp. 2–52. Academic Press, New York.
Galton, V. A. (1970): The physiological role of thyroid hormone metabolism. In: *Recent Advances in Endocrinology,* 8th ed., pp. 181–206. Churchill Press, London.
Galton, V. A., and Ingbar, S. H. (1961): The mechanism of protein deiodination during the metabolism of thyroid hormones by peripheral tissues. *Endocrinology,* 69:30–38.
Galton, V. A., and Ingbar, S. H. (1962*a*): Observations on the relation between the action and

the degradation of thyroid hormones as indicated by studies in the tadpole and the frog. *Endocrinology,* 70:622–632.

Galton, V. A., and Ingbar, S. H. (1962*b*): Observations on the effects and the metabolism of thyroid hormones in *Necturus maculosa. Endocrinology,* 71:369–377.

Galton, V. A., Ingbar, S. H., and von der Heyde, S. (1965): Role of catalases and peroxidases in the deiodination of thyroxine in the frog liver. *Endocrinology,* 76:479–485.

Gorbman, A. (1964): Endocrinology of the amphibia. In: *Physiology of the Amphibia,* edited by J. A. Moore, pp. 371–425. Academic Press, New York.

Griswold, M. D., Fischer, M. S., and Cohen, P. P. (1972): Temperature-dependent intracellular distribution of thyroxine in amphibian liver. *Proc. Natl. Acad. Sci. (USA),* 69:1486–1489.

Hanaoka, Y., Koya, S. M., Kondo, Y., Kobayashi, Y., and Yamamoto, K. (1973): Morphological and functional maturation of the thyroid during early development of anuran larvae. *Gen. Comp. Endocrinol.,* 21:410–423.

Kaltenbach, J. C. (1953*a*): Local action of thyroxin on amphibian metamorphosis. I. Local metamorphosis in *Rana pipiens* larvae effected by thyroxin-cholesterol implants. *J. Exp. Zool.,* 122:21–39.

Kaltenbach, J. C. (1953*b*): Local action of thyroxin on amphibian metamorphosis. II. Development of the eyelids, nictitating membrane, cornea, and extrinsic ocular muscles in *Rana pipiens* larvae effected by thyroxin-cholesterol implants. *J. Exp. Zool.,* 122:41–51.

Kaltenbach, J. C. (1953*c*): Local action of thyroxin on amphibian metamorphosis. III. Formation and perforation of the skin window in *Rana pipiens* larvae effected by thyroxin-cholesterol implants. *J. Exp. Zool.,* 122:449–467.

Kaltenbach, J. C. (1959): Local action of thyroxin on amphibian metamorphosis. IV. Resorption of the tail fin in anuran larvae effected by thyroxin-cholesterol implants. *J. Exp. Zool.,* 140:1–17.

Kaltenbach, J. C. (1968): Nature of hormone action in amphibian metamorphosis. In: *Metamorphosis: A Problem in Developmental Biology,* edited by W. Etkin and L. I. Gilbert, pp. 399–441. Appleton-Century-Crofts, New York.

Kaye, N. W. (1961): Interrelationships of the thyroid and pituitary in embryonic and premetamorphic stages of the frog, *Rana pipiens. Gen. Comp. Endocrinol.,* 1:1–19.

Kollros, J. J. (1943): Experimental studies on the development of the corneal reflex in Amphibia. II. Localized maturation of the reflex mechanism effected by thyroxin-agar implants into the hindbrain. *Physiol. Zool.,* 16:269–279.

Kollros, J. J. (1961): Mechanisms of amphibian metamorphosis: Hormones. *Amer. Zool.,* 1:107–114.

Kollros, J. J., and Kaltenbach, J. C. (1952): Local metamorphosis of larval skin in *Rana pipiens. Physiol. Zool.,* 25:163–170.

Lowry, O. H., Rosebrough, N. J., Farr, A. L., and Randall, R. J. (1951): Protein measurement with the Folin phenol reagent. *J. Biol. Chem.,* 193:265–275.

Moser, H. (1950): Ein Beitrag zur Analyse der Thyroxinwirkung im Kaulquappenversuch und zur Frage nach dem Zustandekommen der Frubereitschaft des Metamorphose-Reaktionssystems. *Rev. Suisse Zool.,* Suppl. 2, 57:1–144.

Nieuwkoop, P. D., and Faber, J. (1956): *Normal Table of Xenopus laevis (Daudin).* North Holland, Amsterdam.

Pesetsky, I., and Kollros, J. J. (1956): A comparison of the influence of locally applied thyroxine upon Mauthner's cell and adjacent neurons. *Exp. Cell Res.,* 11:477–482.

Robinson, H. (1972): An electrophoretic and biochemical analysis of acid phosphatase in the tail of *Xenopus laevis* during development and metamorphosis. *J. Exp. Zool.,* 180:127–140.

Schwind, J. L. (1933): Tissue specificity at the time of metamorphosis in frog larvae. *J. Exp. Zool.,* 66:1–14.

Shaffer, B. M. (1957): Demonstration at 9th International Congress on Cell Biology, St. Andrews.

Shaffer, B. M. (1963): The isolated Xenopus laevis tail: A preparation for studying the central nervous system and metamorphosis in culture. *J. Embryol. Exp. Morphol.,* 11:77–90.

Tata, J. R. (1970): Simultaneous acquisition of metamorphic response and hormone binding in *Xenopus* larvae. *Nature,* 227:686–689.

Tata, J. R. (1971): Hormonal regulation of metamorphosis. *Symp. Soc. Exp. Biol.,* 25:163–181.

Weber, R. (1962): Induced metamorphosis in isolated tails of *Xenopus* larvae. *Experientia,* 18:84–85.

Weber, R. (1967): Biochemistry of amphibian metamorphosis. In: *The Biochemistry of Animal Development,* edited by R. Weber, pp. 227–301. Academic Press, New York.

Weber, R. (1969): Tissue involution and lysosomal enzymes during anuran metamorphosis. In: *Lysosomes in Biology and Pathology,* edited by J. T. Dingle and H. B. Fell, pp. 437–461. North Holland, Amsterdam.

DISCUSSION

Geller: Dr. Robinson, do you know the product of the deiodination?

Robinson: From preliminary chromatography, it appears to be iodine and a compound other than T_3.

Geller: Is the increase in the deiodination due to more iodine coming off the same molecule at later stages?

Robinson: I do not believe so. I must do more chromatography to clarify what compounds are being produced.

Sokoloff: Peroxidation-deiodination reactions have been described before.

Gona: Have you used any of the analogues of thyroid hormone?

Robinson: None other than T_3.

Gona: Did you see a tremendous difference in the rates of deiodination of T_4 and T_3?

Robinson: Both the tail and the liver can deiodinate T_3, but much more slowly than T_4. However, T_3 is much more effective in producing tail regression.

Grave: Did you say that the adult liver is different in its response to T_4 than the tadpole liver and that the adult liver does not respond at all?

Robinson: That statement was based on the work of Galton and Ingbar, who decided, on the basis of work with respiration, that the adult frog liver is unresponsive to T_4.

Thyroid Hormones and Brain Development,
edited by Gilman D. Grave. Raven Press,
New York, 1977.

Aurelia Metamorphosis: Model System for Study of Thyroxine Action

Dorothy Breslin Spangenberg*

Jellyfish are the simplest intact organisms in which to study the effects on development of endogenous as well as exogenous thyroxine. Spangenberg (1967) demonstrated that *Aurelia aurita* (Texas strain) scyphistomae (polyps) respond to iodide by strobilating. She further discovered that the *Aurelia* polyps synthesize thyroxine (T_4) as well as monoiodotyrosine (MIT) and diiodotyrosine (DIT) during the process of strobilation (1971, 1974). Following the synthesis of these compounds, the *Aurelia* segments of the strobilae metamorphose to give rise to ephyrae (immature medusae). Exogenously introduced thyroxine also induces metamorphosis in the *Aurelia* polyps (Spangenberg, 1967). Although the organisms form complicated structures during the transformation from polyp to ephyra tissue, the model involves only seven basic cell types.

The basic cellular structure of the jellyfish is relatively simple; however, its life cycle is more complicated than that of higher organisms. In nature, all of the life stages of *Aurelia* develop within a year. Minute (2 to 3 mm diameter) ephyrae (Fig. 1) grow into large (10 to 12 in. in diameter) medusae (Fig. 2) within a 6-month period. Planula larvae (Fig. 3a) produced by the sexually mature medusae give rise to polyps (Fig. 3b) which overwinter in preparation for their strobilation into ephyrae in the springtime.

The life cycle of *Aurelia* has been completed in the laboratory (Spangenberg, *unpublished results*). Jellyfish polyps are induced to metamorphose with exogenous thyroxine to form strobilae (Figs. 4a and b). The first ephyrae arise from the most distal segment of the strobila and become free-swimming within 6 days (at 30°C). The ephyrae, reared to medusae using brine shrimp (*Artemia*) as their sole nutrient, become sexually mature within 3 months and reproduce giving rise to planula larvae. In the laboratory, a small proportion of the planulae become polyps within a few weeks, completing the entire developmental life cycle in approximately half the time required in nature. Thus far, the role of thyroxine in jellyfish development has been investigated only in the strobilation phase of the life cycle (from polyp to ephyra).

The role of thyroxine in strobilation in *Aurelia* has been emphasized,

---

* Department of Molecular, Cellular, and Developmental Biology, University of Colorado, Boulder, Colorado 80302.

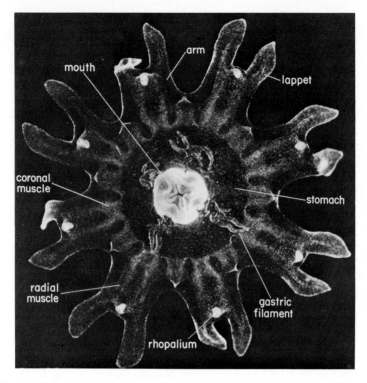

FIG. 1. Ephyrae of *Aurelia,* 4 mm diameter. (Photographed by Howard Cooper.)

a process which is fairly rapid and requires approximately 6 days (at 30°C) to achieve a new free-swimming ephyra from the onset of the development of the first segment of the strobila. The strobilation process has two distinct phases: (1) segmentation, at which time segments are noted, the first segment appearing in 2 to 3 days (at 30°C) after T_4 administration, and (2) metamorphosis, wherein the segment becomes an ephyra. Isolated complete segments develop into ephyrae without the need of contributions of cells or substances from the parent strobila (Spangenberg, 1965). Once completed, the segment is believed to be programmed to give rise to the ephyra. Because T_4 induces strobilation and is present to the first segment stage (and probably longer), the hormone presumably is necessary for the programming for metamorphosis.

During metamorphosis, the programming of the strobila segment is enacted and the relatively sessile polyps give rise to free-swimming ephyrae. Several new structures are formed in the course of metamorphosis, most notably the striated muscles, a more complex nervous system, and statoliths by the induction of mineralization. In addition, a large stomach forms with centralized digestive structures (gastric filaments). Pulsing activity of the

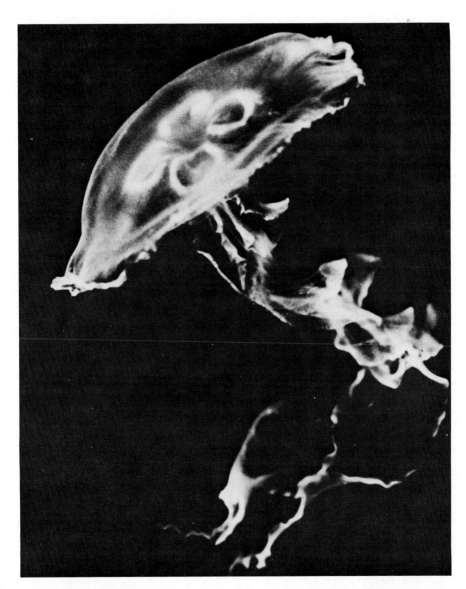

FIG. 2. Medusa of *Aurelia;* bell is 4 in. in diameter; laboratory grown. (Photographed by William Kuenning.)

ephyra occurs before its detachment from the strobila. Although pulsing may not be essential for circulatory purposes in the ephyra, it is quite necessary for circulation of nutrients and gases in the medusae and for swimming activities in both ephyrae and medusae. This pulsing requires considerable coordination of nerves and muscles.

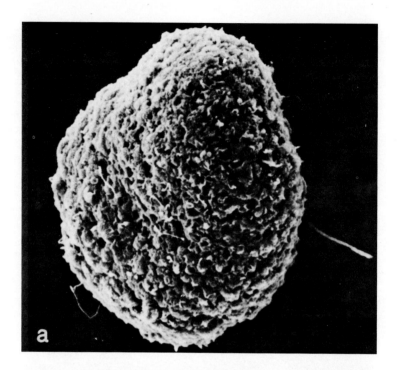

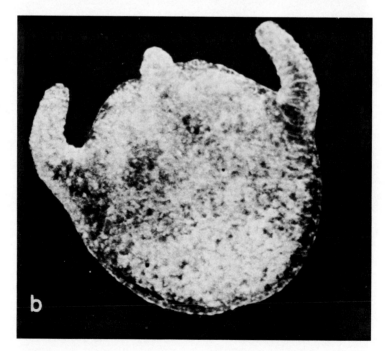

FIG. 3. (a) SEM of Planula Larva of *Aurelia*, ×1,000. **(b)** Developing polyp of *Aurelia*, ×170.

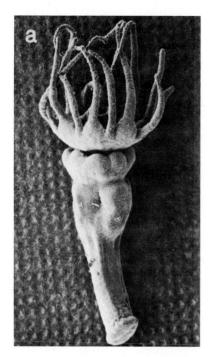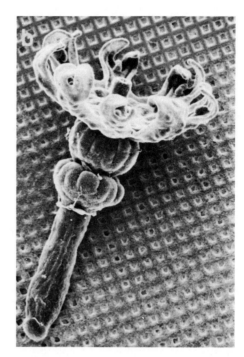

FIG. 4. SEM of strobila of *Aurelia* **(a)** early, ×52; **(b)** late, ×75. (Photographed by Robert McGrew.)

The jellyfish does not form a brain at any stage in its developmental life cycle, although there are complex nerve changes and activities in the various life stages. These changes in nerve function and morphology during the transition from polyp to ephyra are discussed, as well as the differentiation of other new ephyra structures. The role of T_4 in inducing metamorphosis in the *Aurelia*, as well as its role in differentiation of new structures, will also be discussed.

T_4 AND INDUCTION OF METAMORPHOSIS IN *AURELIA*

Spangenberg (1967) reported that low-temperature preconditioned Texas *Aurelia* polyps will strobilate after being placed in low dosages of iodide. Subsequently, she induced *Aurelia* from Woods Hole, the Chesapeake, and Delaware Bays to strobilate with iodide (*unpublished results*). More recently, other investigators have obtained strobilae of *Aurelia* from Texas (Welch, 1973); Puerto Rico (Silvertone, 1974); and Virginia (Olmon and Webb, 1974) using iodide. Jellyfish of different genera were induced to strobilate with iodide when Black and Webb (1973) induced *Chrysaora* and Spangenberg (*unpublished results*) induced *Cyanea* from Mississippi. These results indicated that the iodide response in *Aurelia* is general. However, preconditioning requirements for the iodide response may be more complex for some jellyfish polyps than for others.

When the strobilation response to iodide in *Aurelia* prompted Spangenberg (1971) to test other iodinated compounds in the jellyfish, she found that MIT, DIT, T_3, and thyroglobulin evoked the strobilation response in the Texas *Aurelia*. Welch (1973) and Silverstone (1974) subsequently reported that certain of these compounds also induced strobilation in their Texas and Puerto Rican *Aurelia* strains, respectively.

Radiochromatographic studies of the radioiodide-treated polyps and developing strobilae revealed that the jellyfish synthesized three compounds: MIT, DIT, and T_4 (Spangenberg, 1971). MIT is found within 8 hr after ^{131}I administration, before the detection of DIT or T_4, which appear within 24 hr (Spangenberg, 1974). Also, between 24 and 48 hr, T_4 is excreted into the medium. Welch (1973) confirmed Spangenberg's results in the Texas *Aurelia*. Of special interest was his finding of T_4 12 hr after radioiodide treatment. Black and Webb (1973) found these hormones in strobilating *Chrysaora* polyps and reported the presence of T_4 in segmented strobilae. Olmon and Webb (1974) reported that early strobilae of a Virginia strain of *Aurelia* concentrated iodide against a gradient 30 to 60 times the media concentration. Using acid-alcohol extracted jellyfish tissue, they failed to detect DIT or T_4, but did report minute amounts of MIT.

While T_4 is probably the primary, if not exclusive, natural substance synthesized by the jellyfish for induction of strobilation, other iodinated compounds can induce strobilation in *Aurelia*. Jellyfish respond to exogenously introduced MIT, DIT, T_3, and thyroglobulin (Spangenberg, 1971). Welch (1973) and Silverstone (1974) subsequently confirmed the effects of MIT, DIT, and thyroglobulin on their *Aurelia*. Thus far, no noniodinated compound has evoked strobilation in *Aurelia* in the absence of iodide. Spangenberg tested the effects of dimethyltyrosine (synthesized by Drs. Paul Block, Jr. and Eugene Jorgensen, University of California) to no avail. Spangenberg (*unpublished results*) also obtained negative results using tyrosine, thyronine, bromide, janus green, and neutral red. Silverstone (1974) also obtained no strobilation when testing polyps with bromide.

Administration of low dosages of goitrogens such as thiourea, propyl-thiouracil, and potassium thiocyanate in conjunction with iodide prevents induction of strobilation (Spangenberg, 1974). Radiochromatography of jellyfish given goitrogens and ^{131}I simultaneously revealed a reduced uptake of iodide and an impairment of the synthesis of the iodinated compounds.

When $[^{131}I]T_4$ was administered to the jellyfish and the organisms were radiochromatographed (Spangenberg, 1974), this technique showed that the organisms utilized T_4 directly. Although some of the T_4 was deiodinized, the iodide apparently was not utilized to make precursors of T_4, because no labeled precursors were found. No localized site of intense concentration of ^{131}I or $[^{125}]T_4$ was found in the polyps during initiation of strobilation by autoradiography (Spangenberg, 1971). Both substances were present in greater amounts at the distal, differentiating end of the organisms than at the base, particularly during the early presegmentation strobilation period. Distribution of these two substances within the tissues during strobilation suggests that T_4 may be ingested orally and iodide taken up across the epidermis.

T_4 is synthesized and excreted early in strobilation. Although it was not detected after 48 hr by radiochromatographic techniques in a small tissue sample, further autoradiographic studies indicated that minute amounts of T_4 may still be present in localized areas of the jellyfish at a stage past 48 hr of exposure to T_4. *Aurelia* polyps exposed to 0.25 Ci/ml of $[^{14}C]T_4$ for 48 hr produced ephyrae which when autoradiographed revealed labeling in new structures, such as the rhopalia, nerve and muscle regions, and the gastric filaments. These data imply that minute amounts of T_4 are still present in the ephyrae (radiochromatographic experiments in progress have verified that the labeled material is unmodified T_4). Because ^{131}I was not taken into ephyrae in recordable amounts (Spangenberg, 1974), it is assumed that any T_4 present in the ephyrae is retained from the strobila and does not represent newly synthesized T_4.

In summary, T_4 is believed to be the natural compound responsible for the induction of strobilation because (1) iodide is utilized to synthesize T_4 via a synthetic pathway analogous to that of the mammalian thyroid gland, (2) T_4 is utilized in the minute amounts (excesses are excreted) characteristic of mammalian tissues; (3) when T_4 is administered to jellyfish polyps, it is utilized directly for the induction of strobilation; (4) goitrogens which inhibit synthesis of T_4 (but permit a certain amount of iodide uptake) inhibit metamorphosis; (5) metamorphic cellular events which occur during ephyra formation are consistent with T_4-mediated metamorphosis in amphibians and development in higher organisms.

T_4 AND NEW STRUCTURE FORMATION

During metamorphosis, jellyfish polyps, which are relatively sessile, give rise to ephyrae which are active swimmers. To achieve this, changes must take place in the organisms, most notably those which permit the ephyrae to swim.

Muscle

In the polyps of *Aurelia,* myofibrils composed of thick and thin filaments are found at the base of the epitheliomuscular cells. These cells are large, flagellated, vacuolated, and contain secretory granules. Each cell possesses several myofibrils (Fig. 5a) which join together via specialized junctions to

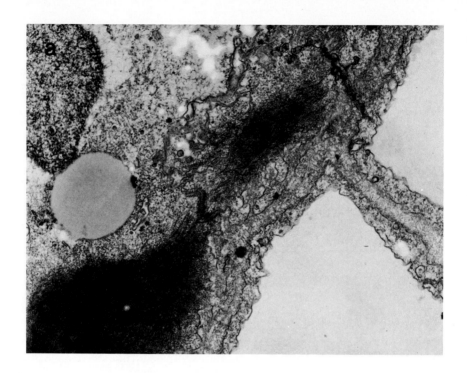

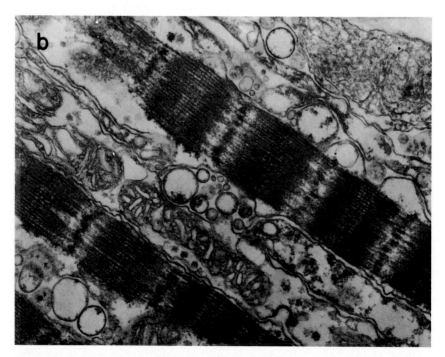

FIG. 5. **(a)** Smooth muscle at base of epitheliomuscular cell in tentacle, ×15,000. **(b)** Striated muscle in arm of ephyra, ×18,720.

form relatively long smooth muscle fibers which permit rapid contraction and relatively slow relaxation of the organisms. During metamorphosis, the smooth muscle is lost and the organisms develop the striated muscle (Fig. 5b) required for the vigorous activity of swimming. Little is known about the mechanisms involved in the loss of the myofibrils and the development of new striated muscle cells, although Spangenberg (*unpublished results*) has recorded the ultrastructural changes associated with the loss of myofibrils in the epitheliomuscular cells at the base of the tentacles during strobilation.

The muscular system of the *Aurelia* ephyra is almost entirely epidermal and is localized in the subumbrellar area. The coronal muscle (Fig. 1) which encircles the stomach region is the major muscle used for swimming. The radial muscles extend from the coronal muscle into the arms of the ephyra. A longitudinal layer of muscle fibers is in the manubrium of the ephyra and the oral arms of the more mature medusae (Hymen, 1940).

Figure 6 depicts a portion of a radial muscle extending into an arm of an ephyra, the ultrastructure of which reveals a striking resemblance to the skeletal and cardiac muscles of mammals. In each myofibril (composed of thick and thin filaments) there are bands corresponding to the Z, A, I, H, and M bands of mammals, and numerous highly developed mitochondria between the myofibrils. A small amount of sarcoplasmic reticulum is present in the muscle cells, but there is no evidence of the complex T-system of mammalian striated muscle. Numerous fat droplets resembling those found in mammalian heart muscle are also found near the myofibrils.

Very little is yet known about the role of T_4 in inducing or mediating muscle changes in the jellyfish. The probable role of lysosomes (Fig. 7) in the degeneration of the smooth myofibrils of the epitheliomuscular cells of the tentacles suggests an involvement of T_4 (Spangenberg, *unpublished results*). In amphibians, T_4 has been implicated in lysosome formation and/or lysosome enzyme activity in tail resorption and in modification of the intestinal tract (Bonneville, 1963; Weber, 1967; Kaltenbach, 1971). A possible involvement of T_4 in striated muscle activity and development is suggested by the work of Minelli and Korecky (1968), who maintain that both T_4 and growth hormone are indispensable for the maintenance of normal growth of the heart. McDevitt, Shanks, and Hadden (1968) also reported that T_4 is directly involved in control of heart beat.

Nerves

Innervation of the muscular systems of jellyfish is poorly understood. The model provided by hydra research may apply to the jellyfish, in which nerve cells have been described at the base of the epitheliomuscular cells in hydra above their muscular processes (Lentz, 1966). Nerves are identified in hydra at the ultrastructural level, primarily because of the presence of

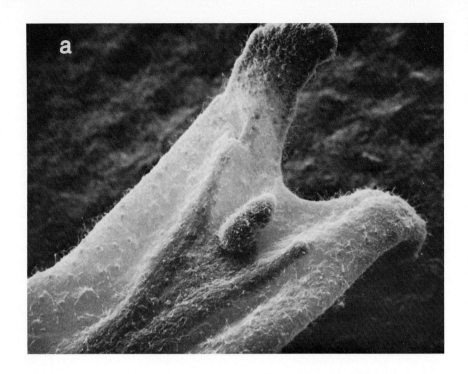

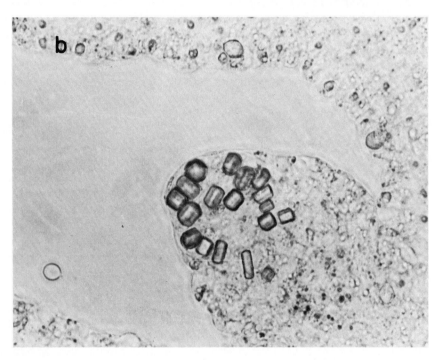

FIG. 6. (a) SEM of arm of ephyra showing rhopalium and radial muscles, ×327. (Photographed by Robert McGrew.) **(b)** Statoliths in the statocyst at the tip of the rhopalium, ×825.

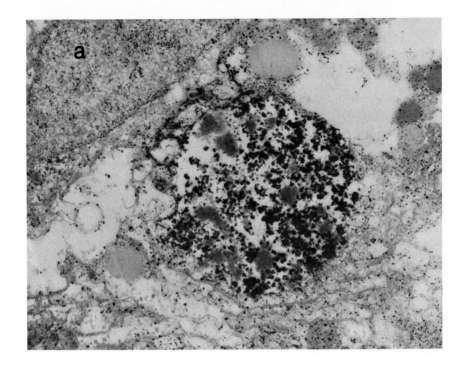

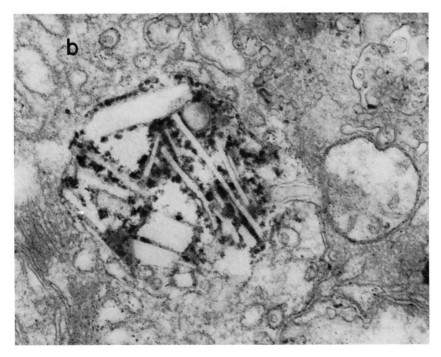

FIG. 7. (a) Lysosome in tentacle of metamorphosing *Aurelia*, ×18,627. **(b)** Calcifying vesicle (lysosome) in rhopalium of *Aurelia* medusa, ×49,750.

microtubules and neurosecretory granules (Davis, 1973). In the *Aurelia*, this identification is more difficult due to the sporadic demonstration of microtubules and the resemblance of nerve cells to other cells of the same size. Recently, Westfall (1973) described synapses in the tentacles of a strain of *Aurelia*.

At the light microscope level, Komai (1942) unsuccessfully attempted to demonstrate the nervous system of the polyps of *Aurelia* using the rongalit white method. Spangenberg more recently stained nerves in *Aurelia* polyp tentacles using the oxidized form of methylene blue (Fig. 8a and b). She found large bipolar nerves in the tentacles and in ephyrae.

Nothing is known about nerve differentiation during metamorphosis of the polyp to form an ephyra. Concerning ephyrae, however, Horridge (1954) reported that the rapid coordination of the beat (pulse) is identified with neurons which spread over the muscles from the marginal ganglia, and that the feeding response and spasm are coordinated by a separate net called the diffuse nerve net which spreads over the entire epithelium. The diffuse net is composed of bipolar cells, presumably sensory, and nonsensory bipolar and multipolar cells. The giant fiber system is composed of large bipolar nerves which are associated with the muscle fibers except where the nerves connect with the marginal ganglia (in rhopalia).

It is not unreasonable to expect that T_4 may be involved in nerve changes in *Aurelia* during metamorphosis from the polyp to the ephyra stage. It is evident that a more complex nervous system evolves during the short time period from the segmented strobila to the ephyra (2 to 3 days at 30°C). A role of T_4 in nerve development in humans and other mammals is clearly established. Sokoloff (1967) emphasized that T_4 has profound effects on the growth, development, and maturation of the nervous system of children. Pesetsky (1962) reported enlarged Mauthner's neurons in anurans following thyroxine administration, and Gorbman and Bern (1966) refer to increased neurosecretory products in the hypothalamus of sharks in response to thyroxine administration.

Rhopalia and Statoliths

Rhopalia (Fig. 6a) development offers an opportunity for the study of complex nerve differentiation and of calcification. At the base of the rhopalia are nerve centers which play a major role in the regulation of the pulse of the jellyfish. At its tip is the statocyst, which is a sac of gypsum crystals (Fig. 6b). The statocyst has been shown to be involved in the "righting reflex" of the medusa. The falling of the rhopalial end weighted with statoliths against the sensory epithelium of the sensory niche apparently provides the stimulus for the "righting" of the medusa bell after it is tilted (Hymen, 1940).

A possible involvement of T_4 in statolith differentiation has been under

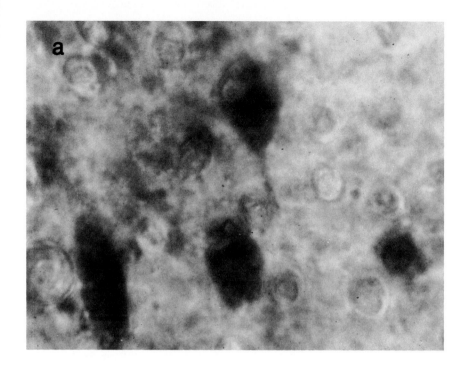

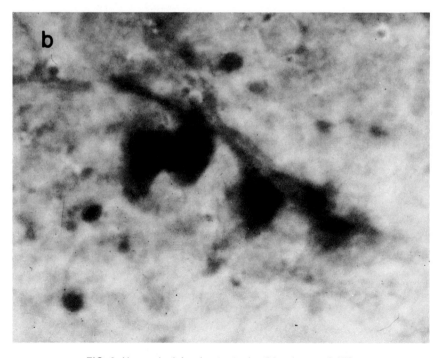

FIG. 8. Nerves in **(a)** polyp tentacle; **(b)** ephyra. ×3,150.

investigation in this laboratory. Spangenberg (1976) reported that the intracellular statoliths originate in acid phosphatase-positive vesicles (Fig. 7b) within the epidermal cells of the rhopalium. These vesicles (1 to 5 μm in length and width) resemble similar vesicles found in developing teeth and bones of mammals (Bonucci, 1967; Bernard, 1972; Eisenmann & Glick, 1972; Anderson, 1973). The calcifying vesicles of jellyfish are probably a modified type of lysosome which is Golgi-derived. The association of T_4 with lysosome formation and function and/or with lysosomal enzyme synthesis in higher animals (Bonneville, 1963; Weber, 1967; Kaltenbach, 1971) suggests a similar association in statolith synthesis in *Aurelia*.

T_4 has been implicated in various mineralization events in higher organisms. Development of bone and teeth is delayed in neonatal hypothyroidism, and enamel hypoplasia occurs in the deciduous teeth of such children (Andersen, 1971). Frieden and Lipner (1971) review the significant role played by T_4 in the metabolism of calcium and the regulation of bone maturation.

In summary, the involvement of T_4 with the initiation of strobilation in *Aurelia* has been established. *Aurelia* polyps synthesize MIT, DIT, and T_4 from iodide prior to metamorphosing. These organisms also respond directly to T_4 introduced into the medium. T_4 may be necessary for the programming of the new ephyra and may also be required during the differentiation and functioning of at least some of the new structures.

Several important new structures develop during differentiation of ephyrae which enable them to swim: striated muscle, a more complicated nervous system, and rhopalia with statoliths. Lysosomes are apparently involved in the degeneration of the smooth myofibrils of the epithelio-muscular cells of polyp tentacles and in the formation of statoliths. T_4 activity has been implicated in higher organisms in the differentiation of nerves, muscle, bones, teeth, and in the synthesis of lysosomes and/or lysosomal enzymes, e.g., cathepsins.

The T_4-induced metamorphosis of jellyfish is the simplest intact system in which to study the effects of T_4. In this rapidly developing system, the role of T_4 in cell programming can be studied and the possible direct effects of T_4 on differentiation of new structures can be investigated. The differentiation of structures closely resembling those of higher organisms provides a useful tool for studying direct effects of T_4 in an intact but simplified organism. The jellyfish model provides new opportunities to determine the action of T_4 in developing biological systems at the molecular, cellular, and organismal levels.

ACKNOWLEDGMENTS

This research was supported by research grants NIH HD 07844 and DE 03796.

REFERENCES

Andersen, H. J. (1971): Prenatal damage in hypothyroidism. In: *Hormones in Development,* edited by M. Hamburgh and E. J. W. Barrington. Appleton-Century-Crofts, New York.

Anderson, H. C. (1973): Calcium-accumulating vesicles in the intercellular matrix of bone. In: *Hard Tissue Growth, Repair, and Remineralization.* Elsevier, New York.

Bernard, G. W. (1972): Ultrastructural observations of initial calcification in dentine and enamel. *J. Ultrastruct. Res.,* 41:1.

Black, R. E., and Webb, K. L. (1973): Metabolism of ^{131}I in relation to strobilation of *Chrysaora quinquecirrha* (Scyphozoa). *Comp. Biochem. Physiol.,* 45A:1023.

Bonneville, M. A. (1963): Fine structural changes in the intestinal epithelium of the bullfrog during metamorphosis. *J. Cell Biol.,* 18:579.

Bonucci, E. (1967): Fine structure of early calcification. *J. Ultrastruct. Res.,* 20:33.

Davis, L. (1973): Structure of neurosecretory cells with special references to the nature of the secretory product. In: *Biology of Hydra,* edited by A. Burnett, pp. 319–342. Academic Press, New York.

Eisenmann, D. R., and Glick, P. L. (1972): Ultrastructure of initial crystal formation in dentin. *J. Ultrastruct. Res.,* 41:18.

Frieden, E., and Lipner, H. (1971): *Biochemical Endocrinology of the Vertebrates.* Prentice-Hall, Englewood Cliffs, N.J.

Gorbman, A., and Bern, H. (1966): *A Textbook of Comparative Endocrinology.* John Wiley & Sons, New York.

Horridge, A. (1954): Observations on the nerve fibres of *Aurellia aurita. Quart. J. Microsc. Sci.,* 95:85.

Hymen, L. H. (1940): *The Invertebrates,* Vol. I. McGraw-Hill Book Company, New York.

Kaltenbach, J. C. (1971): Histochemical patterns in the tail of the metamorphosing tadpole. In: *Hormones in Development,* edited by M. Hamburgh and E. J. W. Barrington. Appleton-Century-Crofts, New York.

Komai, T. (1942): The nervous system in some Coelenterate types. 2. Ephyra and scyphula. *Ann. Zool. Jap.,* 21:25.

Lentz, T. L. (1966): *The Cell Biology of Hydra.* John Wiley & Sons, New York.

McDevitt, D. G., Shanks, R. G., and Hadden, D. R. (1968): The role of the thyroid in the control of heart-rate. *Lancet,* 1:998.

Minelli, R., and Korecky, B. (1968): Effect of growth hormone and thyroxine on isometric contractile mechanics of cardiac muscle. *Can. J. Physiol. Pharmacol.,* 47:545.

Olmon, J. E., and Webb, K. L. (1974): Metabolism of ^{131}I in relation to strobilation of *Aurelia aurita,* L. (Scyphozoa). *J. Exp. Mar. Biol. and Ecol.,* 16:113.

Pesetsky, I. (1962): The thyroxine-stimulated enlargement of Mauthner's neuron in Anurans. *Gen. Comp. Endocrinol.,* 2:229.

Silverstone, M. P. (1974): Studies on the mechanism of strobilation initiation in *Aurelia aurita.* Master's thesis. University of Puerto Rico, Mayaguez, Puerto, Rico.

Spangenberg, D. B. (1965): A study of strobilation in Aurelia under controlled conditions. *J. Exp. Zool.,* 160:1.

Spangenberg, D. B. (1967): Iodine induction of metamorphosis in *Aurelia. J. Exp. Zool.,* 165:441.

Spangenberg, D. B. (1971): Thyroxine induced metamorphosis in *Aurelia. J. Exp. Zool.,* 178:183.

Spangenberg, D. B. (1974): Thyroxine in early strobilation in *Aurelia. Am. Zool.,* 14:825.

Spangenberg, D. B. (1977): Intracellular statolith synthesis in *Aurelia aurita.* In: *International Symposium on the Mechanisms of Mineralization in Invertebrates and Plants.* University of South Carolina Press (*in press*).

Sokoloff, L. (1967): Action of thyroid hormones and cerebral development. *Am. J. Dis. Child.,* 114:498.

Weber, R. (1967): Biochemistry of amphibian metamorphosis. In: *The Biochemistry of Animal Development,* edited by R. Weber, Vol. 2, p. 227–298. Academic Press, New York.

Welch, W. J. (1973): Production of iodinated compounds and the effect on strobilation in *Aurelia aurita.* Master's thesis. Morehead State University, Kentucky.

Westfall, J. A. (1973): Ultrastructural evidence for neuromuscular systems in Coelenterates. *Am. Zool.,* 13:237.

DISCUSSION

Hamburgh: Is the molecule of T_4 absorbed by the cells of both the epiderm and the gastroderm in both the polyp and the medusa? Do these cells make T_4?

Spangenberg: I cannot say whether each cell type is absorbing T_4. At the light microscopic level, I have found ^{131}I labeling, which I believe to represent $[^{131}$I$]T_4$ throughout the polyp and the early strobila. Recently, I found ^{14}C labeling, which I believe to be $[^{14}$C$]T_4$, throughout the ephyrae (after $[^{14}$C$]T_4$ administration to the polyps). I plan to investigate the location of T_4 in polyps and ephyrae at the ultrastructural level by using electron microscope autoradiography after labeling with $[^{14}$C$]T_4$.

Hamburgh: What about making T_4?

Spangenberg: Synthesis is another question which remains open. I know neither if there are specific cells that synthesize T_4 nor the identity of these cells. At the moment I am studying utilization of T_4, rather than its synthesis.

Sokoloff: Do you know if any of those cells concentrate iodine?

Spangenberg: I was not able to identify specific cells in association with iodine by light microscopy. Since the cells are quite small, the answer should be available at the ultrastructural level by electron microscopy.

Sokoloff: The biosynthesis of thyroid hormones is itself very complex, and the thyroid gland is highly specialized to accomplish the task.

Spangenberg: Aurelia do not have such organs as glands (although they do have glandular cells). The organisms have only seven specific types of cell, and activities such as the biosynthesis of thyroid hormone must be carried out at the cellular level. Which cells are synthesizing the hormone can ultimately be determined.

Grave: Can your polyps live in sea water that has no iodine in it?

Spangenberg: They can, although I feed them brine shrimp (*Artemia salina*) which contain minute amounts of iodine.

Grave: Can you keep a polyp so that it never metamorphoses into a medusa?

Spangenberg: We have a culture of *Aurelia* that has been in existence for 50 years in the polyp form. One has to work very hard, in fact, to condition them to respond to iodide by metamorphosing. Presumably, if the organisms are never exposed to minimal doses of iodine or T_4, they will never form medusae.

Grave: Must you work hard to get all strains of *Aurelia* to metamorphose?

Spangenberg: The cold-water British strain is harder to induce than the American *Aurelia*. Importantly, the Texas *Aurelia* (warm-water strain) responds to T_4 consistently by 100% strobilation and the production of ephyrae within 6 days. It is a very well-ordered process.

Grave: Will they strobilate if you give them just iodine?

Spangenberg: Yes, but they utilize iodine to synthesize T_4 and its precursors, MIT and DIT.

Timiras: Mammals have a very specialized series of functions for producing thyroid hormones. Therefore, it would be useful to learn whether T_4 is responsible for the effect described, or whether a similar effect could be obtained by administering some analogues of T_4 with similar structure but with different functions or no functions at all.

Spangenberg: I am aware that amphibia are very responsive to analogues of T_4. I do not claim a specificity of response for T_4 alone in *Aurelia* (although T_4 is the naturally occurring compound in the jellyfish). But one must question the specificity of T_4 in mammals as well. According to the recent work of Jorgensen and his colleagues (1974), non-iodine-containing analogues of T_4 are functional in reversing thiouracil-induced goiter in the rat and increasing amino acid uptake in a rat thymocyte *in vitro*. The compounds are methylated in the place of iodine, such as 3′,5′-dimethyl-ʟ-thyronine.

Sokoloff: Is there no iodine on the inner ring (the α ring) of these analogues?

Spangenberg: That is right. There are no iodine atoms in the entire molecule.

Sokoloff: One of the most active of all the thyroactive analogues is the isopropyl derivative in which isopropyl groups replace iodine atoms in the β ring adjacent to the phenolic group. I have not heard of any thyroactive compounds in which alkyl groups replace the iodine atoms of the α ring. That is very interesting.

Kollros: Do you imply also that there is no iodine-containing compound in the tissue culture medium?

Spangenberg: There is a recent paper by Frieden and Yoshizato (1974), who tested these compounds in amphibia, in which they get a percentage effect compared with T_4. Use of these compounds has led to some interesting effects in mammals and amphibia (although dimethyl-tyrosine was not effective in jellyfish) and leads to the speculation that tissue response to T_4 in these systems is not specific.

Kollros: What about the propionic and formic acid analogues? If they are placed in pellets and put into the tail, as Kaltenbach (1968) has done, they have a local effect there.

Sokoloff: The side chain is not important for activity. There may be quantitative differences because of effects on binding to plasma proteins, transport, etc., but the side chain is not a structural requirement for activity. The benzoic acid side chain, the acetic acid, and the propionic acid side chain will all work.

As simple as the molecule of T_4 appears, we still do not know all of its structural requirements for activity. We have always thought that the phenolic group is essential for activity, but Lardy put a methyl group on T_4 and made a methyl ether. He found that this ether is not demethylated, which means there is no phenolic group there at all, yet he observed some biologic activity. Even the oxygen bridge can be replaced by sulfur, and some activity remains. There are quantitative differences, but the absolute requirement for activity of the molecule is not really known.

DISCUSSION REFERENCES

Frieden, E., and Yoshizato, K. (1974): Thyromimetic activity of methyl-thyronines in the bullfrog tadpole. *Endocrinology,* 5:188–194.

Jorgensen, E. C., Murray, W. J., and Block, P. (1974): Thyroxine analogs. 22. Thyromimetic activity of halogen-free derivatives of 3,5,-dimethyl-ʟ-thyronine, *J. Am. Chem. Soc.,* 17: 434–439.

Kaltenbach, J. (1968): Nature of hormone action in amphibian metamorphosis. In: *Metamorphosis,* edited by W. Etkin and L. I. Gilbert, p. 399. Appleton-Century-Crofts, New York.

Thyroid Hormones and Brain Development,
edited by Gilman D. Grave. Raven Press,
New York, 1977.

Brain Myelination in Experimental Hypothyroidism: Morphological and Biochemical Observations

N. Paul Rosman* and Michael J. Malone**

The association of congenital hypothyroidism with mental subnormality remains poorly understood; knowledge of the pathophysiological mechanisms by which thyroid deficiency alters brain function is incomplete. The relationship is important because the fundamental abnormality is biochemical and potentially reversible.

The anatomical basis for the developmental retardation that commonly accompanies congenital hypothyroidism is uncertain, despite writings on the subject that date back to the sixteenth century. Morphological studies of the brains of such patients have been few and findings have varied. Recorded abnormalities have included lowered brain weight, a reduction in cells in the cerebral cortex, malformed convolutions with poor differentiation of the cortical layers, and delayed myelination of brain (Mott, 1917; Marinesco, 1924; Benda, 1946; Beierwaltes, Carr, Raman, Spafford, Aster, and Lowrey, 1959).

The changes recorded in the brains of laboratory animals made hypothyroid include altered brain shape, reduced brain weight, decreased size and increased density of cortical neurons, simplification of neuronal dendrites, decreased numbers of cortical axons, delayed disappearance of the cerebellar external granular layer, and retarded myelination of brain (Barrnett, 1948; Eayrs and Taylor, 1951; Eayrs, 1954, 1955, 1964, 1966; Hamburgh, Lynn, and Weiss, 1964). Biochemical studies in such brains have shown increased concentration of DNA with lowered RNA per unit DNA (Geel and Timiras, 1967), and a reduction in myelin lipids (Balázs, Brooksbank, Davison, Eayrs, and Wilson, 1969; Walravens and Chase, 1969). A general criticism of these studies is their failure to consider to take into account the possible contribution of coexisting malnutrition. A reduction in brain weight and axon density, with increased density of nerve cell bodies (Eayrs and Horn, 1955; Horn, 1955) and impaired brain myelination (Benton, Moser, Dodge, and Carr, 1966) have been found in animals made nutritionally deficient.

It thus appeared that further study of the effects of hypothyroidism on

* Departments of Pediatrics and Neurology (Pediatric Neurology), Boston University School of Medicine, Boston City Hospital, Boston, Massachusetts 02118.
** Geriatric Research Educational and Clinical Center, Veterans Administration Hospital, Bedford, Massachusetts 01730.

myelinogenesis could provide additional understanding of an important biochemical cause of impaired brain maturation. We decided to study first the effects of neonatal hypothyroidism on myelin development, using a complementary morphological and biochemical approach.

WHOLE BRAIN STUDIES

Experimental Hypothyroidism

MATERIALS AND METHODS

Five methods of producing hypothyroidism in Sprague-Dawley white rats were tried. These included surgical thyroidectomy, administration of ^{131}I to pregnant female rats, injection of ^{131}I through the uterine wall into individual fetuses, administration of parenteral methimazole to pregnant female rats, and intraperitoneal injection of ^{131}I to newborn rats (Goldberg and Chaikoff, 1949). The last method proved to be the most satisfactory.

Rats at midterm of pregnancy were placed on an iodine-deficient diet and within 24 hr after whelping one-half of their pups were radiothyroidectomized by intraperitoneal injection with 100 μCi of ^{131}I. The remaining pups were injected intraperitoneally with normal saline.

The animals were weighed every 2 days. Two experimental animals and 2 control littermates were killed daily. The thyroid glands were removed and fixed in formalin. The whole brains were removed, weighed, and cut sagittally; one-half was fixed in formalin and the other half was weighed and frozen for chemical analysis.

After fixation, thyroid glands of rats from 6 to 31 days were embedded in paraffin, sectioned, and stained with hematoxylin-eosin.

The half-brains of animals sacrificed on days 11 through 31 were embedded in paraffin, sectioned coronally in a semiserial fashion, and stained with hematoxylin-eosin, cresyl violet, and by the Loyez method for myelin. Biochemical measurements of brain lipid hexose and proteolipid were made in experimental and control animals using standardized techniques (Folch-Pi, 1955; Radin, 1958; Lowry, Rosebrough, Farr, and Randall, 1951).

RESULTS

Total body weights of the hypothyroid rats were less than those of their control littermates (Fig. 1); this weight difference increased with age. Body growth of the hypothyroid rats ceased after 24 days (Fig. 2). The brains of these animals were smaller than those of their littermates, especially after 14 days. This difference increased with age, but at all ages the difference in brain weights was less marked than the disparity in body weights (Fig. 3).

The thyroid glands of all control animals were normal, with well-formed follicles and colloid deposition in specimens older than 6 days. Radiothyroidectomized rats from 6 days on showed total destruction of thyroid tissue with effacement of the normal follicular pattern and extensive loss of cells. At 11 days most of the thyroid gland was replaced by connective tissue, and by 21 days the gland was hyalinized (Fig. 4).

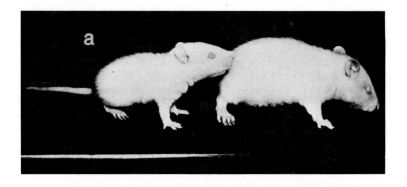

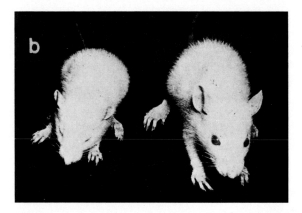

FIG. 1. (a) Six-week-old rat littermates. **Left:** hypothyroid (31 g); **right:** control (79 g).
(b) Seven-week-old rat littermates. **Left:** hypothyroid (17 g); **right:** control (40 g).

In brain sections stained for myelin, a consistent distinction could be made after 14 days between hypothyroid and control specimens. The brains of hypothyroid animals showed less myelination than those of their control littermates. Myelination of all tracts was delayed by approximately 3 to 6 days in the hypothyroid animals. Myelination in the 19-day-old hypothyroid animals resembled that in 16-day-old controls; in 28-day-old hypothyroid animals it was comparable to that in 22-day-old controls. The sequence of myelination in different tracts was identical in both groups. There was no evidence of myelin breakdown (Figs. 5 and 6).

After 12 days, total lipid hexose and proteolipid, which in the brain occur principally in myelin, differed significantly in control and hypothyroid brains. In the latter, these biochemical indices of myelination were delayed in appearance and failed to reach the levels present in mature control animals. The pattern of proteolipid increase followed a sigmoid curve of maturation between 12 and 24 days in the control animals. This critical period was delayed in the hypothyroid rats until 18 to 26 days, and total accumulation of these myelin lipids was decreased (Fig. 7). These differences were even

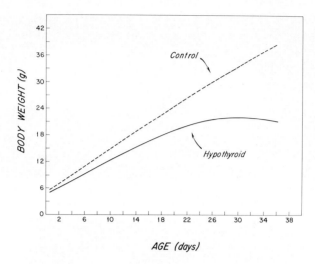

FIG. 2. Body growth in hypothyroid and control rats. (Reproduced with permission from *Neurology*.)

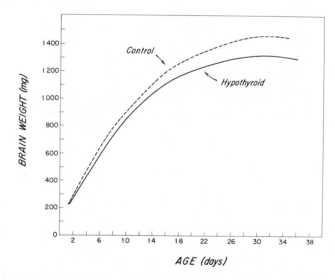

FIG. 3. Brain growth in hypothyroid and control rats. (Reproduced with permission from *Neurology*.)

more striking in the lipid hexose measurements, where the critical period in the hypothyroid rats was delayed until days 20 to 30 (Fig. 8) (Rosman, Malone, Helfenstein, and Kraft, 1972).

Experimental Malnutrition

Because it is well known that myelination is impaired in nutritionally deprived newborn rats (Benton et al., 1966; Chase, Dorsey, and McKhann, 1967; Bass, Netsky, and Young, 1970), one could question whether the

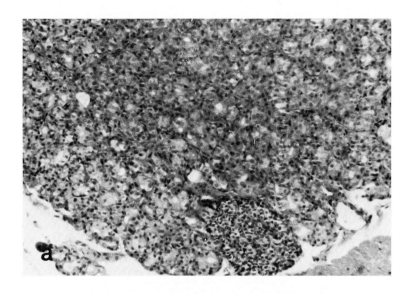

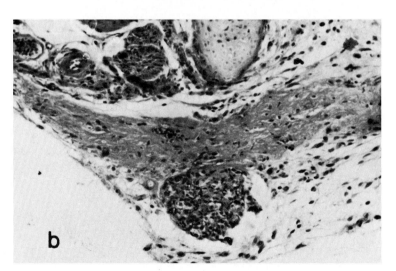

FIG. 4. Thyroid glands in 21-day-old control **(a)** and hypothyroid **(b)** rat littermates. Hematoxylin and eosin, ×35.

changes in brains of the hypothyroid animals might be caused by malnutrition rather than by a deficiency of thyroid hormone. Did the hypothyroid animals who weighed less than their control littermates compete ineffectively for food and develop nonspecific malnutritional changes in brain?

MATERIALS AND METHODS

To answer this question, malnourished rats were raised whose weights at all ages approximated those of the hypothyroid rats investigated earlier.

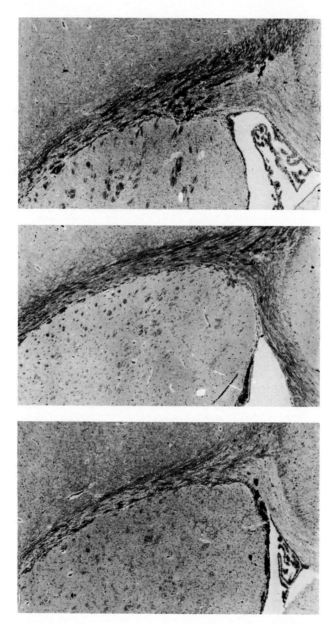

FIG. 5. Brain myelination in 22-day-old control, malnourished, and hypothyroid rats. **Top:** control rat. Normal myelination of radiation of corpus callosum. **Middle:** malnourished rat. Slightly reduced myelination of radiation of corpus callosum. **Bottom:** hypothyroid rat (littermate of 4a). Considerably reduced myelination of radiation of corpus callosum. Loyez stain, ×30. (Reproduced with permission from *Neurology*.)

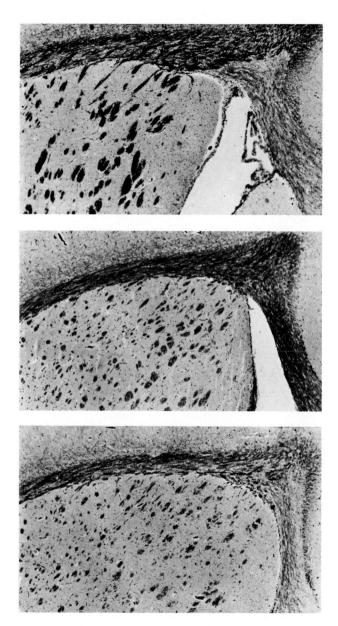

FIG. 6. Brain myelination in 31- and 32-day-old control, malnourished, and hypothyroid rats. **Top:** control rat (31 days old). Normal myelination of corpus striatum and radiation of corpus callosum. **Middle:** malnourished rat (32 days old). Slightly reduced myelination of corpus striatum and radiation of corpus callosum. **Bottom:** hypothyroid rat (31 days old; littermate of 5a). Considerably reduced myelination of corpus striatum and radiation of corpus callosum. Loyez stain, ×30. (Reproduced with permission from *Neurology*.)

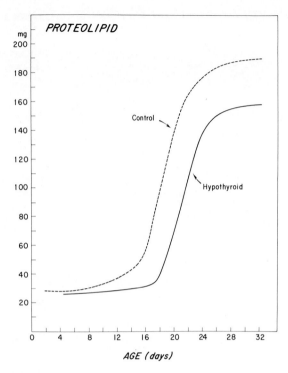

FIG. 7. Brain proteolipid in hypothyroid and control rats. (Reproduced with permission from *Neurology*.)

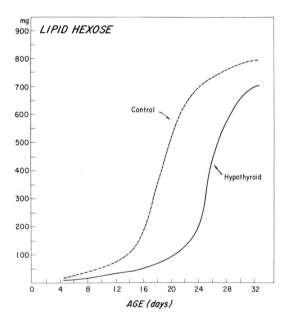

FIG. 8. Brain lipid hexose in hypothyroid and control rats. (Reproduced with permission from *Neurology*.)

Pregnant rats were fed an iodine-deficient diet beginning at midterm. On the day of whelping the offspring from 4 to 5 litters were pooled; from this pool, groups of 20 newborns were placed with foster mothers. Because each foster mother had only a limited amount of milk for her large number of pups, the newborns became nutritionally deprived. A number of newborn rats were kept in reserve and used as necessary to supplement the malnourished groups. In this way, the mean body weights of these groups could be controlled; the more numerous the suckling rats, the lower their mean body weight.

The animals were weighed several times each week. Two malnourished animals were killed every other day. Histological preparations and biochemical analyses of brains were performed as before. Data obtained from these animals were compared with those obtained previously on hypothyroid and control animals.

RESULTS

Mean total body weights of the malnourished animals were slightly lower than those of the hypothyroid rats of the same ages until the 28th day, then rose slightly. There was no cessation of total body growth as in the hypothyroid animals after 24 days, and by the end of the experiment at 34 days, the malnourished curve had not leveled off (Fig. 9). The brain weights of the malnourished rats were approximately equal to those of the hypothyroid animals, slightly less until day 16, and then slightly greater. As in the hypothyroid animals, brain growth of the malnourished animals was less severely retarded than was total body growth (Fig. 10).

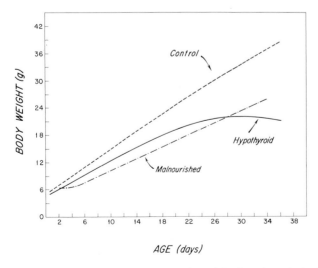

FIG. 9. Body growth in hypothyroid, malnourished, and control rats.

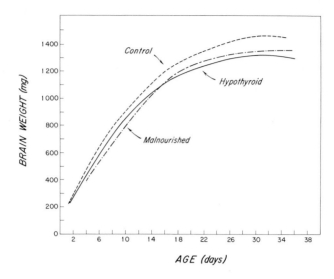

FIG. 10. Brain growth in hypothyroid, malnourished, and control rats.

Sections of malnourished rat brains stained for myelin disclosed less myelin than in the control brains. These changes were obvious by 16 days of age and were present in all white matter tracts. At all ages, however, myelination in malnourished rat brains was greater than in the hypothyroid rat brains (Figs. 5 and 6).

Proteolipid content was slightly greater in malnourished than in control brains until 15 days. From 16 to 28 days the appearance of proteolipid in malnourished brains followed a sigmoid curve, slightly below control values but well above the amounts present in hypothyroid brains. Thereafter, the proteolipid values in malnourished brains were somewhat higher than in the controls (Fig. 11). Total lipid hexose was slightly less in malnourished than in control brains until age 19 days. Lipid hexose values in malnourished brains then overlapped the control curve until 22 days, after which values from the malnourished brains were slightly elevated over control values. At all ages, lipid hexose content in the malnourished brains was considerably greater than in the hypothyroid brains (Fig. 12).

Thus myelination in malnourished animals, as determined histologically and biochemically, was intermediate between that in control animals and that in hypothyroid animals. Neonatal hypothyroidism therefore causes a delay in myelinogenesis which cannot be explained simply by malnutrition (Rosman and Malone, 1973).

The preceding investigations were carried out on whole brains, containing both myelin and nonmyelin constituents. In order to study more specifically the effects of hypothyroidism on developing myelin, we next analyzed preparations of purified myelin.

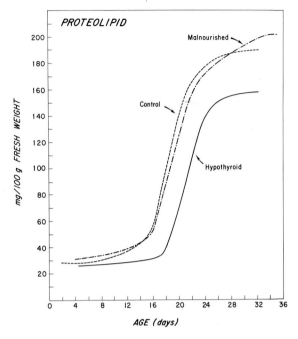

FIG. 11. Brain proteolipid in hypothyroid, malnourished, and control rats.

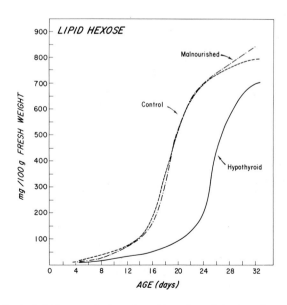

FIG. 12. Brain lipid hexose in hypothyroid, malnourished, and control rats.

MYELIN STUDIES

Study A

MATERIALS AND METHODS

Newborn rats were rendered hypothyroid with intraperitoneal ^{131}I as before. Hypothyroid animals were killed in groups of 8 on alternate days,

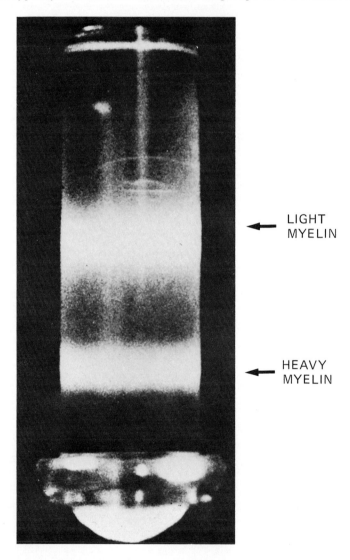

FIG. 13. Preparation of purified myelin with separation of light myelin and heavy myelin components.

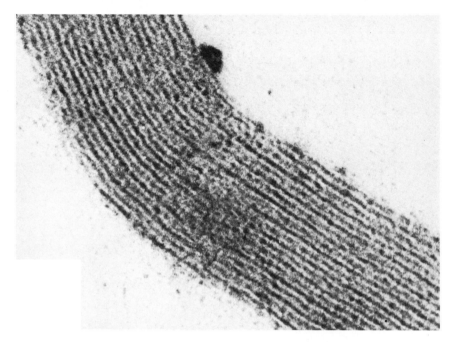

FIG. 14. Ultrastructure of pure myelin, ×108,750.

from ages 12 to 24 days. The larger control animals were killed in groups of 5 on the same days.

Pooled whole brains for each age were homogenized, and purified myelin was prepared by a slight modification of the method of Poduslo and Norton (1973), using preparative ultracentrifugation on a sucrose gradient. Two fractions were obtained, one designated light myelin and the other heavy myelin (Fig. 13). Electron microscopic examination of these fractions showed no evidence of contamination (Fig. 14). Biochemical analyses were then done on the light and heavy myelin fractions obtained from the hypothyroid and control animals.

RESULTS

Total myelin increased rapidly postnatally, particularly between ages 20 and 24 days, and especially in the heavy myelin fraction. This increase was depressed two- to fourfold in the hypothyroid animals, specifically in the heavy myelin fraction (Fig. 15). Hypothyroidism appeared to have no effect on synthesis of total protein (Fig. 16) or glycolipid (Fig. 17). Synthesis of phospholipid was reduced, but only in the light myelin fraction from the hypothyroid brains (Fig. 18). Synthesis of cholesterol (Fig. 19) and proteolipid (Fig. 20) was decreased in both the light and heavy myelin fractions

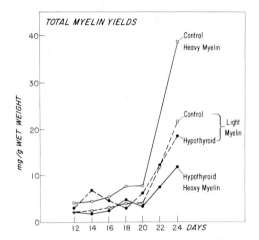

FIG. 15. Total myelin yields from brains of hypothyroid and control rats.

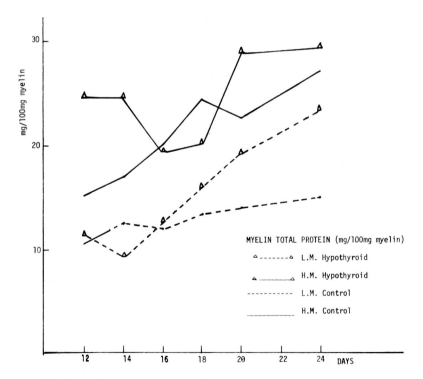

FIG. 16. Myelin total protein from brains of hypothyroid and control rats.

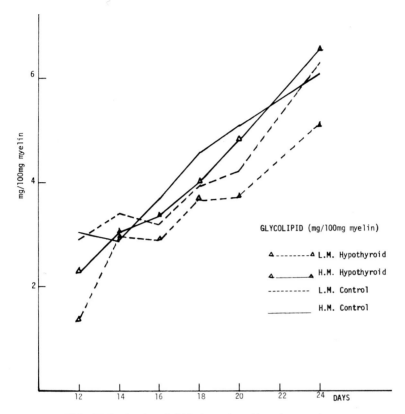

FIG. 17. Brain glycolipid in hypothyroid and control rats.

from the hypothyroid animals. The most striking biochemical alteration in the hypothyroid brains was seen in myelin basic protein. In control animals, heavy myelin basic protein appeared at 12 days; light myelin basic protein appeared at 14 days (Fig. 21). In hypothyroid animals, light myelin basic protein did not appear until 16 days, and by 24 days, there still was no basic protein in the heavy myelin fraction, as determined by precipitation and acid-gel electrophoretic techniques (Fig. 22).

It thus appeared that neonatal hypothyroidism interfered with total myelin yield, and seemed to cause impaired synthesis of cholesterol, proteolipid and basic protein (Malone and Rosman, 1973).

Study B

MATERIALS AND METHODS

We decided next to extend these studies beyond 24 days and to study individual myelin proteins using the SDS acrylamide gel system of Chan

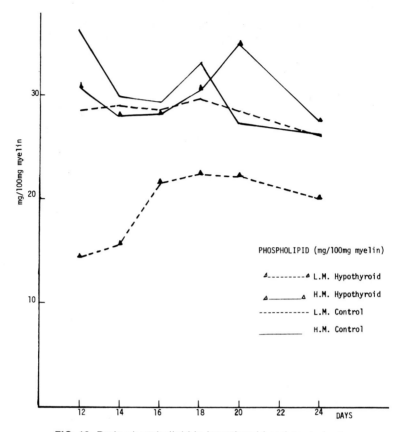

FIG. 18. Brain phospholipid in hypothyroid and control rats.

and Lees (1974). Again, newborn rats were rendered hypothyroid with [131]I. Hypothyroid animals were killed every 4 days in groups of 8, from days 16 to 40; control littermates were killed in groups of 5 on the same days. As before, preparations of light and heavy myelin were obtained from hypothyroid and control animals (Fig. 23).

RESULTS

Total myelin increased rapidly postnatally, particularly after 20 days, and total myelin synthesis was depressed in the hypothyroid animals. After 24 days, however, myelin yields from the hypothyroid specimens increased sharply, and by 40 days the myelin yields from hypothyroid and control animals were similar (Fig. 24). Hypothyroid animals showed a persistence of high molecular weight protein (A) compared with controls. Proteolipid protein (B) showed little change with development, whereas

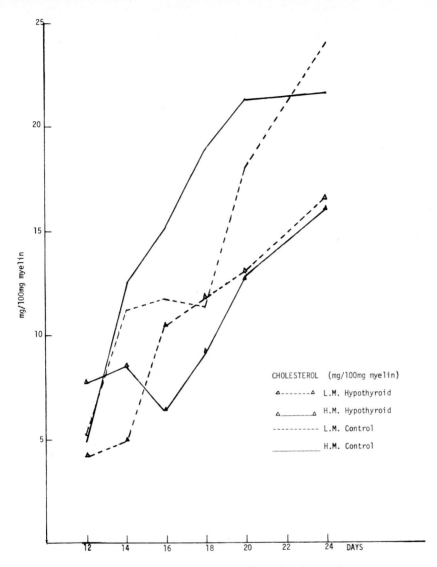

FIG. 19. Brain cholesterol in hypothyroid and control rats.

MYELIN PROTEOLIPID PROTEIN (mg/100mg myelin)

DAYS	HYPOTHYROID L.M.	HYPOTHYROID H.M.	CONTROL L.M.	CONTROL H.M.
12	.480	1.695	2.0	9.6
14	.906	2.057	6.9	9.1
16	2.028	1.940	8.3	8.0
18	2.969	2.976	9.6	12.2
20	1.563	5.415	13.1	14.3
24	3.946	2.684	8.4	10.0

FIG. 20. Brain myelin proteolipid protein in hypothyroid and control rats.

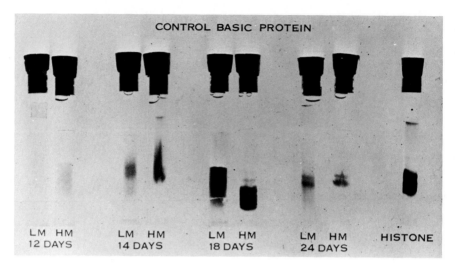

FIG. 21. Brain myelin basic protein in control rats.

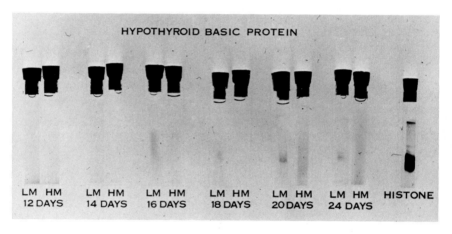

FIG. 22. Brain myelin basic protein in hypothyroid rats.

the DM-20 protein fraction increased. Two minor bands, designated X and Y, that appeared on our disk gels between the DM-20 and basic proteins were less prominent in the hypothyroid animals but showed no consistent changes with development. Basic protein appeared in two well-defined bands (D_1, D_2) which were present as major components in light and heavy myelin isolates from hypothyroid and control animals at each of the ages studied (Figs. 25 through 30).

Thus, although both of our studies of purified myelin showed that early hypothyroidism causes a reduction in total myelin yield, study B demon-

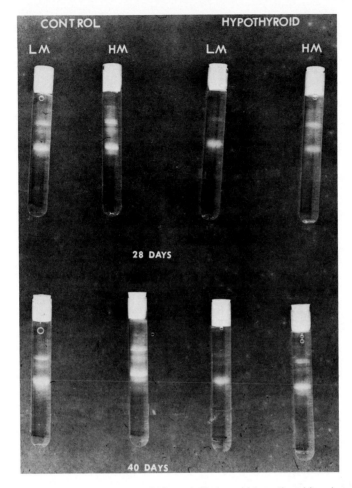

FIG. 23. Purified myelin from brains of 28- and 40-day-old hypothyroid and control rats.

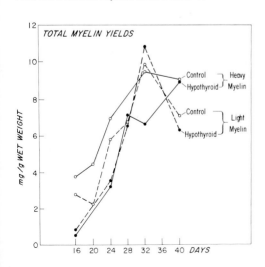

FIG. 24. Total myelin yields from brains of hypothyroid and control rats.

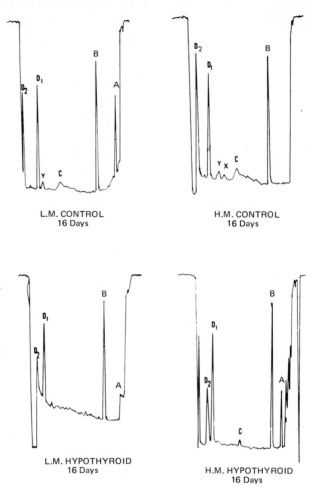

FIG. 25. Components of purified myelin from 16-day-old hypothyroid and control rats. A, high-molecular-weight protein; B, proteolipid protein; C, DM-20 protein; X, Y; D_1, D_2, basic protein.

strated that the hypothyroid animal has the capacity during later develop-ment to increase its synthesis of myelin and eventually to produce myelin at a rate comparable to that in control animals. This finding is analogous to the delayed "catch-up" growth seen in malnutrition (Rosman, 1972).

In sharp contrast to study A of purified myelin, study B demonstrated basic protein to be present as a major component in all myelin isolates from hypothyroid and control animals. In study A we utilized precipitation techniques for protein fractionation and cathodal disk gel electrophoresis

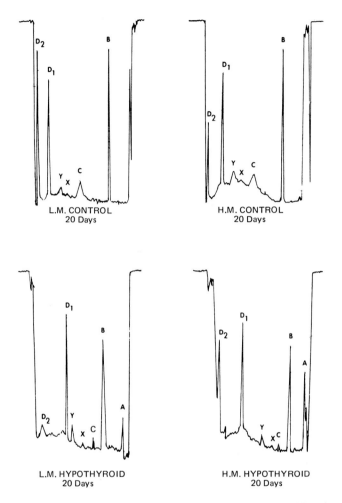

FIG. 26. Components of purified myelin from 20-day-old hypothyroid and control rats. For key, see Fig. 25.

in an acidic buffer for identification of basic protein material. Under these circumstances, basic protein may have been precipitated out with the high-molecular-weight insoluble protein material, resulting in spuriously low values for basic protein.

Myelin basic protein has been thought to play a central role in myelino-genesis (Malone and Rosman, 1973), and indeed the findings in study A of purified myelin were consistent with that view. Study B does not support that contention, however, and indicates that the effects of early hypothy-

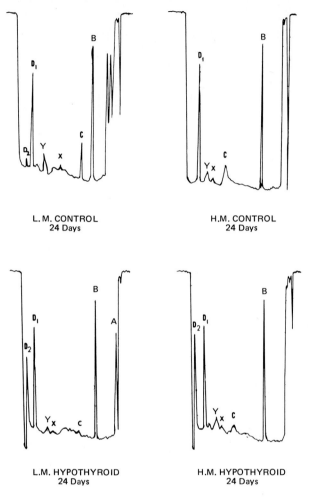

FIG. 27. Components of purified myelin from 24-day-old hypothyroid and control rats. For key, see Fig. 25.

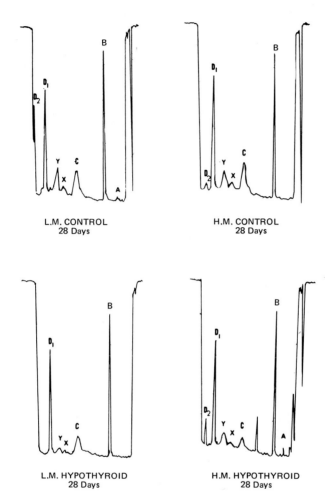

FIG. 28. Components of purified myelin from 28-day-old hypothyroid and control rats. For key, see Fig. 25.

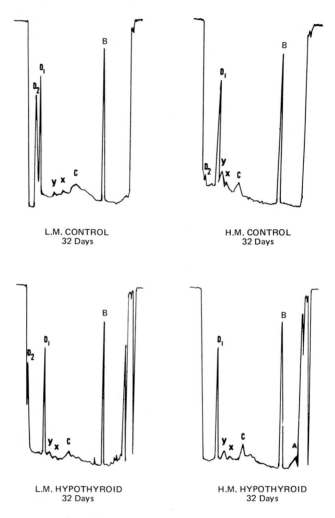

FIG. 29. Components of purified myelin from 32-day-old hypothyroid and control rats. For key, see Fig. 25.

roidism on synthesis of myelin proteins, including basic protein, are less specific than our earlier work had indicated.

In summary, neonatal hypothyroidism causes a nonselective reversible delay in myelinogenesis and provides a model that may have considerable utility for the detailed "slow-motion" study of stages in brain development.

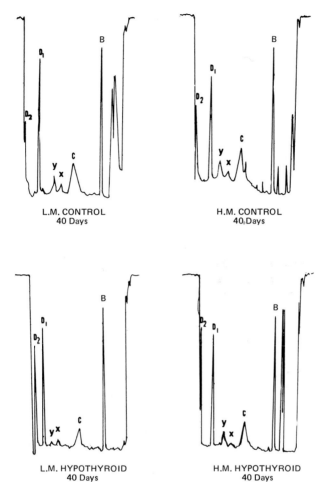

FIG. 30. Components of purified myelin from 40-day-old hypothyroid and control rats. For key, see Fig. 25.

REFERENCES

Balázs, R., Brooksbank, B. W., Davison, A. N., Eayrs, J. T., and Wilson, D. A. (1969): The effect of neonatal thyroidectomy on myelination in the rat brain. *Brain Res.*, 15:219.

Barrnett, R. J. (1948): In: *The Hormones*, edited by C. Pinkus and K. V. Thimann. Academic Press, New York.

Bass, N. H., Netsky, M. G., and Young, E. (1970): II. Microchemical and histological study of myelin formation in the rat. *Arch. Neurol.*, 23:303.

Beierwaltes, W. W., Carr, E. A., Raman, G., Spafford, N. R., Aster, R. A., and Lowrey, G. E. (1959): Institutionalized cretins in the State of Michigan, *J. Mich. State Med. Soc.*, 58:1077.

Benda, C. E. (1946): *Mongolism and Cretinism.* Grune & Stratton, New York.

Benton, J. W., Moser, H. W., Dodge, P. R., and Carr, S. (1966): Modification of the schedule of myelination in the rat by early nutritional deprivation. *Pediatrics*, 38:801.

Chan, D. S., and Lees, M. B. (1974): Gel electrophoresis studies of bovine brain white matter proteolipid and myelin proteins. *Biochemistry*, 13:2704.

Chase, H. P., Dorsey, J., and McKhann, G. M. (1967): The effect of malnutrition on the synthesis of a myelin lipid. *Pediatrics*, 40:551.

Eayrs, J. T. (1954): The vascularity of the cerebral cortex in normal and cretinous rats. *J. Anat.*, 88:164.

Eayrs, J. T. (1955): The cerebral cortex of normal and hypothyroid rats. *Acta Anat.*, 25:160.

Eayrs, J. T. (1964): Effects of thyroid hormones on brain differentiation. *Ciba Foundation Study Group #18*. Little, Brown, Boston, p. 60.

Eayrs, J. T. (1966): Thyroid and central nervous development. In: *The Scientific Basis of Medicine Annual Reviews*, p. 317.

Eayrs, J. T., and Horn, C. (1955): The development of cerebral cortex in hypothyroid and starved rats. *Anat. Rec.*, 121:53.

Eayrs, J. T., and Taylor, S. H. (1951): The effect of thyroid deficiency induced by methyl thiouracil on the maturation of the central nervous system. *J. Anat.*, 85:350.

Folch-Pi, J. (1955): Composition of the brain in relation to maturation. In: *Biochemistry of the Developing Nervous System*, edited by H. Waelsch, p. 121. Academic Press, New York.

Geel, S. E., and Timiras, P. S. (1967): The influence of neonatal hypothyroidism and of thyroxine on the ribonucleic acid and deoxyribonucleic acid concentrations of rat cerebral cortex. *Brain Res.*, 4:135.

Goldberg, R. C., and Chaikoff, I. L. (1949): A simplified procedure for thyroidectomy of the newborn rat without concomitant parathyroidectomy. *Endocrinology*, 45:64.

Hamburgh, M., Lynn, E., and Weiss, E. P. (1964): Analysis of the influence of thyroid hormone on prenatal and postnatal maturation of the rat. *Anat. Rec.*, 150:147.

Horn, G. (1955): Thyroid deficiency and inanition. *Anat. Rec.*, 121:63.

Lowry, O. H., Rosebrough, N. J., Farr, A. L., and Randall, R. J. (1951): Protein measurement with the Folin phenol reagent. *J. Biol. Chem.*, 193:265.

Malone, M. J., and Rosman, N. P. (1973): Hypothyroidism and myelinogenesis. In: *Proceedings of the 2nd National Meeting of the Child Neurology Society*, Nashville, abstract, p. 19.

Marinesco, M. G. (1924): Contribution a l'étude des lesions du myxedema congenital (iodiotic myxodemateuse du Bourneville). *Encephale*, 19:265.

Mott, F. W. (1917): The changes in the central nervous system in hypothyroidism. *Proc. Roy. Soc. Med.*, 10:51.

Poduslo, S. E., and Norton, W. T. (1973): The characterization of the plasma membrane and myelin fractions obtained from isolated oligodendroglia. In: Proceedings of the 4th Meeting, American Society for Neurochemistry, Columbus, Ohio, No. 123.

Radin, N. S. (1958): Glycolipid determination. In: *Methods of Biochemical Analysis*, Vol. 6, edited by D. Glick, p. 163. Interscience, New York.

Rosman, N. P. (1972): The neuropathology of congenital hypothyroidism. In: *Human Development and the Thyroid Gland, Relation to Endemic Cretinism: Advances in Experimental Medicine and Biology*, Vol. 30, edited by J. B. Stanbury and R. L. Kroc, p. 337. Plenum Press, New York.

Rosman, N. P., and Malone, M. J. (1973): The comparative effects of thyroid deficiency and malnutrition on myelination of brain: A morphologic and biochemical study. *Neurology*, 23:442 (abstract).

Rosman, N. P., Malone, M. J., Helfenstein, M., and Kraft, E. (1972): The effect of thyroid deficiency on myelination of brain. *Neurology*, 22:99.

Walravens, P., and Chase, H. P. (1969): Influence of thyroid on formation of myelin lipids. *J. Neurochem.*, 16:1477.

DISCUSSION

Timiras: Elizabeth Einstein (Dalal, Valcana, Timiras, Einstein, and Csejtey, 1971) published similar data several years ago while collaborating with workers in my laboratory. She will be particularly interested in your comments on the effects of hypothyroidism on the basic proteins, a subject on which we have a recent publication (Valcana, Einstein, Csejtey, Dalal, and Timiras, 1975). I think we arrived at somewhat different results: At 13 days both basic proteins are higher in the hypothyroid than in the control rat. At 22 days, however, the slow-moving basic protein is lower in hypothyroids, whereas the fast-moving protein is not significantly different from controls. By 37 days, the slow-moving protein remains lower, but the fast-moving protein is higher. This latter agrees with your findings. We differ in regard to both the slow-moving basic protein and to interpretation of events during early myelin formation (between 10 and 13 days).

Rosman: The youngest animals in which we studied purified myelin were 16 days of age.

Valcana: Do you have any idea as to why one of the proteins is more effective than the other?

Rosman: I do not know. Although two basic protein fractions (D_1, D_2) were identifiable at each of the ages studied, one fraction was not consistently more or less prominent than the other. In our second study (Rosman, Malone, and Szoke, 1975) the findings were strikingly different from those we had obtained earlier (Malone, Rosman, Szoke, and Dairs, 1975). As with basic protein, synthesis of proteolipid was found to be impaired in early hypothyrodism in our first study but not in our subsequent investigation.

Valcana: We also find depressed amounts of proteolipid by 22 days.

Rosman: It may be that methodological differences account for the differing results. The most impressive effect of hypothyroidism on the immature brain is a general retardation in brain maturation, producing a model of brain development in slow motion. It would be surprising to learn of a specific brain constituent, either lipid or protein, that was selectively and irreversibly altered by deficiency of thyroid hormone.

Sokoloff: Evidently hypothyroidism results in a change of developmental tempo and not really in qualitative differences.

Balázs: In thyroid deficiency, there is a retardation in a number of developmental processes, and myelination is not an exception. However, ultimately the composition (although not the total amount) of myelin seems to be very similar to that in controls. Since there is a shift in the developmental curve, it depends on the age of the animal whether one observes differences from the controls. Legrand's groups studied myelination with morphological techniques and found that the normal relationship between axon diameter and number of myelin lamellae remains normal in thyroid deficiency but abnormal in undernutrition (Clos and Legrand, 1969, 1970). They also reported that the ultrastructure of the Schwann cells in the peripheral nerves is severely affected in undernutrition, whereas it is apparently normal in thyroid deficiency. Thus, it seems that, in comparison with thyroid deficiency, undernutrition has a more severe effect on myelination.

Pesetsky: Dr. Rosman, when you say that hypothyroidism causes only a slowdown in rate of development, you wouldn't include morphological changes, would you? Many morphological changes have been demonstrated to be of a seemingly permanent nature.

Rosman: However, many of the morphological alterations reverse in time. An example would be the delayed disappearance of the cerebellar external granular layer.

Pesetsky: I am not aware that the Purkinje dendritic tree, for example, is ever entirely restored to normal in hypothyroid animals. And Drs. Lauder and Altman have shown that Bergman cells in hypothyroid rats increase in number. This change, too, seems to be permanent. LeGrand has demonstrated that the Bermann glial profiles around the Purkinje dendritic tree increase and that also seems to be permanent.

Altman: We must not forget that myelination is dependent on glial cells. There is evidence from other models that if you retard cell proliferation, there is a recovery in glial cells but not other components. For instance, in the hippocampus, there is no neuronal recovery after low-level X-irradiation, but there is a gradual glial recovery.

Bass: The delayed recovery is not seen when one looks at specific areas of the cerebral cortex and at subcortical white matter. We found irreversible changes such as a lack of both migration and differentiation of glial cells. The problem inherent in doing chemical analyses on subcellular fractions of pathological material must be considered in terms of disturbed myelinogenesis; the fractions may not be exactly the same in control and hypothyroid animals. We all realize, also, that different areas of brain develop asynchronously, but in analyzing a whole hemisphere, you are dealing with a critical period that is averaged for the whole organ. Thus, our work cannot be directly compared with yours because we are examining one specific area of cortex. Nevertheless, our evidence shows irreversible changes. Even thyroid replacement therapy in our experiments has failed to establish normal cortical and subcortical architecture.

Timiras: We were very fortunate to have Dr. Chaikoff in our department, so that his methods of producing hypothyroidism were ready for us to adopt. When you induce hypothyroidism by injecting a dose of radioactive iodine at birth, one of the main consequences is that by day 45 most of the hypothyroid animals show a marked hypertrophy in the area of the thyroid. They have difficulty in breathing and in eating and die around 50 days of age as a result of respiratory infection and malnutrition due to local mechanical compression of the goiter.

Rosman: Why would a goiter develop in an animal given radioiodine?

Timiras: Because the radioactive material accumulates very early and results in a very marked enlargement of the area.

Sokoloff: What kind of cells comprise the goiter?

Timiras: Connective tissue, maybe some thyroid remnants which undergo hypertrophy.

Pesetsky: Has that been the experience of other people who use radioactive iodine for thyroidectomy?

Bass: They do not develop goiters at all.

Valcana: This is not a goiter. It appears to be damage to the laryngeal nerve.

Bass: We have not seen anything like that in our animals.

Grave: How old are your animals, Dr. Bass?

Bass: Fifty days.

Lauder: I use propylthiouracil and inject it up to 90 days of age, and I have not had that problem.

Timiras: But that is quite different from a massive injection of radioiodine at birth.

Lauder: You would expect to see more of a goiter in that case.

Bass: Yes, that would cause a goiter.

Timiras: But it might not be just a goiter. I used the word "goiter" in a very unspecific way, but it remains as in Dr. Chaikoff's day, that these animals die around 50 or 60 days of age from advanced malnutrition or severe pulmonary respiratory infections.

Hamburgh: No doubt there is mortality, and it is striking around 40 days; but my empirical observation is that you can get good viability if you get litters born from young, preferably virgin mothers. But in litters from mothers that are too old the mortality is very high. This is just an empirical observation. I have no explanation for it.

Weichsel: When does the animal treated by the Chaikoff method become hypothyroid by measurements of serum T_4?

Bass: At 3 days of age there is only 13% of normal circulating T_4 in the blood, after ^{131}I is given at birth.

Rosman: Dr. Bass, how do you measure T_4 in animals 3 days of age?

Bass: It takes a lot of blood.

Rosman: More than the animal can spare.

Bass: We have to pool it, but we are interested in this particular feature as well as the histological disappearance of the thyroid gland.

Lauder: Maybe one of the mortality problems has to do with malnutrition in terms of the split litter design. If you have hypothyroid animals in the same litter as control animals, they are much more apt to be malnourished than if you have a whole litter of hypothyroid animals. I design my experiments to try to avoid the malnutrition effect.

Timiras: In terms of what they eat, the malnutrition effect does not occur after 21 days.

Lauder: No, but there may be such an effect. If you give too high a dose of propylthiouracil, the animals become dehydrated and generally die by 45 days of age.

Timiras: The only point I wanted to bring up is that, at later ages, the factor of malnutrition due to mechanical obstruction should be considered carefully.

Altman: Dr. Rosman, you tried to dissociate malnutrition and hypothyroidism by having a malnourished group. Have you tried the opposite: taking hypothyroid animals and artificially trying to make them grow? Can you at least cut down on some of the so-called hypothyroid effects?

Rosman: That is a good idea.

Pesetsky: In our histochemical studies of various kinds, we find that we can reverse the effects of hypothyroidism by giving them propylthiouracil plus thyroid hormone. These animals, presumably, would be equally malnourished, but the thyroid hormone seems to restore the histochemically demonstrable enzyme levels to normal or above normal.

Lauder: I have animals that are 90 days old, and I have noted in them an interesting phenomenon. One has said hypothyroids stop growing after 15 to 21 days. If they are healthy, this is not true. If you continue to inject propylthiouracil from 60 to 90 days, they start to grow again. It is possible that there is some kind of catch-up growth if they are healthy once they start to eat well.

Pesetsky: Hypothyroid rats that we have kept for almost a year do not catch up in weight; they are always at least 100 to 150 g lighter than normal controls.

Timiras: In your experiments that may also be due to the dose of propylthiouracil.

Lauder: I am just saying that they start to grow again.

Timiras: Yes, but the fact that you see better growth might be secondary to the animals becoming more used to the treatment, and less receptive to the effect of propylthiouracil.

Lauder: But it still produces morphological changes.

Timiras: In the experiments in which Drs. Valcana and Einstein gave replacement therapy with T_4, all of the changes described by Drs. Rosman and Balázs on total lipids, on myelin lipids, and on proteins were reversed.

Grave: What does a brain from a 90-day cretinous animal look like if it is sectioned and stained for myelin? Can you tell the difference between that and one taken from a control animal at that late stage?

Rosman: There was some demonstrable myelin at 10 or 11 days. The first time we were sure of a difference was at 14 days. We did not carry out morphological studies beyond 32 days.

Grave: Presumably you would expect to see no difference in adult rats after the myelin catch-up that you are speaking of.

Rosman: I would judge that to be correct. As indicated by the myelin yields at 40 days, the hypothyroid animals seemed to have nearly caught up with the control animals.

Sokoloff: To draw that conclusion, one needs some kind of quantification.

Timiras: The yield of myelin is a very poor index.

Lauder: We are currently studying this long-term effect on myelin in my laboratory. Dr. Victor Friedrich has done a quantitative morphological study of myelin in several different tracts.

Balázs: The techniques of biochemistry are probably better tools than those of morphology to answer the question as to whether or not there is a catch-up in myelination in thyroid deficiency. It is possible to get a reliable quantitative estimate by determining cerebrosides or other chemical constituents which seem to be localized predominantly in myelin, but it would be a very complicated task to obtain a quantitative morphological estimate concerning overall myelination in the brain.

Altman: What I had in mind was taking a cross section of a particular tract. If you take the fornix, for instance, cut it in cross section for electron microscopy, and count the number of fibers, you could get some index which might be better quantifiable.

Balázs: Dr. Bass, it is very much up to you to substantiate further your claim, which is at variance with most of the results in the literature, namely, that in thyroid deficiency oligodendroglial functions in terms of normal myelin formation are permanently impaired. The important question here is whether or not a differentiated function of a particular cell type is persistently influenced by thyroid deficiency.

DISCUSSION REFERENCES

Clos, J., and Legrand, J. (1969): Influence of thyroid deficiency and of undernutrition on growth and replication of the nervous fibres in the cervical spinal cord and the sciatic nerve of the white rat. *Arch. Anat. Microsc. Morphol. Exp.,* 58:339–354.

Clos, J., and Legrand, J. (1970): Effects of thyroid deficiency and underfeeding on growth and myelination of the sciatic nerve fibres in the young rat for electron microscopic study. *Brain Res.,* 22:285–297.

Dalal, K. B., Valcana, T., Timiras, P. S., Einstein, E. R., and Csejtey, J. (1971): Effects of thyroid hormone on myelinogenesis. In: *Third International Meeting of the International Society for Neurochemistry,* Budapest.

Malone, M. J., Rosman, N. P., Szoke, M., and Davis, D. (1975): Myelination of brain in experimental hypothyroidism: An electron-microscopic and biochemical study of purified myelin isolates. *J. Neurol. Sci.,* 26:1.

Rosman, N. P., Malone, M. J., and Szoke, M. (1975): Reversal of delayed myelinogenesis in experimental hypothyroidism. *J. Neurol. Sci.,* 26:159.

Valcana, T., Einstein, E. R., Csejtey, J., Dalal, K. B., and Timiras, P. S. (1975): Influence of thyroid hormones on myelin proteins in the developing rat brain. *J. Neurol. Sci.,* 25:19–27.

Thyroid Hormones and Brain Development,
edited by Gilman D. Grave. Raven Press,
New York, 1977.

Defective Maturation of Cerebral Cortex: An Inevitable Consequence of Dysthyroid States During Early Postnatal Life

Norman H. Bass,* E. Williams Pelton, II,*·** and Elizabeth Young*

Thyroid hormones exert regulatory control on the mitosis and differentiation of neural cells, suggesting their role as a biological timing mechanism for the complex sequence of normal brain maturation (Hamburgh, Lynn, and Weiss, 1964; Hamburgh, 1968). In the human fetus, the thyroid gland begins to function after the first trimester of gestation, and although maternal T_4 (thyroxine) crosses the placenta, its rate of passage is extremely limited (Grumbach and Werner, 1956; Osorio and Myant, 1962; New England Journal of Medicine, 1967). Thyroid hormones are therefore probably not essential for such important neuroembryologic events as neural tube formation and closure. However, during the last 6 months of human gestation, in association with the maximal increments of intrauterine brain growth, hormones are increasingly synthesized and released from the thyroid gland (Raiti and Newns, 1971; New England Journal of Medicine, 1967). This occurs in response to thyroid-stimulating hormone (TSH) produced by differentiating basophilic cells in the anterior pituitary gland. These cells, in turn, are regulated by thyrotropin-releasing hormone (TRH) secreted by differentiating hypothalamic neurons. During the first year of postnatal life, circulating T_4 is transiently elevated, reaching values that would be considered excessive for older children and adults (O'Halloran and Webster, 1972; Davies, Lawbon, and Waring, 1974; Graham, Baertl, Claeyssen, Suskind, Greenberg, Thompson, and Blizzard, 1973). During this period further increments of brain growth occur, which are not only equivalent to those found *in utero,* but which also involve regional structures, such as the cerebral cortex, the functional maturation of which is essential for normal intellectual achievement.

Although thyroid deficiency is the most common endocrine disorder of childhood (Klein, Meltzer, and Kenny, 1972), the clinical signs of hypothyroidism are not apparent in athyrotic cretins until several months after

* Department of Neurology, University of Virginia School of Medicine, Charlottesville, Virginia 22901.
** Present address: Department of Neurology, The Albany Medical College of Union University, Albany, New York 12208.

birth (Raiti and Newns, 1971). Nonspecific symptoms, such as constipation, feeding problems, and lethargy, occur in only half of such newborn infants. Although umbilical hernias are present in 68% of cases, more specific clinical signs of cretinism, such as typical facies, enlarged tongue, coarse, thickened, and cool skin, decreased muscle tone, and bradycardia are found in only one-quarter of patients (Raiti and Newns, 1971). To complicate the diagnostic problem further, body weight and neurological status of cretins at birth are usually within normal limits, and sufficient time must elapse before deviation from norms becomes obvious (Wilkins, 1957).

The fact that early diagnosis and hormonal replacement in cretins is essential for achieving therapeutic success was recognized as early as 1915 by Tredgold, and has been verified by many contemporary workers (Blaim and Ignaciuk, 1967; Smith, Blizzard, and Wilkins, 1957; Klein et al., 1972; Maenpaa, 1972). It has been found that administration of T_4 during the early newborn period significantly improves the intellectual capacity of these children (Collipp, Kaplan, Kogut, Tasem, Plachte, Schlamm, Boyle, Ling, and Koch, 1965; Blaim and Ignaciuk, 1967; Raiti and Newns, 1971; Klein et al., 1972). In fact, beginning therapy after 4 months of age is associated with a dismal mental prognosis that is nearly identical to untreated cases (Smith et al., 1957; Maenpaa, 1972) (Fig. 1).

The failure to achieve a normal range of intellectual function, despite treatment with thyroid hormone often within hours after birth, has provoked speculation that: (1) irreversible brain damage may have occurred during the late stages of intrauterine life; or (2) mental retardation and congenital hypothyroidism may be unrelated diseases that occur in the same patient (Wilkins, 1957). However, clinical methods for so-called thyroid replacement may be inadequate during the early newborn period (Collipp et al., 1965). This conclusion is based on the facts that clinical signs of thyroid deficiency or excess are difficult to assess during replacement therapy (Wilkins, 1957), and that a chemically hyperthyroid state is physiologically normal during early postnatal life (O'Halloran and Webster, 1972; Graham et al., 1973; Davies et al., 1974). Most clinicians have treated cretinism with either a fixed and inadequate dosage schedule (Collipp et al., 1965) or with rapidly increasing doses individually titrated but complicated by hyperthyroidism with loss of hair and body weight (Klein et al., 1972).

The present experimental study in rats indicates that an excess of thyroid hormone, administered chronically to either normal or hypothyroid infant animals, results in abnormal development of cerebral cortex. Hence, we suggest that only precise restoration of a chemically euthyroid state during early postnatal development will optimize the intellectual achievements of human cretins.

The developmental period of maximally increasing brain weight occurs

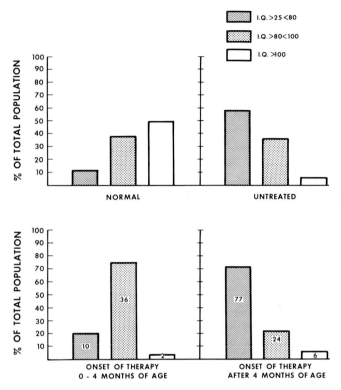

FIG. 1. Effects of early treatment of children with congenital hypothyroidism. Note improved mental prognosis when T_4 is administered before 4 months of age. (*) Data compiled from: Klein et al., *J. Pediatr.*, 81:912, 1972; Raiti and Newns, *Arch. Dis. Child.*, 46:692, 1971; Collipp et al., *Am. J. Ment. Defic.*, 70:432, 1965; Blaim and Ignaciuk, *Pol. Med. J.*, 6:1267, 1967.

entirely postnatally in the rat (Davson and Dobbing, 1968), beginning at birth in association with the onset of thyroid hormone secretion, and continuing for 24 postnatal days (Geloso, Hemon, Legrand, and Jost, 1968; Samel, 1968; Conklin, Schindler, and Hall, 1973). Similarly, maximal increments of brain in man (Davson and Dobbing, 1968) correlate with functional maturation of the thyroid gland, but begin during the last half of gestation and continue for approximately 1 year of postnatal life (Klein et al., 1972). The extreme immaturity of the rat brain at birth and its subsequent rapid rate of growth may preclude exact correlations with human brain development. Nevertheless, in both species, functional, biochemical, and structural maturation of the cerebral cortex occurs postnatally, such that the developmental stage of human cerebral cortex at birth is comparable to that found in the rat at 10 postnatal days (Bass, Netsky, and Young, 1969*a,b*). Hence, the rat is a particularly good laboratory animal for com-

parative ontogenetic studies of the effects of dysthyroid states on developing cerebral cortex.

Four major changes in the normal sequence of cortical maturation have
been previously reported from our laboratory, using quantitative histochemical techniques (Bass et al., 1969*a,b*). First, between birth and 10
postnatal days, there is an extensive proliferation of large-diameter neuronal
processes resulting in the replacement of large extracellular clefts with
neuropil and a doubling of cortical thickness to reach normal adult width.
Second, between 15 and 25 days postnatally, there is further neuronal
differentiation, characterized by the proliferation of small-diameter
axodendritic fibers and the formation of synapses. Third, between 10 and
50 days postnatally there is a continuous migration of neuroglial cells from
the subependymal zone through the white matter into the cerebral cortex.
Fourth, these glial cells continuously differentiate, some yielding mature
oligodendrocytes which form myelin at a maximal rate between 30 and 50
postnatal days. In summary, the maturation of rat cerebral cortex consists
of an orderly sequence of neuronal and glial events involving phases of
cell proliferation, migration, and differentiation. The completion of each
event sets the stage for the next in order of complexity, resulting in a series
of cellular events that are all critical and interdependent (Fig. 2).

Rats made hypothyroid at birth may somewhat resemble human patients

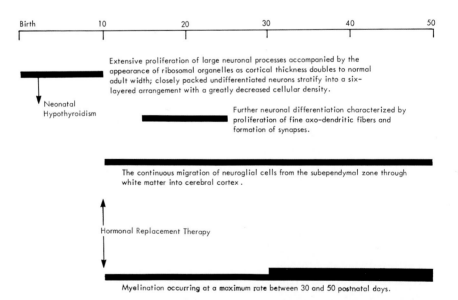

FIG. 2. Schematic representation of four processes contributing to the normal maturation
of the somatosensory area of rat cerebral cortex during 50 days of postnatal development.
The thyroid gland was completely destroyed by radioactive iodine on day 3; hormonal
replacement with T_4 was started on day 10.

who are born without a thyroid gland (athyrotic cretinism), and in whom pathological cortical development may begin during perinatal life. Although the exact mechanism by which thyroid hormone regulates normal brain maturation remains unknown, available evidence suggests that dysthyroid states may inhibit or stimulate mitotic activity in some cells, and lead still others to degenerative changes (Balázs, Kovaks, Teichgraber, Cocks, and Eayrs, 1968; Hamburgh, 1968; Maenpaa, 1972). Because the timing of cellular events is critical to normal cortical maturation, disruptions of early stages of neuronal organization may inexorably derange subsequent stages of myelinogenesis in association with faulty differentiation of glial cells. In the present series of experiments, Bass and Young (1973) and Pelton and Bass (1973) used microchemical assays of DNA (a quantitative index of postmitotic cell density) and cholesterol and cerebrosides (quantitative indices of myelin mass) to monitor the effects of dysthyroid states on maturation of the somatosensory area of rat cerebral cortex.

Experiment 1. A single injection of 150 μCi of carrier-free ^{131}I into rats at birth causes selective destruction of the thyroid gland and decreases serum levels of thyroid hormone by 87% within 3 days after intraperitoneal administration (Geloso et al., 1968; Samel, 1968). Animals become dwarfed, show infantile facial features, brachycephaly with reduced skull size, delayed development of teeth, and retention of short, soft, fine hair (Eayrs and Lishman, 1953). They achieve only 40% of the body weight of age-matched controls (Fig. 3) and show retarded behavioral development (Eayrs and Lishman, 1953), impaired learning ability (Eayrs and Levine, 1963), and electroencephalographic abnormalities (Bradley, Eayrs, and Schmalbach, 1960).

The highest cellular density in *normal* cerebral cortex is found at birth, when DNA values per unit volume are 20% greater than those of the 50-day-old adult. Between birth and 10 days, as cortical thickness doubles in response to proliferation of large axodendritic processes, DNA levels per unit volume decrease by 90%. Between 10 and 50 days, DNA progressively increases as glial cells migrate from the subependymal zone into cortex and white matter (Bass et al., 1969a). In the *hypothyroid* rats, DNA decreased at a normal rate between birth and 10 days of age. However, there was no subsequent increase to adult values normally found between 10 and 50 days. At 50 days of age, DNA was 49% lower in the cortex, and 44% lower in subcortical white matter than in age-matched controls, suggesting that the lack of thyroid hormone resulted in a metabolic derangement which interfered with the sequential migration of glial cells from the subependymal zone into cerebrum (Bass et al., 1969a; Bass and Young, 1973) (Fig. 4). Associated with the normal influx of glial cells, myelin begins to form at 10 days and accumulates most rapidly between 30 and 50 days (Bass et al., 1969b). During this time, the plasma membranes of undifferentiated oligodendrocytes proliferate rapidly and progressively

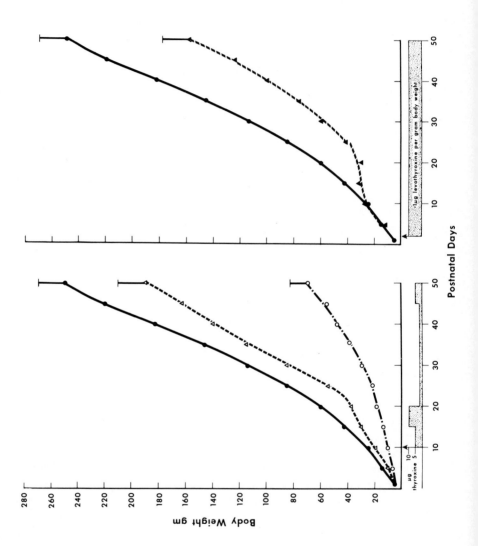

ensheath the axons to produce fibers with complex lamellation. In hypothyroid rats, the rates of accumulation of myelin lipids were markedly decreased, resulting in values that were 50 to 80% below 50-day-old control specimens (Fig. 4). These findings were correlated with decreased numbers of mature oligodendroglia and poorly stained myelin. Evidently, a deficiency of thyroid hormone during early postnatal life disturbed myelinogenesis in developing rat cerebral cortex by inhibiting the migration and differentiation of glial cells (Balázs, Brooksbank, Davison, Eayrs, and Wilson, 1969; Walravens and Chase, 1969; Bass and Young, 1973).

Experiment 2. Na^+-L-T_4 was injected daily beginning on the tenth day of postnatal life, titrated at 5-day intervals in an attempt to achieve normal body growth in rats rendered athyrotic at birth (Pelton and Bass, 1973). Morphologic features of the rat cerebral cortex at 10 postnatal days of age resemble those found in the human at birth (Bass et al., 1969a), coinciding with the earliest period in which the diagnosis and treatment of athyrotic cretinism can be instituted. This regimen proved successful in restoring the growth spurt and produced a mean body weight at 50 days of age that was 80% of age-matched controls (Fig. 3). Moreover, the characteristic cretinoid features in the young adult rat disappeared, and rehabilitated athyrotic animals could not be phenotypically distinguished from saline-injected controls (Eayrs, 1961). However, these apparently normal young adult rats disclosed chemical and histologic abnormalities of cortical maturation identical to those in the untreated hypothyroid animal (Fig. 5). We must conclude that our method of hormonal replacement was ineffective in normalizing myelinogenesis in developing cerebral cortex (Pelton and Bass, 1973).

During this therapeutic failure, it was observed that animals intermittently showed behavioral signs of hyperthyroidism, manifested by hyperactivity, tremulousness, and diarrhea. Although hormonal replacement therapy implies the accurate titration of thyroid hormone to a euthyroid state, such a condition during early postnatal development has rarely been achieved in either experimental hypothyroidism or human cretinism (Evered, Young, Orniston, Menzies, and Smith, 1973). In fact, overdosage is preferred to undertreatment with T_4 in an effort to accelerate the rate of body growth (Collipp et al., 1965). Hence, it was considered essential to assess the vulnerability of the developing cerebral cortex to excess thyroid hormone and the possibility that the administered agent may itself impede normal brain development.

FIG. 3. Body growth of normal albino rats (●——●) compared with those subjected to chronic hypothyroidism (○——○) and chronic hyperthyroidism (▲——▲) on the third day of postnatal life. Hormonal replacement therapy for hypothyroid rats (△——△) was instituted at 10 days of age: in an attempt to achieve normal body growth, daily doses of T_4 were adjusted as indicated by the bar under the abscissa. Bracketed vertical lines at 50 days represent standard errors of the means. Shaded area represents 1 μg per gram body weight.

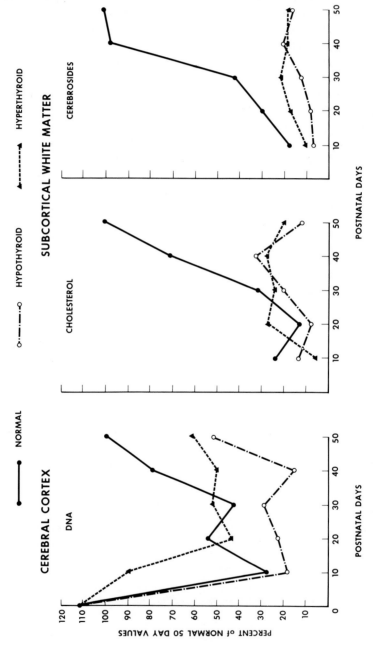

FIG. 4. Adverse effects of dysthyroid states on the biochemical maturation of rat cerebrum. The ordinate represents amounts of DNA, cholesterol, and cerebrosides expressed as percentage of the amount in normal specimens at 50 days.

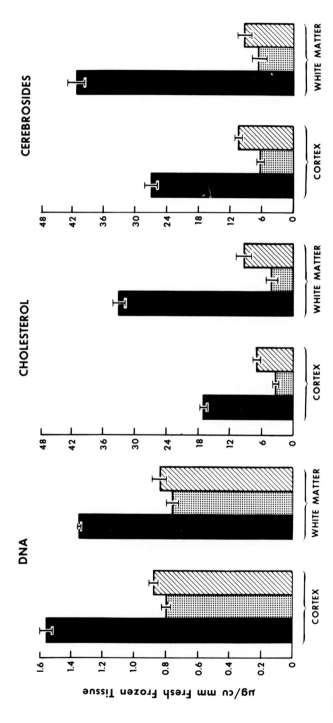

FIG. 5. Effects of hormonal replacement therapy on biochemical components in the cerebrum of 50-day-old rats subjected to neonatal hypothyroidism. The ordinate represents mean values for DNA, cholesterol, and cerebrosides expressed as micrograms per cubic millimeter of fresh frozen tissue. Bracketed vertical lines at the top of each bar represent standard errors of the means.

Experiment 3. Albino rats were made severely hyperthyroid beginning on the second day after birth, with daily subcutaneous injections of 1.0 $\mu g/g$ of body weight of Na^+-L-T_4 (Pelton and Bass, 1973). The dose and schedule of injections were empirically determined in an effort to produce observable behavioral signs of hyperthyroidism, and were sustained throughout postnatal life. Although such massive doses of T_4 resulted in a 40% mortality, our intent was to avoid reactive hypothyroidism, a criticism of previously reported studies in which lower doses and intermittent schedules of administration were used (Eayrs and Holmes, 1964; Bakke and Lawrence, 1966; Best and Duncan, 1969). Similarly triiodothyronine (T_3) could not be used, for despite its increased penetration into brain from the systemic circulation, its short half life of 9 hr could induce reactive hypothyroidism (Eayrs and Holmes, 1964).

Animals chronically treated with high doses of T_4 showed increased agility and exaggerated responses to noxious stimuli. This was thought to relate to hypermetabolic effects of excess thyroid hormone and not to reflect an accelerated rate of behavioral development (Schapiro, 1966). The rate of body growth for thyrotoxic animals paralleled that found for hypothyroid rats with hormonal replacement: body weights were significantly decreased throughout development and reached 60% of normal values by 50 days (Fig. 3). Abnormalities in the accumulation profiles for both DNA and myelin lipids in thyrotoxic animals were similar to those found in the cortex of hypothyroid rats. The failure of DNA concentrations to increase between 10 and 50 days postnatally (reaching only 60% of normal adult values), suggested that excess thyroid hormone can diminish the rate of glial cell migration into cortex in a manner similar to that found in rats subjected to a lack of the hormone (Fig. 4). Moreover, the defect of glial cell migration in thyrotoxic animals was also accompanied by a failure of oligodendroglia to form myelin. This was shown by a marked reduction of myelin lipids resulting in concentrations reaching only 10 to 30% of normal adult values (Fig. 4).

Thyroid hormone therefore exerts potent pharmacologic effects on the postnatal development of rat cerebral cortex; both deficient and excess hormone produce biochemical and morphologic abnormalities (Bass and Young, 1973; Pelton and Bass, 1973). Hence, it may be argued that any deviation from the euthyroid state can interfere with the normal sequence of maturational events, thereby deranging the complex organizational pattern necessary for optimal cortical function. The demonstrated failure of hormonal replacement therapy in the hypothyroid rat may be ascribed not only to delayed onset of treatment, but to a direct toxic effect of the hormone on developing cerebral cortex when delivered in amounts exceeding physiologic requirements.

Both early diagnosis and optimal hormonal replacement in human cretinism are essential to achieve maximal intellectual capabilities associated with functional maturation of the cerebral cortex. Based on the facts that (1) the diagnosis of congenital hypothyroidism under 4 months of age is difficult (Wilkins, 1957; Raiti and Newns, 1971), (2) early treatment can definitely improve mental prognosis (Tredgold, 1916; Collipp et al., 1965; Blaim and Ignaciuk, 1967; Raiti and Newns, 1971; Klein et al., 1972), and (3) that the disorder is not rare (an estimated incidence of 1 per 5,000 or 10,000 births) (Klein et al., 1972), a laboratory screening program for newborn infants utilizing such variables as levels of thyroxine and/or TSH in serum can be strongly recommended (Klein, Augustin, and Foley, 1974). However, even if the diagnosis is established at birth, the problem of titration to a euthyroid state and avoiding excess hormone administration becomes equally important (Collipp et al., 1965; Evered et al., 1973; Pelton and Bass, 1973). Standard laboratory tests of thyroid function in human infants have been notoriously unreliable, and normal values for thyroxine and TSH in serum only recently have been reported (O'Halloran and Webster, 1972; Graham et al., 1973; Davies et al., 1974). Until such factors are used routinely to assess the adequacy of hormonal replacement, therapy will fail to achieve the euthyroid state essential for normal brain maturation. Moreover, if response to treatment is monitored only by crude signs such as body growth and clinical appearance, defective maturation of cerebral cortex will be the inevitable consequence.

REFERENCES

Bakke, J. L., and Lawrence, N. (1966): Persistent thyrotropin insufficiency following neonatal thyroxine administration. *J. Lab. Clin. Med.*, 67:477.

Balázs, R., Brooksbank, B. W. L., Davison, A. L., Eayrs, J. T., and Wilson, D. A. (1969): The effect of neonatal thyroidectomy on myelination in the rat brain. *Brain Res.*, 15:219.

Balázs, R., Kovaks, S., Teichgraber, P., Cocks, W. A., and Eayrs, J. T. (1968): Biochemical effects of thyroid deficiency on the developing brain. *J. Neurochem.*, 15:1335.

Bass, N. H., Netsky, M. G., and Young, E. (1969a): Microchemical studies of postnatal development in rat cerebrum, 1. Migration and differentiation of cells. *Neurology (Minneap.)*, 19:258.

Bass, N. H., Netsky, M. G., and Young, E. (1969b): Microchemical studies of postnatal development in rat cerebrum, 2. Formation of myelin. *Neurology (Minneap.)*, 19:405.

Bass, N. H., and Young, E. (1973): Effects of hypothyroidism on the differentiation of neurons and glia in developing rat cerebrum. *J. Neurol. Sci.*, 18:155.

Best, M. M., and Duncan, C. H. (1969): Accelerated maturation and persistent growth impairment in the rat resulting from thyroxine administration in the neonatal period. *J. Lab. Clin. Med.*, 73:135.

Blaim, A., and Ignaciuk, A. (1967): Analysis of the development of children with congenital hypothyroidism after many years of treatment. *Polish Med. J.*, 6:1267.

Bradley, P. B., Eayrs, J. T., and Schmalbach, K. (1960): The electroencephalogram of normal and hypothyroid rats. *Electroenceph. Clin. Neurophysiol.*, 12:467.

Collipp, P. A., Kaplan, S. A., Kogut, M. D., Tasem, W., Plachte, F., Schlamm, V., Boyle, D. C., Ling, S. M., and Koch, R. (1965): Mental retardation in congenital hypothyroidism. Improvement with thyroid replacement therapy. *Am. J. Ment. Defic.*, 70:432.

Conklin, P. M., Schindler, R. J., and Hall, S. F. (1973): Hypothalamic thyrotropin releasing factor activity and pituitary responsiveness during development in the rat. *Neuroendocrinology*, 11:197–211.

Davies, R. H., Lawbon, K., and Waring, D. (1974): Thyroxine levels in normal newborn infants. *Arch. Dis. Child.,* 49:410.

Davison, A. N., and Dobbing, J. (1968): The developing brain. In: *Applied Neurochemistry,* edited by A. N. Davison and J. Dobbing, p. 253. Davis, Philadelphia.

Eayrs, J. T. (1961): Age as a factor determining the severity and reversibility of the effects of thyroid deprivation in the rat. *J. Endocrinol.,* 22:409.

Eayrs, J. T., and Holmes, R. L. (1964): Effect of neonatal hypothyroidism on pituitary structure and function in the rat. *J. Endocrinol.,* 29:71.

Eayrs, J. T., and Levine, S. (1963): Influence of thyroidectomy and subsequent replacement therapy upon conditioned-avoidance learning in the rat. *J. Endocrinol.,* 25:505.

Eayrs, J. T., and Lishman, W. A. (1953): The maturation of behavior in hypothyroidism and starvation. *Anim. Behav.,* 3:17.

Evered, D., Young, E. T., Orniston, B. J., Menzies, R., and Smith, P. A. (1973): Treatment of hypothyroidism—a reappraisal of thyroxine therapy. *Br. Med. J.,* 3:131.

Geloso, J. P., Hemon, P., Legrand, C., and Jost, J. P. (1968): Some aspects of thyroid physiology during the perinatal period. *Gen. Comp. Endocrinol.,* 10:191.

Graham, G. G., Baertl, J. M., Claeyssen, G., Suskind, R., Greenberg, A. H., Thompson, R. G., and Blizzard, R. M. (1973): Thyroid hormonal studies in normal and severely malnourished infants and small children. *J. Pediatr.,* 83:321.

Grumbach, M. M., and Werner, S. C. (1956): Transfer of thyroid hormone across the human placenta at term. *J. Clin. Endocrinol.,* 16:1392.

Hamburgh, M. (1968): An analysis of the action of thyroid hormone on development based on *in vivo* and *in vitro* studies. *Gen. Comp. Endocrinol.,* 10:198.

Hamburgh, M., Lynn E., and Weiss, E. P. (1964): Analysis of the influence of thyroid hormone on prenatal and postnatal maturation of the rat. *Anat. Rec.,* 150:147.

Klein, A. N., Agustin, A. V., and Foley, T. P. (1974): Successful laboratory screening for congenital hypothyroidism. *Lancet,* 2:77–79.

Klein, A. N., Meltzer, S., and Kenny, F. M. (1972): Improved prognosis in congenital hypothyroidism treated before age three months. *J. Pediatr.,* 81:912.

Maenpaa, J. (1972): Congenital hypothyroidism, aetiological and clinical aspects. *Arch. Dis. Child.,* 47:914.

New England Journal of Medicine (1967): Transplacental passage of thyroid hormones. 277:486.

O'Halloran, M. T., and Webster, H. L. (1972): Thyroid function assays in infants. *J. Pediatr.,* 81:916.

Osorio, C., and Myant, M. B. (1962): The binding of thyroxin by human fetal serum. *Clin. Sci.,* 23:277.

Pelton, E. W., and Bass, N. H. (1973): Adverse effects of excess thyroid hormone on the maturation of rat cerebrum. *Arch. Neurol.,* 29:145.

Raiti, S., and Newns, G. H. (1971): Cretinism: Early diagnosis and its relation to mental prognosis. *Arch. Dis. Child.,* 46:692.

Samel, M. (1968): Thyroid function during postnatal development in the rat. *Gen. Comp. Endocrinol.,* 10:229.

Schapiro, S. (1966): Metabolic and maturational effects of thyroxine on the infant rat. *Endocrinology,* 78:527.

Smith, D. W., Blizzard, R. M., and Wilkins, L. (1957): The mental prognosis in hypothyroidism in infancy and childhood, review 128 cases. *Pediatrics,* 19:1011.

Tredgold, A. F. (1916): *Mental Deficiency (Amentia),* 2nd ed., p. 285. Wood, Baltimore.

Walravens, P., and Chase, H. P. (1969): Influence of thyroid on formation of myelin lipids. *J. Neurochem.,* 16:1477.

Wilkins, L. (1957): *The Diagnosis and Treatment of Endocrine Disorders in Childhood and Adolescence.* Blackwell, Oxford.

DISCUSSION

Weischel: I agree that cretinism is difficult to diagnose during early postnatal life; however, the astute clinician is frequently alerted to this possibility by the presence of a low-pitched cry and constipation. Is it necessary to establish laboratory screening programs for neonatal hypothyroidism?

Bass: The frequency of neonatal hypothyroidism has been shown to be 1 in 7,000 births. The incidence of phenylketonuria, a metabolic disorder now subject to mass biochemical screening, is about 1 in 18,000 births. If diagnosed early and properly treated, mental retardation can be prevented in both instances. Radioimmunoassay of thyroxine can be performed on blood-soaked disks at a cost of approximately $0.50 per test. Because neonatal hypothyroidism is usually not diagnosed until a significant degree of irreversible mental retardation has occurred, it is clearly worthwhile to detect each case at birth.

Salas: Although your data are in general agreement with ours, can you comment on malnutrition as an additional variable affecting brain development in hypo- and hyperthyroid rats?

Bass: The variable of malnutrition is difficult if not impossible to dissect from our experimental design. Hypothyroidism is characterized by a lowered metabolic rate, and decreased food intake may result in relative malnutrition. Hyperthyroidism is characterized by an accelerated metabolic rate, and increased food intake may not keep pace with increased metabolic requirements. Hence, both animal models may be associated with a relative degree of malnutrition. However, data presented by Rosman in this symposium indicate that the brain of hypothyroid rats is more severely affected than weight-matched, underfed controls, indicating that total caloric undernutrition cannot account for the impairment of brain maturation in experimental cretinism.

Valcana: What is the incidence of hyperthyroidism in human newborns? Are such children mentally retarded?

Bass: Neonatal hyperthyroidism is rare and occurs only in infants of thyrotoxic mothers. The mother secretes long-acting thyroid stimulator (LATS) from the hypothalamus. LATS crosses the placenta, produces intrauterine hyperthyroidism, and the infant is born in a clinically hyperthyroid state. Since it is a rare condition, I have been unable to find any follow-up studies which describe the intellectual achievement of such patients. Probably, it is more common to find cases of cretinism among patients who become hyperthyroid during postnatal life as a result of overtreatment with thyroxine and subsequently fail to achieve normal intellectual function.

Sokoloff: I certainly agree that it may be unrealistic to expect clinicians to titrate the dose of thyroid hormone carefully enough to bring patients with no functioning thyroid gland to the normal euthyroid state. The thyroid is not a static gland that lies in the neck and dispenses a daily dose of hormone. It is a dynamic organ, and its output of thyroid hormone varies in response to physiologic demands. Many years ago Baumann found that after he fed a protein meal, there was a loss of iodine content of the thyroid gland. This resulted from secretion of the hormone in response to apparent needs that were established by a protein meal. So a theoretically optimal titration of thyroid hormone may have to be based on *hourly* requirements rather than *daily* dosage.

Bass: Although I concur with Dr. Sokoloff's statement, I believe that more optimum daily hormonal replacement for hypothyroid neonates can be achieved. There are two presently accepted clinical methods to replace thyroid hormone in newborn cretins. One is simply to monitor body weight and height and administer enough hormone to achieve a relatively normal growth profile. Of course, we know that the major period of brain maturation antedates the body growth spurt, thereby rendering it possible to achieve a normal body configuration in association with mental retardation. Another method of thyroid hormone replacement is to rapidly increase hormone dosage to the toxic range during early postnatal life. However, this technique may also have adverse consequences for brain maturation as suggested by our experimental studies. I propose that more optimal therapy for neonatal hypothyroidism can be achieved by daily monitoring of hormonal replacement with assays of TSH in blood. This method would be particularly important during the first few weeks after birth when normal values for thyroxine are in a range that would be considered thyrotoxic for the adult.

Balázs: Your studies are most welcome. Instead of the whole brain or a greater part of the brain such as the entire forebrain, where the complexities are enormous, you have concentrated on a well-defined area of the cerebral cortex. However, your results differ sufficiently from previous observations, making it compulsory to discover the reasons for the discrepancies. One of the differences relates to the acquisition of new cells in terms of DNA estimates in untreated animals. The DNA content of the rat forebrain reaches a constant level, characteristic of the adult, by about day 21. On the other hand, your results show that cell migration into the cerebral cortex continues well beyond that time. This suggests a persistent and significant acquisition of new cells destined for the adult cortex, which must be balanced by a corresponding loss of cells from some other part of the forebrain, since the overall cell number does not change. These results are unexpected and require an explanation.

The other important difference relates to the effect of thyroid hormone deficiency on myelination. Most previous results on the whole forebrain are consistent with the view that, in comparison with controls, the main effect is a retardation of myelinogenesis (Balázs, Lewis, and Patel, 1975). However, your observations on the cerebral cortex seem to show an irreversible impairment. Therefore, you should study these effects with conventional "macrotechniques" in the whole forebrain of one group of animals and with your sophisticated "microtechniques" in the cerebral cortex of another group under identical conditions.

Bass: Neurochemists have assembled a large body of data on developing whole brain or gross parts such as the entire cerebral hemisphere ("forebrain") in many animal species including man. Although of great value, these observations do not permit detailed morphological or physiological correlations because different regions of developing brain mature, and even different areas of cerebral cortex mature and involute asynchronously. Based on this fact, it is not possible to speak of a single maturational profile or critical period for developing brain or cerebral hemisphere, unless we completely neglect the fact that the brain is exquisitely partitioned into a variety of systems whose rates of morphological and functional maturation are entirely different.

During the past 20 years, many laboratories have performed detailed neurochemical studies on relatively minute parts of brain. In my laboratory we have concentrated our efforts on one cubic millimeter of rat somatosensory cortex or area 9 of human frontal isocortex in an attempt to directly relate a given chemical determination to the morphological and physiological integrity of the tissue in health and disease. The "microtechniques," classically referred to as quantitative histochemistry, utilize conventional neurochemical methods of analysis which are simply adapted to the small dimensions of tissue involved, usually micrograms or less, and their accuracy and reproducibility are equivalent to macroscale neurochemical studies as performed by Dr. Balázs and others. The advantage of our technique, as compared with conventional methods, is that our ability to interpret biochemical data on cerebrosides (components of myelin membranes) and DNA (components of cell nuclei) is strengthened by our own parallel morphological observations (light and electron microscopy, as well as autoradiographic studies) and physiological observations (EEG or more detailed neurophysiological studies). Due to the formidable heterogeneity of the tissue analyzed by Dr. Balázs and others, their chemical determinations merely denote an average effect that cannot be subject to interdisciplinary verification either by themselves or others.

Although certain quantitative histochemical indices of brain ultrastructure are better than others, I am delighted that Dr. Balázs chose to focus his attention on the interpretation of chemical changes in DNA. We have shown that by combining differential cell counts in fixed stained tissue with DNA assay of fresh tissue, an accurate quantitative profile of the neuron and glial cell population of cerebral cortex expressed as a function of tissue volume or dry weight can be obtained. DNA is assayed in microtome-prepared frozen sections (15 to 30 μg dry weight) by the microfluorometric method of Kissane and Robins, yielding a precision of $\pm$ 3% standard deviation. Our data are in close agreement with more tedious but classical anatomic methods of cell counting (Chalkey method), and our values in rat somatosensory isocortex have been confirmed by independent neuroanatomic investigations. Similar neuroanatomic correlations cannot, of course, be made on the entire cerebral hemisphere or whole brain.

Dr. Balázs and others have shown that the number of postmitotic brain cell nuclei, as assessed by the DNA content of normal rat forebrain, reaches adult values by approximately 21 postnatal days. Although this observation cannot be disputed, its interpretation in terms of the dynamics of cell acquisition is subject to large problems. Firstly, average values for DNA in rat forebrain not only represent numerous areas of asynchronously developing isocortex, but include functionally diverse regions such as hippocampus, thalamus, basal ganglia, etc. All of these brain regions have sequences of cell acquisition that have not been individually assessed and may in fact encompass time intervals ranging from days to months of postnatal development. Our detailed studies on a well-defined but minute area of isocortex (6 mm^2 of surface area) not only provide a description of the chemical maturational sequence, but include parallel morphological observations that lend credence to our interpretation. Secondly, the plateau in DNA content of whole forebrain at 21 days or similar data in whole cerebellum should not be subject to overinterpretation based on cytological data such as that derived by Dr. Altman on a single lobule of cerebellar vermis. Neural maturation is a complex process that involves not only continuous acquisition and death of cells (turnover of glia probably greater than neurons) but the continuous dispersion of cells by the proliferation of axodendritic and glial processes which include myelin. To cytologically interpret chemical data on DNA content during forebrain maturation without histological control is hazardous and becomes even more speculative under conditions where maturation has been deranged. Hence, it is Dr. Balázs's overinterpretation of his data that leads to his so-called unexpected conclusions.

The somatosensory area of rat cerebral cortex is one of the last structures of all those included in the forebrain to complete myelinogenesis. The 50-day-old Sprague-Dawley rat (body weight of 250 g) is a very young adult animal. We now know that myelinogenesis is a process that does not cease, but continues at small but significant increments throughout adult life. Hence, the arbitrary termination of our experiment at 50 days may be misleading in that we may have shown the period of maximal insult and failed to examine possible later stages of recovery between 50 and 300 days of postnatal life.

Balázs: I am glad that you have used the word "man," since hitherto we have been considering animal models, especially the hypothyroid rat. I do not think that the hypothyroid rat is a good model of the human disorder. The relationship between the timing of the development of the neuroendocrine system, including the thyroid gland, and that of the CNS are greatly different in man and the rat. It would be worthwhile to consider more appropriate animal models of human cretinism.

Bass: Although interspecies comparisons are always hazardous, biochemical, morphological, and physiological data exist on the distribution of neurons and their complex interarticulation of processes in rat and human isocortex. From these observations, it has been concluded that despite the more complex elaboration of neuronal processes seen in human isocortex, the relatively simple rat cortex may have general significance for a clearer understanding of human cortical function. From the point of view of developmental neurobiology, the rat provides an excellent experimental model for the following reasons: (1) It is more accessible to experimental assessment of early maturation since it is born with a histologically immature brain comparable to a stage of development during the last trimester of human gestation; (2) months to years of human brain development are compressed into 50 days of postnatal growth in the rat; (3) the metabolic rate of rat brain is higher than that of man so that induced biochemical errors will manifest themselves in tissue pathology in days and weeks as compared to months and years in the human; (4) the brain of the rat can be removed from the skull with great speed and quickly frozen insuring the preservation of biochemical constituents; and (5) the nonconvoluted cerebral cortex of the rat allows accurate reproducible microsampling.

From the point of view of developmental neuroendocrinology, the rat thyroid gland begins to function at about the 18th day of gestation (last trimester). This can be compared with human thyroid function which begins at the beginning of the second trimester of gestation. Since the newborn rat is equivalent to a premature human infant, this difference may indeed be more apparent than real. Nevertheless, it may be suggested that the newborn human cretin may have been subject to abnormalities of neurogenesis *in utero* and that ideal replacement therapy in man may require its initiation prior to birth. However, in our studies of thyroid hormone replacement, we have attempted to produce the insult at birth (a stage analogous to the third trimester of human cortical development) and have begun treatment at 10 days (a stage analogous to human cortical development at birth). Nevertheless, I agree that if cost were no factor, the rhesus monkey might provide a more ideal experimental model for human cretinism.

DISCUSSION REFERENCE

Balázs, R., Lewis, P. D., and Patel, A. J. (1975): Effects of metabolic factors on brain development. In: *Growth and Development of the Brain,* edited by M. A. B. Brazier. Raven Press, New York.

Thyroid Hormones and Brain Development,
edited by Gilman D. Grave. Raven Press,
New York, 1977.

Effect of Thyroxine on Neurotransmitter Uptake into Rat Cerebral Synaptosomes During Development

Edward Geller*

We have been continuing the observations made by Schapiro and his colleagues (1971*a,b*) on the effects of neonatal hormone injection on brain development of the infant rat.

The first set of experiments (Schapiro, Vukovich, and Globus, 1973) were performed on 76 Sprague-Dawley rats of both sexes bred in the laboratory: 41 served as controls; 17 were given thyroxine (T_4, 1 μg/g) intraperitoneally on postnatal days 2, 3, and 4; and 18 received a subcutaneous injection of hydrocortisone acetate (1.0 mg) on the first postnatal day. They were maintained under the usual laboratory conditions within their own litters and were killed at various times within 1 month. The brains were stained using the rapid Golgi method working with a block of tissue (3 mm wide) cut through the visual-auditory cortex. This method stains the entire soma-dendritic complex, including the dendritic spine. The number of spines per linear micrometer was determined with the aid of a reticle. Only pyramidal cells were counted, the cell bodies of which lay in layer IV of the visual cortex and the dendritic processes of which were completely visible. Four dendritic areas were counted. The pyramidal cell soma gives rise to lateral basilar dendrites and, at the vertex, an apical dendrite which rises toward the pia, divides, and spreads into the subpial arches, called terminal dendrites. Oblique dendrites arise from the apical dendrite along its course and near layer I (Figs. 1, 2, and 3). The differences in spine density are obvious to the eye, and are confirmed by the spine counts shown in Figs. 4 through 7 for apical dendrites, oblique dendrites, basilar dendrites, and for composite densities. Thus, anatomical evidence indicates that T_4 accelerates and hydrocortisone retards the development of important synaptic structures.

A further set of experiments suggests that the anatomical changes seen can be functional (Salas and Shapiro, 1970). These experiments (see also Chapter 15) involve the recording of evoked potentials to sensory stimulation in areas of the cortex in hormone-treated animals and demonstrate that cortical responsivity is accelerated in T_4-treated animals and retarded in

---

* Neurobiochemistry Laboratory, Brentwood Veterans Administration Hospital and the Department of Psychiatry and Brain Research Institute, UCLA School of Medicine, Los Angeles, California 90073.

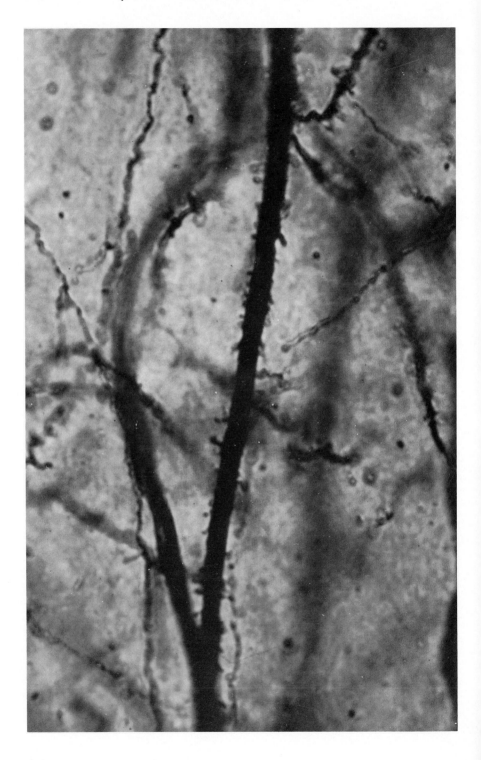

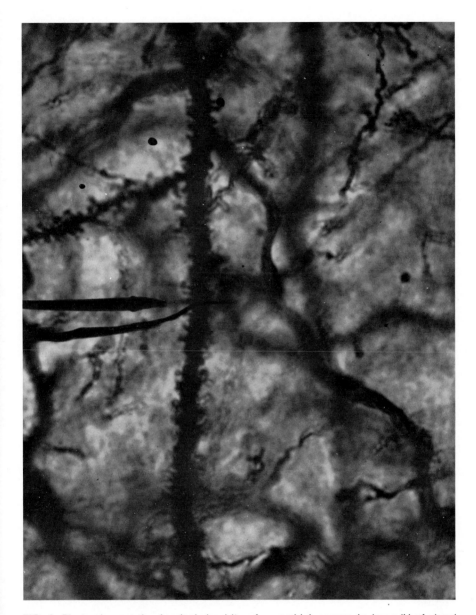

FIG. 2. Photomicrograph of apical dendrite of pyramidal neuron in layer IV of visual cortex (×250) from 15-day-old T₄-treated rat.

FIG. 1. Photomicrograph of apical dendrite of pyramidal neuron in layer IV of visual cortex (×250) from 15-day-old control rat.

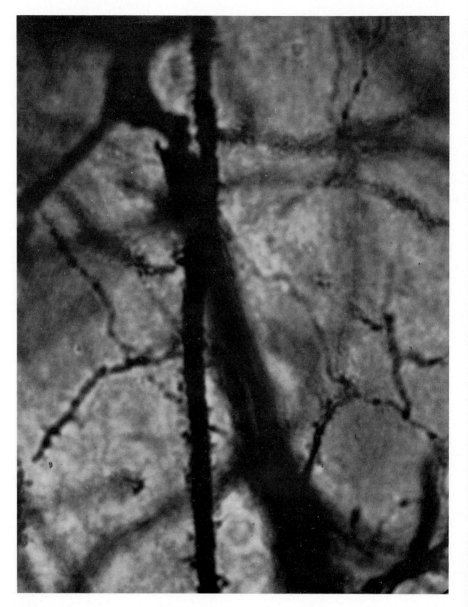

FIG. 3. Photomicrograph of apical dendrite of pyramidal neuron in layer IV of visual cortex (×250) from 15-day-old HCA-treated rat.

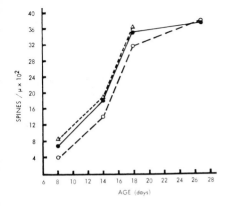

FIG. 4. Developmental changes in the number of spines on the apical dendrite. Spines were counted at 450× at various ages. ● = controls; ○ = HCA-treated; △ = T₄-treated. (From Schapiro et al., 1973, with permission of the authors.)

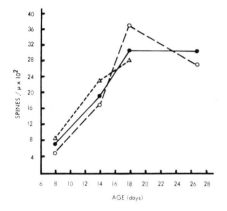

FIG. 5. Maturational changes in spine density along oblique dendrites. The number of spines on the oblique dendrite per linear micrometer were counted at 450× at various ages. ● = controls; ○ = HCA-treated; △ = T₄-treated. (From Schapiro et al., 1973, with permission of the authors.)

cortisol-treated animals. Other studies not shown here indicate similar patterns of altered development following hormonal treatment in other organized behaviors, including startle response, eye opening, swimming behavior, total body activity, and a few simple learning tasks (Schapiro, 1971*a,b*).

The thrust of these studies has been to demonstrate that early hormone administration leads to changes in postsynaptic structures and that these changes are mirrored by demonstrable functional changes. We expect similar alterations in presynaptic structures and perhaps in the involved neurotransmitter systems.

The actions of a number of neurotransmitters are partly terminated by a reuptake of the transmitter across the presynaptic membrane and reincorporation of the transmitter into synaptic vesicles. Many previous studies of reuptake have utilized the synaptosome, an artificial organelle created by gentle fracture of the nerve ending (Gray and Whittaker, 1962). We found, however, that it is difficult to prepare synaptosomes in good yield from brains of neonatal rats (particularly after hormone treatment), presumably

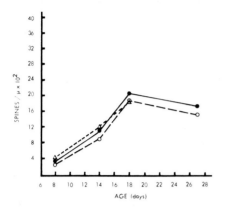

FIG. 6. Maturational changes in spine density along basilar dendrites. The number of spines on the basilar dendrite per linear micrometer counted at 450× at various ages. ● = controls; ○ = HCA-treated; △ = T_4-treated. (From Schapiro et al., 1973, with permission of the authors.)

because the lipids needed to reseal the pinched-off nerve ending are not present in sufficient quantity. As a consequence, during the discontinuous sucrose-gradient centrifugations used in the isolation of the synaptosomes, many are lost, and those that survive do not appear, morphologically, to have the same membrane integrity as synaptosomes isolated from a more mature animal.

This problem may be circumvented by measuring uptake of L-norepinephrine (L-NE) by particulate fractions of crude homogenates or by slightly

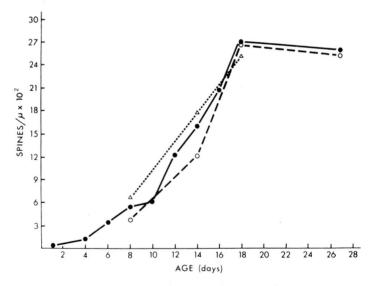

FIG. 7. Maturational changes in composite spine density. The composite is the sum of the average of the apical, terminal, oblique, and basilar dendrites divided by 4. ● = controls; ○ = HCA-treated; △ = T_4-treated. (From Schapiro et al., 1973, with permission of the authors.)

purified homogenates. We have confirmed the work of Kuhar (1973), using sucrose-density gradient centrifugation that, following incubation of homogenates with L-NE, almost all of the bound transmitter is in the synaptosomal fraction. Accordingly, we examined the uptake of L-NE by homogenates of rat cortex at different ages following treatment at birth with either L-T_4 or hydrocortisone acetate, as a means of relating the physiological effects of such treatment to the development of the presynaptic transmitter storage system.

Coyle and Axelrod (1971) have studied some developmental aspects of NE uptake into particulate fractions of homogenates of whole rat brain. However, their study was directed toward kinetic analysis of the process and utilized initial rates of uptake, measured over short periods of time. We now have examined the total storage capacity of the homogenate, calculated by Scatchard analysis, following attainment of equilibrium after longer periods of incubation.

Sprague-Dawley rats originally obtained from Charles River Laboratory were bred in the laboratory. Two days before anticipated date of delivery, gravid females were placed in separate metal cages containing pine shavings as nest material. Animals were checked daily at 0800 and 1700 hours for delivery, and newborns were designated as being zero days old. Hormone-treated neonates were injected at 0800 hours if they were born between 1700 and 0800, and at 1700 if they were born between 0800 and 1700. Hydrocortisone acetate (HCA) treated animals were removed from their mothers at day 0 and injected subcutaneously with 20 μl of a solution containing 1 mg of HCA in a carboxymethylcellulose vehicle (Cortef acetate). Injections were made by inserting a 31-gauge needle under the loose skin at the base of the skull and depositing 20 μl of suspension with a Hamilton syringe under the skin beneath the shoulder blade. T_4-treated animals were injected intraperitoneally with 1 μg/g of L-T_4 (1 μg/μl) dissolved in water with 1 N NaOH. Injections were on days 0, 1, and 2. Animals were kept warm under an incandescent lamp during the less than 5 min required for the injection procedure per litter, then returned to their mothers. Mothers were maintained on a diet of Purina Chow and water. The animal room was maintained on a 0500-to-1700 light cycle and was temperature-controlled.

At the appropriate age sufficient animals from one litter were decapitated to yield about 1 g of cortex. The brains were removed quickly and the cortices carefully peeled off the subcortical structures. The tissue was kept on ice until about 1 g was accumulated, then homogenized in 9 volumes 0.32 M sucrose at 0°C using a homogenizer with a 0.025-mm pestle clearance. The homogenate was centrifuged for 10 min at 800 × g at 0 to 2°C to remove large particles that tend to clog the filters.

Uptake of NE was measured by adding 0.1 ml of homogenate to a tube containing 0.9 ml of buffer (final concentration after additions: sodium, 125 mM; potassium, 2.4 mM; magnesium, 1.1 mM; phosphate, 10 mM; sulfate,

1.1 mM; chloride, 118 mM; glucose, 1.0 mM; pargyline, 0.05 mM; pH 7.0), 5 μl of L-[7-³H]NE and 100 μl of unlabeled L-NE, both appropriately diluted to give a final concentration between 4×10^{-9} M and 6×10^{-7} M. All tubes were prepared in duplicate and incubated at 37°C for the desired times: for measurement of uptake kinetics (not reported) 5 min; for equilibrium to be established, 2.5 hr. To correct for binding of L-NE to the filters, two tubes were prepared at an intermediate NE concentration and filtered immediately after addition of homogenate. A second set of tubes was always prepared and treated identically to the first set except that they were kept at 0°C for the incubation time.

To be more certain that NE uptake and not membrane binding was being measured, identical sets were occasionally prepared and lysed by the addition of 9 ml of H_2O before filtration. Very low counts were found in these, indicating that the bulk of the NE was not membrane-bound but was incorporated in a form that was filterable after lysis.

Millipore filters (HAWP02500) with a pore diameter of 0.45 μm were soaked in 0.32 M sucrose containing 1 mM L-NE for at least 5 min before use and placed in a Millipore 3025 sampling manifold. At the appropriate time, the contents of each tube were poured onto a filter, the tube rinsed with 0.9 ml of 0.32 M sucrose, and the wash poured on the filter. The filters were then washed again twice with 0.9 ml of 0.32 M sucrose, dried under infrared lamps, and placed in a scintillation vial to which was added 10 ml of scintillation cocktail made up of 5 g of 2,5-diphenyloxazole (PPO) in 300 ml of Triton-X100 and 500 ml of toluene. To measure efficiency of counting under these conditions, 5 μl of each NE dilution were directly added to counting vials, and dpm determined by automatic external standard calibration curves prepared for the Packard 3375 Scintillation Spectrometer. Duplicate 5-μl aliquots were dried on Millipore filters and counted. A simple calculation yields the efficiency of counting on the filters; this differed little for the different NE concentration. Proteins in each homogenate were measured by the method of Lowry as described by Layne (1957).

Figure 8 shows the uptake of norepinephrine as a function of time in the control cortex. Following a very rapid initial uptake, equilibrium is reached after about 2 hr; therefore, the following experiments were done using a 2.5 hr incubation. By knowing the counts on the filter, the predetermined efficiency of counting on the filters, and the known specific activity in the incubation mixture, it was possible to calculate the concentration of L-NE in the synaptosomes after the incubation. Then a Scatchard plot (1949) of NE-bound/NE-free versus NE-bound was made for animals at different ages. Figure 9 shows the appearance of a Scatchard plot of values obtained from cortex of an adult rat treated with T_4 at birth. The intercept on the x-axis was used as a measure of the number of binding sites per unit of protein, and the slope of the line as an indication of the association constant. Figure 10 is a similar plot from cortex of a 2- to 3-day-old rat treated with T_4 to show

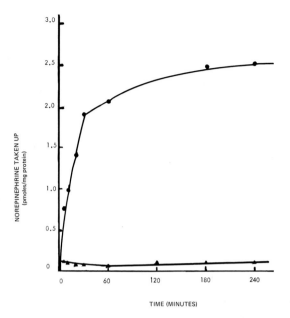

FIG. 8. Uptake of [³H]NE by homogenates of cortex from adult control rat. ●———●, 37°C; ▲———▲, 0°C.

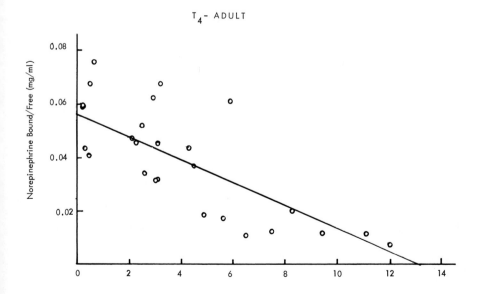

FIG. 9. Scatchard plot of uptake of [³H]NE after 2.5 hr incubation by homogenates of cortex from adult T₄-treated rat. Each point represents an individual determination and the line is calculated by a least-squares procedure.

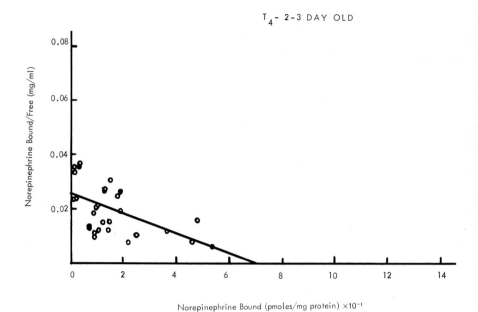

FIG. 10. Scatchard plot of uptake of [³H]NE after 2.5 hr incubation by homogenates of cortex from 2- to 3-day-old T₄-treated rat. Each point represents an individual determination and the line is calculated by a least-squares procedure.

the type of data on which measurements of binding sites were based. The slope is not greatly different, indicating similar binding constants at different ages, but the intercepts are different, showing an altered number of binding sites.

Figure 11 summarizes the data from control animals. The slopes show a trend toward tighter binding with increasing age, and the intercepts suggest a somewhat greater number of binding sites per milligram of protein in the older animals. From the data on T₄ (Fig. 12), the number of binding sites is seen to increase with increasing age. The slopes are more uniform, but there is still a trend toward tighter binding in the older animals. Figure 13 shows similar results from HCA-treated animals.

Table 1 summarizes the three previous figures. All three groups exhibit the same type of development, but both the T₄- and HCA-treated animals are delayed in the achievement of control levels of binding sites and may not reach control levels even as adults.

This result is surprising in view of the advanced appearance of the anatomical and physiological measure for T₄-treated animals. We cannot explain this discrepancy except to speculate that the number of binding sites in the isolated synaptosomes may represent more than is needed for good function and so may not be a good measure of presynaptic development. The decrease in number of sites in the treated animals may be the result of

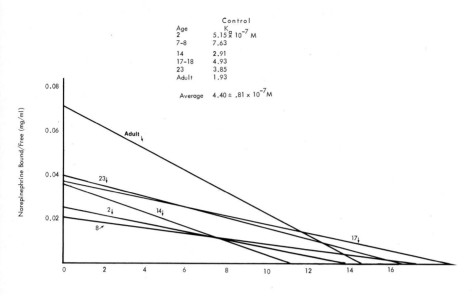

FIG. 11. Least-square lines from Scatchard plots of uptake of [³H]NE by cortex homogenates from control rats of different ages (indicated in days at each line). K_a's calculated from the slopes of the lines are also given.

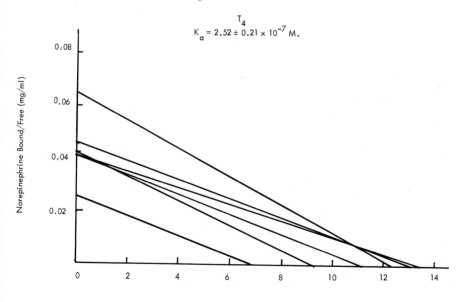

FIG. 12. Least-square lines from Scatchard plots of uptake of [³H]NE by cortex homogenates from T_4-treated rats of different ages. Ages are as in Fig. 11. A K_a calculated from the mean of the slopes is also given.

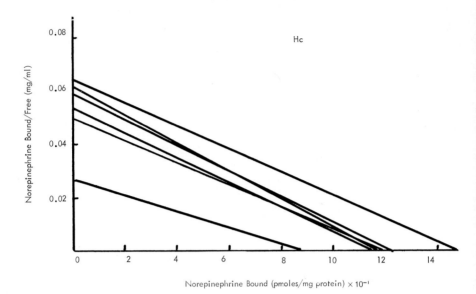

FIG. 13. Least-square lines from Scatchard plots of uptake [³H]NE by cortex homogenates from HCA-treated rats of different ages. Ages are as in Fig. 11.

TABLE 1. *Concentration of binding sites calculated from intercepts of lines on Figs. 11, 12, and 13 (uptake column) and K_a calculated from slopes of the same lines on those figures*

Age (days)	Control Uptake (pmoles/mg protein)	K_a × 10⁻⁷ M	T₄ Uptake (pmoles/mg protein)	K_a × 10⁻⁷ M	HCA Uptake (pmoles/mg protein)	K_a × 10⁻⁷ M
2	134.6	5.15	68.1	2.73	88.2	3.34
8	168.6	7.63	90.3	2.14	117.8	2.37
13–14	109.4	2.91	132.2	3.34	116.3	1.89
17–18	188.2	4.93	111.8	3.69	146.8	2.29
23	153.9	3.85	123.0	1.90	116.3	2.06
Adult	142.8	1.93	129.0	2.31	123.6	2.10

different processes in the two hormonal conditions. T₄ is known to stimulate protein synthesis and so may stimulate nonreceptor protein accumulation; thus there may be an apparent reduction in sites per total protein, whereas the hydrocortisone may more specifically reduce the amount of binding protein. Further experiments may be able to distinguish between the two processes.

ACKNOWLEDGMENTS

This work was supported by the Medical Research Service of the Veterans Administration and, in part, by U.S. Public Health Service grant

HD-04364. The author also thanks Ms. Carol Siporin for her excellent technical assistance.

REFERENCES

Coyle, J. T., and Axelrod, J. (1971): Development of the uptake and storage of L-(^{3}H)-norepinephrine in the rat brain. *J. Neurochem.*, 18:2061–2075.

Gray, E. G., and Whittaker, J. P. (1962): The isolation of nerve endings from brain — an electron microscopic study of all fragments derived by homogenization and centrifugation. *J. Anat.*, 96:79–88.

Kuhar, M. J. (1973): Neurotransmitter uptake: A tool in identifying neurotransmitter-specific pathways. *Life Sci.*, 13:1623–1634.

Layne, E. (1957): Spectrophotometric and turbidometric methods for measuring protein. In: *Methods in Enzymology*, Vol. 3, edited by S. P. Colowick and N. O. Kaplan, pp. 447–454. Academic Press, New York.

Salas, M., and Schapiro, S. (1970): Hormonal influences upon the maturation of the rat brain's responsiveness to sensory stimulation. *Physiol. Behav.*, 5:7–11.

Scatchard, G. (1949): The attraction of protein for small molecules and ions. *Ann. N.Y. Acad. Sci.*, 51:660–672.

Schapiro, S. (1971*a*): Hormonal and environmental influences on rat brain development and behavior. In: *Brain Development and Behavior*, edited by M. B. Sterman, D. J. McGinty, and A. M. Adinolfi, pp. 307–334. Academic Press, New York.

Schapiro, S. (1971*b*). Influence of hormones and environmental stimulation of brain development. In: *Influence of Hormones on the Nervous System*, edited by D. H. Ford, pp. 63–73. S. Karger, Basel.

Schapiro, S., Vukovich, K., and Globus, A. (1973): Effects of neonatal thyroxine and hydrocortisone administration on the development of dendritic spines in the visual cortex of rats. *Exp. Neurol.*, 40:286–296.

Whittaker, J. P., and Barker, L. A. (1972): The subcellular fractionation of brain tissue with special reference to the preparation of synaptosomes and their component organelles. In: *Methods of Neurochemistry*, Vol. 2, edited by R. Fried, pp. 1–52. Marcel Dekker, New York.

DISCUSSION

Ford: Were you thinking in terms of Dr. Schapiro's hypothesis about the relative effects of T_4 versus cortisone on cerebral differentiation, namely that T_4 propels cells into early differentiation, whereas cortisone maintains them in proliferation?

Geller: That is a good, concise summary of Dr. Schapiro's viewpoint. He thought that T_4 pushed the animal through differentiation so fast that it had too little time for experiential factors to influence cerebral cortical development, whereas cortisol-treated animals went through differentiation more slowly and were able fully to incorporate experiential input. Such may well be the case.

Timiras: Those of us dealing with mammalian brains work with complex systems involving many different development schedules. We are also dealing with complex endocrinological systems. When we speak of high doses of T_4 and try to interpret in terms of other events, we always think of malnutrition. But we must not forget that the endocrine system works as a whole, and whenever you alter markedly a certain endocrine function you produce a constellation of alterations in other endocrine functions. For example, we know that hormones other than thyroid influence development. When we try to interpret some of the long- and short-term effects of thyroid hormones, we must consider them in light of other endocrine functions.

In our laboratory, we continue to find that hypothyroidism alters the normal development and sequence not only of TSH (Cons, Umezu, and Timiras, 1976) but LH and FSH (Umezu, Cons, and Timiras, 1976), and probably also ACTH (which we have not measured). Even though you restore thyroid levels, you are still faced with impairment of gonadal and other endocrine functions. In turn, we know that gonadal hormones have an influence on brain development.

In the case of steroid hormones, the age and the maturational state at the time of administration play important roles. For example, with cortisol you produce a different effect depending on whether you inject it within the first 3 days or after 12 days (Vernadakis and Woodbury, 1964). No matter how well you succeed in achieving euthyroidism, you may overlook some other important endocrine factor.

Bass: Cortisol administered in the first days of extrauterine life presents a false signal to the developing hypothalamic-pituitary axis; the model that Dr. Schapiro and Dr. Geller developed is unique because it operates during such a brief period of time.

Thyroid hormones produce their effects over a broader period of time. The runting effect seen after neonatal cortisol injections is a total endocrinopathy that is induced in the developing thyroid via the hypothalamic-pituitary axis following a single injection of cortisol.

We understand very little yet about the ways we can jolt the developing hypo-thalamic-hypophyseal axis. I do not think we are dealing solely with the effect of cortisone in the runting situation.

Geller: I must correct the general feeling that there is a single injection; we inject cortisol acetate, which is barely soluble. It is injected as a suspension, which remains at the site of injection for a period of time, while it is gradually hydrolyzed and utilized. We are now measuring how long it remains at the injection site by injecting radioactive cortisol acetate; I think we produce a sustained rather than a single stimulus.

Bass: We have duplicated the experiment with dexamethasone, which disappears rapidly from the circulation. Its effective period of time is even narrower than what you describe. In fact, the effect can be produced only by day 3 and 4 of postnatal life, not before, or not after.

Pelton: Hormones other than thyroid may be involved in disorders of brain development. Such effects could be caused by abnormal amounts of either a single hormone (such as cortisol), or multiple hormones (such as a decrease of both thyroid and growth hormones). Dr. Bass and I have pursued the question of the effect of abnormal amounts of growth hormone (GH) in brain development, particularly as that may relate to thyroid disorders.

Since the early work of Goldberg and Chaikoff (1949), numerous studies have reported the interrelationship between GH and thyroid hormone (Eayrs and Holmes, 1964; Schooley, Friedkin, and Evans, 1966; Iwatsubo, Miyai, Abe, Kumahara, Omori, Okada, and Fukuchi, 1967; Daughaday, Peake, Birge, and Mariz, 1968). In both cretinism and hyperthyroidism, pituitary eosinophils are degranulated, and plasma GH is diminished. Despite this, and despite the effects of GH on biosynthetic activity and cellular proliferation (McGarry and Beck, 1972), it appears that GH plays little or no role in perinatal brain development alone or in conjunction with thyroid deficiency. Fetal hypophysectomy (by decapitation) does not change birth lengths (Tanner, 1972); brains of animals with induced cretinism are not benefited by exogenous GH (Eayrs, 1961; Campbell and Eayrs, 1965; Hamburgh, 1966; Geel and Timiras, 1971); perinatal exogenous GH causes little and inconstant effect (Zamenhof and van Marthens, 1971); and, in rats dwarfed by intraventricular injection of 6-hydroxydopamine (a catecholamine toxin), the resulting hyposomatotrophic appearance is not changed by GH therapy (Breese and Traylor, 1972).

Most studies in humans report normal intelligence in GH-deficient patients. However, Laron dwarves, who are unresponsive to GH, are also not normal intellectually (Laron, Pertzelan, and Frankel, 1971). In animal experiments other factors may play roles: GH preparations are often impure; injected GH has a short half-life and therefore causes unsustained effects; and other hormones may be influenced *in vivo* by GH treatment.

We have investigated a unique animal model of exclusive and selective GH deficiency. During postnatal days 2 through 5, newborn albino rats were given intraperitoneal injections of a highly specific antibody to rat GH. This antibody had been prepared by immunizing adult rhesus monkeys to highly purified rat GH (containing no TSH) and then concentrating the serum GH antibody (Ellis, Nuenke, and Grindeland, 1968). Controls were given nonimmune monkey serum.

Infant rats treated with this monkey antirat GH serum (MARGHS) displayed impaired body growth, particularly after 21 days, reaching a 30% decrease by 50 days of age. Brain weights were similarly diminished by 10%.

The effect of the MARGHS was a selective GH deficiency (Table 1). The anterior lobe of the pituitary weighed 46% less than the controls; eosinophils were selectively diminished by differential cell count; and pituitary GH content was reduced by 67% in concentration and 82% in total content at adulthood. In contrast to these data were the normal results for gonadal and adrenal weights (per gram of body weight); thyroid uptake of ^{131}I; plasma prolactin; and ability to mate. Thus, the rats treated with MARGHS had a selective GH deficiency.

Histological and chemical studies of the adult cerebral somatosensory cortex in this model disclosed findings similar to those found in cretin and hyperthyroid animals, although more restricted (Fig. 1). In the subcortical white matter of the adult, we found severe deficits of DNA (65% decrease), cerebrosides, and cholesterol

TABLE 1. *Hormonal effects of treatment with monkey antirat growth hormone serum (MARGHS)*

	Age (days)	Antiserum treated		Decrease (%)	Controls	
Ant. pituitary lobe (mg/100 g body wt.)	78		2.56 ± 0.16[a]	46	4.75 ±	0.19
Pituitary cell count	41					
Acidophils		(♂)	29.3 ± 0.9[a]	27	40.3 ±	1.1
Basophils		(♂)	19.6 ± 0.7[b]		17.0 ±	0.6
Chromophobes		(♂)	51.1 ± 1.3[c]		42.7 ±	1.3
GH concentration (μg/mg wet wt.)	78		4.7 ± 1.8[a]	67	14.3 ±	1.9
GH content/gland (μg/mg wet wt.)	50		10.7 ± 9.5	82	19.2 ±	1.7
Gonadal weight (mg/100 g body wt.)	41	(♂) 917	± 57		965	±18
Adrenal weight (mg/100 g body wt.)	41	(♂)	17.8 ± 1.3		10.0 ±	1.0
Thyroid ^{131}I uptake (nCi/mg tissue wt.)	41		13.1 ± 1.8		10.8 ±	0.8
Prolactin (ng/ml plasma)	41		30 ± 4.5		31 ±	6.5

[a] $p < 0.001$.
[b] $p < 0.01$.
[c] $p < 0.05$.

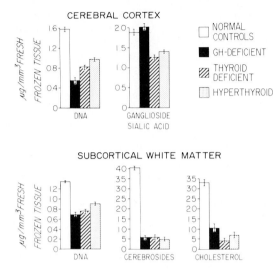

FIG. 1. Effects of neonatal dyshormonal states on somatosensory cortex in adult rats. The ordinate represents mean values of the substances shown in the figure. The bracketed vertical lines at the top of each bar indicate standard error of the mean.

(70 to 88% reduction). Although the cortex displayed a deficit of DNA, there was no abnormality of ganglioside sialic acid, a chemical marker of neurons. Thus, the abnormality in this GH-deficient model was restricted to glial cells and consequently to myelin production. In support of this interpretation, histologic studies demonstrated the persistence of glial cell precursors in the subependymal zone in the adult; those cells should have disappeared as glia migrate into the cortex during maturation.

This deficit differs from both cretin and hyperthyroid animals, which show neuronal as well as glial damage. The reason for this difference may relate to the phase of cerebral maturation at which the insult occurs. In the cretin and hyperthyroid models, the insult (hormone change) occurs almost immediately after birth (within 2 to 3 days), while cortical neurons are still actively differentiating. In the GH-deficient animal, the disappearance of GH probably occurs between 10 and 20 days, during the phase in cortex of glial cell migration, oligodendroglial differentiation and myelin formation.

In this model, selective GH deficiency is clearly associated with abnormal development of myelin in the somatosensory cerebral cortex. There is some similarity between this model and the dysthyroid rats. Perhaps the GH deficiency known to accompany dysthyroid states contributes to the abnormal maturation of the cerebral cortex in those conditions.

Ford: When we make an animal hypothyroid at birth, we are creating an effect prior to the differentiation of many cells of the hypothalamus. This time interval has been called the critical period for development of normal thyroid, gonadal, and adrenal feedback control systems. Each of us has produced animals in which the hypothalamic-pituitary axes have been disturbed. The degree to which normal differentiational changes can now occur in the hypothalamus is unknown. The whorls which we see in the hypothalamus may represent a pathologic response to the initial hormonal insult. Have we created animals in which the hypothalami are permanently unable to regulate pituitary function in a normal manner? Can we ever really provide adequate replacement therapy? We have interfered with the development of a part of the brain at a very significant time. Since the hypothalamus controls systems other than endocrine, numerous other physiologic functions may be permanently altered or damaged.

Geller: Our single injection of cortisol acetate disturbs the later development of the adrenal system, but not in an obvious manner. The stress response of the animal which develops later is relatively normal; i.e., if you stress the animal, you will get a reasonably normal adrenal output. However, there is a disturbance in the later development of the normal diurnal rhythm of circulating corticoids.

Nobody has mentioned thyroid-releasing factor (TRF). There have been reports in the literature recently that TRF has an effect on the mood of depressed patients; I was wondering if anybody knows what TRF does to the brain, if anything.

Timiras: TRF has also been used for treatment of hyperactive children, apparently with some success.

Geller: It has been tried with some autistic children; it does no apparent good.

Rosman: An important clinical study by Pharoah and co-workers (1971) suggests that the neurological damage in congenital hypothyroidism is attributable to iodine deficiency in the first trimester. A study was initiated in New Guinea, where alternate families were injected with either iodized oil or saline and followed for 4 years. Of 534 children born to mothers who had received saline, 26 were hypothyroid; but of 498 children born to mothers who had received iodized oil, only 7 were hypothyroid, and 6 of their 7 mothers were known to have been already pregnant at the time the injection of iodine was given.

Pharoah's study is worth mentioning, in view of Dr. Bass's comment about lack of placental transfer of T_4. The situation is not quite as bleak as he suggests with regard to early hypothyroidism and later intellectual development, as illustrated by three clinical studies. The first was by Smith and co-workers (1957), who showed that if you treat congenitally hypothyroid children with replacement therapy within the first 6 months of life, 45% of them achieve normal intelligence. In 1969, Skorodok in Russia showed that 60% of such children later were intellectually normal. Raiti, in a study from Great Britain in 1971, showed that correction of congenital thyroid deficiency within the first 3 months of life resulted in normal intelligence in 70% of the children.

One might seek an alternative explanation for Dr. Bass's failure to correct with thyroid hormone the biochemical abnormalities he found in the brains of his hypothyroid animals. To explain his lack of success satisfactorily, it would be necessary to know the serum levels of thyroid hormone in his treated animals. In order to obtain such measurements on individual animals it is necessary to employ a microtechnique. We have done this in our own studies. Our method is a modification of one developed originally by Hordynsky and collaborators in 1969, which permits measurement of protein-bound iodide (PBI) on as little as 25 μl of serum. This has made it possible for us to quantify the severity of hypothyroidism in individual animals rendered hypothyroid by the injection of ^{131}I. Even though the thyroid glands of such animals are morphologically abnormal, their PBI levels vary. This may explain why different investigators, using similar methodologies, not uncommonly obtain differing results when studying the effects of thyroid dysfunction on the developing brain.

I suspect that animals assumed to be hypothyroid are not uniformly so (and some may not be hypothyroid at all), even though they may have been given seemingly adequate doses of ^{131}I or propylthiouracil. Another potential source of error relates to the intraperitoneal injection of ^{131}I. When one injects intraperitoneally, not uncommonly a drop or two of the fluid leaks out onto the abdomen; and since the total volume to be injected (isotope plus diluent) may be only 0.05 ml, the loss of 1 or 2 drops can result in a significant difference in the amount of radioisotope delivered.

Finally, I come to a defense of the study of the whole brain as a means of assessing the central neurological effects of experimental hypothyroidism. Dr. Bass's criticisms are valid, since any study of whole brain aliquots is somewhat crude in contrast to his approach which involves analysis of very small portions of brain. One can only hope that the areas he is sampling are, in fact, representative of the developing brain as a whole; if they are not, his elegant work may have limited relevance.

Bass: In the latest textbooks on current etiology, one sees that iodine is actually contraindicated in pregnant mothers. Iodine is commonly slipped into commercial preparations that are sold over the counter; pregnant women can unwittingly get a good deal of iodine that way. The mechanism of the effect is unknown, but it has been clinically well described.

The next question related to giving the dose of ^{131}I. We have been very careful how we administer this potentially dangerous gamma emitter. It is not proper for anyone to leave a gamma emitter with that high a dose for a technician to inject; most of the investigators here probably inject it themselves. Intraperitoneal injection poses a methodologic problem in all experiments.

Whether 2 mm of cerebral cortex is representative of all of the cerebral cortex (it certainly is not representative of all of the brain) is something I cannot answer. The developmental sequence, as I have described it, for rat somatosensory cortex is similar but not identical to that of other areas of cerebral cortex. The visual cortex, for instance, does not develop in the same temporal sequence as the somatosensory cortex, which we studied, and which we can sample reproducibly. The cerebral cortex is not a perfectly synchronous organ. However, what happens in one area of cerebral cortex following a systemic insult can be assumed to happen in other areas of cortex.

Pelton: Dr. Bass and I agree that the story is not as bleak as it could be. Those patients who were treated early did better than those who either were not treated, or who were treated later. However, in the studies to which you refer, normal IQ is considered to be 80 or above. I do not consider 80 to be normal (nor is it by definition). These children are intellectually impaired, in many cases in spite of early treatment.

In regard to Pharoah's study, there is more than one kind of hypothyroidism. His study concerns iodine-deficient hypothyroidism, but we were talking about athyreotic hypothyroidisms. These may not be comparable conditions. Nevertheless, successful prophylactic treatment of the former type with iodine prior to pregnancy emphasizes the need for diagnosis and immediate treatment at birth.

Ford: Does the level of PBI reflect thyroid function adequately?

Pelton: Measurement of thyroid-stimulating hormone (TSH) is superior to PBI in evaluating thyroid requirements of cretin children. Measurement of TSH is successful, economically feasible, and requires only 25 μl of serum. Measurement of TRF may prove to be another useful test in this situation.

Bass: The protein-binding properties of man and rat differ, and they differ in the pregnant mother and her fetus in both species. The pregnant mother has an estrogen-induced elevation of thyroid-binding globulin. The mother not only binds excessive amounts of her own thyroid hormones, but may also accomplish a net transfer of free T_4 from her fetus. However, the transfer of the available free T_4 in a thyroid-deficient fetus would be in the reverse direction if the mother were euthyroid. The most reliable tests for measuring the thyroid status of the newborn are TSH and free T_4.

Hamburgh: Two questions: First, is there evidence that some forms of hypothyroidism are linked genetically to mental retardation? The other question is directed to the myelin experts: Are there any studies which indicate when biochemical markers such as proteolipids, sphingomyelin, and ceramide appear in the developing brain? Myelin seems to become visible rather suddenly. During the critical period of brain maturation everything happens together: axons sprout, the nucleus becomes vesicular, and many enzymes make their appearance. What concentration of myelin lipids or myelin proteins are present prior to the time when myelin becomes visible by light or electron microscopy?

Rosman: Most cases of congenital hypothyroidism in the United States are due to agenesis or dysgenesis of the thyroid gland and appear not to be genetically determined. In contrast, the rare cases of sporadic cretinism caused by impaired enzymatic synthesis of thyroid hormone must be of genetic origin.

In answer to your question Dr. Hamburgh, the accumulation of myelin markers begins slowly and then accelerates quickly. The rate of their accumulation parallels closely the morphological evidence of myelin accumulation in brain.

I did not want to leave the impression that I regard the PBI as the best test of thyroid function, but it is a good test in the absence of iodine contamination. In humans in whom one can obtain several milliliters of serum, a free T_4 or a TSH determination would be preferable.

DISCUSSION REFERENCES

Breese, G. R., and Traylor, T. D. (1972): Developmental characteristics of brain catecholamines and tyrosine hydroxylase in the rat: Effects of 6-hydroxydopamine. *Br. J. Pharmacol.,* 44:210–222.

Campbell, H. J., and Eayrs, J. T. (1965): Influence of hormones on the central nervous system. *Br. Med. Bull.,* 21:81–86.

Cons, J. M., Umezu, M., and Timiras, P. S. (1976): Developmental patterns of pituitary and plasma TSH in the normal and hypothyroid female rat. Endocrinology *(in press).*

Daughaday, W. H., Peake, G. T., Birge, C. A., and Mariz, I. K. (1968): The influence of endocrine factors on the concentration of growth hormone in rat pituitary. In: *Growth Hormone,* Proceedings of the International Symposium, Milan, Italy, September 11–13, 1967, p. 238. Excerpta Medica Foundation, New York.

Eayrs, J. T. (1961): Protein anabolism as a factor ameliorating the effects of early thyroid deficiency. *Growth,* 25:175–189.

Eayrs, J. T., and Holmes, R. L. (1964): Effect of neonatal hyperthyroidism on pituitary structure and function in the rat. *J. Endocrinol.,* 29:71–81.

Ellis, S., Nuenke, J. M., and Grindeland, R. E. (1968): Identity between the growth hormone degrading activity of the pituitary gland and plasmin. *Endocrinology,* 83:1029–1042.

Geel, S. E., and Timiras, P. S., (1971): The role of thyroid and growth hormones on RNA metabolism in the immature brain. In: *Hormones in Development,* edited by M. Hamburgh and E. J. W. Barrington, pp. 391–401. Meredith, New York.

Goldberg, R. C., and Chaikoff, I. L. (1949): A simplified procedure for thyroidectomy in the newborn rat without concomitant parathyroidectomy. *Endocrinology,* 45:64–70.

Hamburgh, M. (1966): An analysis of the action of thyroid hormone on development based on *in vivo* and *in vitro* studies. *Gen. Comp. Endocrinol.,* 10:198–213.

Hordynsky, W. E., King, G. A., McDonald, T. A. et al. (1969): An ultramicromethod for PBI. *Clin. Chem.,* 15:244.

Iwatsubo, J., Miyai, K., Abe, H., Kumahara, Y., Omori, K., Okada, Y., and Fukuchi, M. (1967): Human growth hormone secretion in primary hypothyroidism before and after treatment. *J. Clin. Endocrinol.,* 27:1751–1754.

Laron, Z., Pertzelan, A., and Frankel, J. (1971): Growth and development in the syndromes of familial isolated absence of HGH or pituitary dwarfism with high serum concentration of an immunoreactive but biologically inactive HGH. In: *Hormones in Development,* edited by M. Hamburgh and E. J. W. Barrington, Meredith, New York.

McGarry, E. E., and Beck, J. C. (1972): Metabolic effects of human growth hormone. In: *Human Growth Hormone,* edited by A. S. Mason, pp. 25–38. William Heinemann Medical Books, Chichester.

Pharoah, P. O., Butterfield, I. H., and Hetzel, B. S. (1971): Neurological damage to the fetus resulting from severe iodine deficiency during pregnancy. *Lancet,* 1:308–310.

Raiti, S., and Newns, G. H. (1971): Cretinism: Early diagnosis and its relation to mental prognosis. *Arch. Dis. Child.,* 46:692–694.

Schooley, R. A., Friedkin, S., and Evans, E. S. (1966): Reexamination of the discrepancy between acidophil numbers and growth hormone concentration in the anterior pituitary following thyroidectomy. *Endocrinology,* 79:1053–1057.

Skorodok, L. M. (1969): Vlianie zamestitel'noi gormonal'noi terapil na umstvennoe razvitie dete bol'nykh gipotireozom. *Pediatriia,* 48:81–86.

Smith, D. W., Blizzard, R. M., and Wilkins, L. (1957): The mental prognosis of hypothyroidism in infancy and childhood. *J. Pediat.,* 19:1011–1022.

Tanner, J. M. (1972): Human growth hormone. *Nature,* 237:433–439.

Umezu, M., Cons, J. M., and Timiras, P. S. (1976): Developmental patterns of FSH, LH, and TSH in the hypothyroid female. *(In press.)*

Vernadakis, A., and Woodbury, D. (1964): Effects of cortisol and diphenylhydantoin on spinal cord convulsions in developing rats, *J. Pharmacol. Exp. Ther.,* 144:316–320.

Wurtman, R. J., and Fernstrom, J. D. (1974): Nutrition and the brain. In: *The Neurosciences,* 3rd Study Program, edited by F. O. Schmitt and F. G. Worden, pp. 685–694. MIT Press, Cambridge, Mass.

Zamenhof, S., and van Marthens, E. (1971): Hormonal and nutritional aspects of prenatal brain development. In: *Cellular Aspects of Neural Growth and Differentiation,* edited by D. C. Pease, pp. 329–359. University of California Press, Los Angeles.

Thyroid Hormones and Brain Development,
edited by Gilman D. Grave. Raven Press,
New York, 1977.

Effects of Thyroid State on Development of Rat Cerebellar Cortex

Jean M. Lauder*

The necessity of thyroid hormone for normal brain development became apparent from clinical studies of cretins (Kerley, 1936). Subsequently, thyroid hormone was shown to influence both general somatic and brain development during a certain "critical period" (Salmon, 1936, 1941; Scow and Simpson, 1945; Hamburgh and Vicari, 1957).

Subsequent to these early studies many investigations were begun in an effort to specify the effects and mechanisms of this profound influence on neural development. Early postnatal hypo- and hyperthyroidism were both shown to decrease adult cerebral and cerebellar weights in the rat, but for apparently different reasons (Eayrs and Taylor, 1951; Eayrs and Horn, 1955; Eayrs 1961; Ghittoni and Gomez, 1964; Pasquini, Kaplún, García Argiz, and Gómez, 1967; Balázs, Cocks, Eayrs, and Kovacs, 1971a,b). In hypothyroidism this effect resulted mainly from a decrease in cell size and increase in cellular packing density (Eayrs and Taylor, 1951; Geel and Timiras, 1967; Pasquini et al., 1967; Balázs, Kovacs, Teichgräber, Cocks, and Eayrs, 1968; Krawiec, García Argiz, Gómez, and Pasquini, 1969; Geel and Timiras, 1971), whereas in hyperthyroidism the deficit involved a decrease in cell numbers (Balázs et al., 1971a,b; Zamenhof, van Marthens, and Bursztyn, 1971). These studies raised the possibility that thyroid hormone might be important for normal cell acquisition and neuropil accumulation in the postnatal development of the brain.

More specifically, the growth and disappearance of the external granular layer (EGL) of the developing cerebellum was shown to be greatly influenced by hypothyroidism. In this condition the EGL was found to persist for a longer period (Legrand, 1965, 1967) and to retain its capacity to incorporate [³H]thymidine (Hamburgh, Mendoza, Burkart, and Weil, 1971), indicating that these cells were still proliferating. This prompted Hamburgh et al. (1971) to propose that thyroid hormone might act as a "time clock" in the developing nervous system to signal the termination of cell proliferation.

Effects of thyroid hormone on neuropil development were demonstrated in rat cerebral and cerebellar cortices. These effects involved: changes in

---

* Department of Biobehavioral Sciences, University of Connecticut, Storrs, Connecticut 06268.

the amount and composition of the neuropil in hypothyroid sensorimotor cortex (Eayrs and Taylor, 1951; Eayrs and Horn, 1955; Eayrs, 1961); decreased number of synapses in hypothyroid visual cortex (Cragg, 1970); delayed maturation of the Purkinje cell dendritic tree; retarded development of glomeruli in hypothyroid cerebellar cortex (Legrand, 1967; Geloso, Hemon, Legrand, Legrand, and Jost, 1968); and accelerated development of acetylcholinesterase and cholinesterase staining in hyperthyroid cerebellar cortex (Lefranc, George, and Tusques, 1968). Cocks, Balázs, Johnson, and Eayrs (1970) and Patel and Balázs (1971) reported that the development of glutamate compartmentation, presumably reflecting the maturation of dendritic processes and nerve terminals, was changed in hypo- and hyperthyroidism. Likewise, Geel and Timiras (1967) found a significant reduction in acetylcholinesterase activity in both cerebral cortex and hypothalamus of rats made hypothyroid from birth.

In order to explore the effects of altered thyroid states on cell proliferation, differentiation, and synaptogenesis during postnatal neurogenesis, Altman and I undertook a detailed autoradiographic and electron microscopic study in the developing cerebellar cortex of the hypo- and hyperthyroid rat (Nicholson and Altman, 1972a,b,c). We chose the cerebellum because it undergoes extensive postnatal neurogenesis, had previously been shown to be influenced by thyroid hormone during this period, and allows precise quantitative analyses of hormonally induced changes.

CELL PROLIFERATION AND ACQUISITION IN THE EGL

The effects of hypo- and hyperthyroidism on body, brain, and cerebellar weights are shown in Figs. 1 and 2. The time course of EGL growth (cell

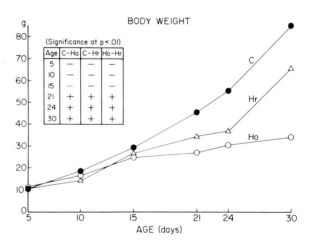

FIG. 1. Body weight. Statistical significance given in inset (Duncan's multiple range test). C, controls; Ho, hypothyroids; Hr, hyperthyroids.

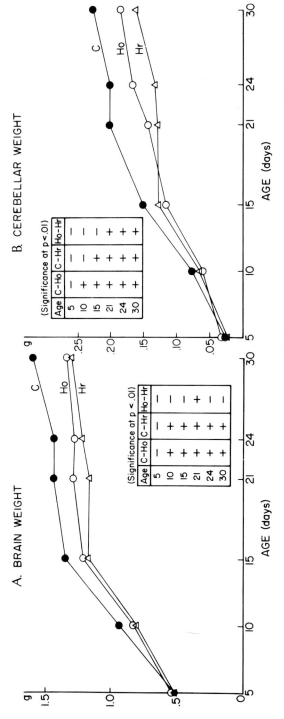

FIG. 2. A: Brain weight. **B:** Cerebellar weight. Statistical significance given in insets (Duncan's multiple range test). C, controls; Ho, hypothyroids; Hr, hyperthyroids. (From Nicholson and Altman, 1972a.)

acquisition) is given in Fig. 3, where the retardation and acceleration effects of hypo- and hyperthyroidism can be seen clearly.

Cell proliferation in the proliferative zone of the EGL was initially studied using short survival [³H]thymidine autoradiography to examine the effects of thyroid hormone on the proportion of cells dividing on a given day of postnatal development (Fig. 4A). In controls, cell proliferation was already underway by 5 days, continued through 15 days, then rapidly declined. Hypothyroidism caused cell proliferation to continue at high levels through 24 days, corresponding to the prolonged presence of the EGL, especially the proliferative zone (Figs. 3 and 4B). Cell proliferation rapidly decreased after 5 days and ceased prematurely in hyperthyroidism (Fig. 4A), accompanied by early disappearance of the proliferative zone (Fig. 4B).

These results indicated that proper levels of thyroid hormone are important for the normal time course of cell proliferation in the EGL, and are consistent with recent biochemical studies in which the activity of thymidine kinase and DNA content were examined in hyperthyroidism. Weichsel (1974) reported that the activity of thymidine kinase was elevated in the cerebellum at 1 to 5 days in hyperthyroid animals. Higher DNA content was also demonstrated at 2 to 6 days, indicating increased cell production, a finding also reported by Gourdon, Clos, Coste, Dainat, and Legrand (1973). These results are in agreement with our finding that the proportion of proliferating cells is increased at 5 days in the hyperthyroid rat (Fig. 4A).

These biochemical and morphological data indicate that excess thyroid hormone initially stimulates cell proliferation in the EGL when cells are rapidly proliferating. It is interesting in this regard to note that a sharp

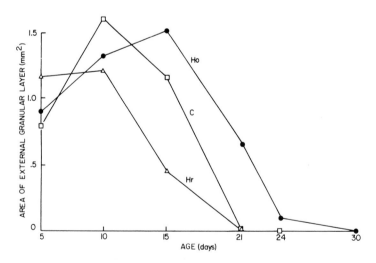

FIG. 3. Area of the EGL of the vermis (sagittal plane). C, controls; Ho, hypothyroids; Hr, hyperthyroids. (From Lauder, Altman, and Krebs, 1974.)

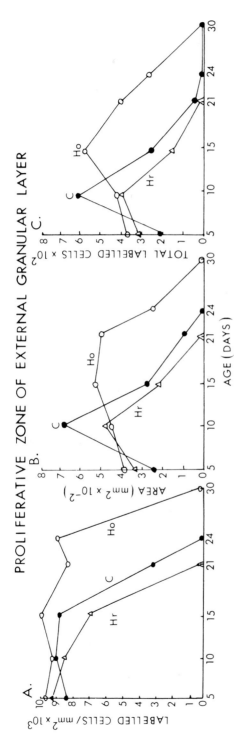

FIG. 4. Cell proliferation in the EGL of the pyramis (sagittal plane). **A:** Proportion of cells incorporating [³H]thymidine in the proliferative zone (2-hr survival). **B:** Area of the proliferative zone. **C:** Total labeled cells in the proliferative zone. C, controls; Ho, hypothyroids; Hr, hyperthyroids. (Revised from Nicholson and Altman, 1972a.)

peak of serum thyroxine has been reported to occur at 1 to 2 days in the normal rat (Samel, 1968). Such a sharp rise in serum levels of thyroid hormone might provide a stimulus for rapid cell proliferation in the EGL, which begins to increase in size at this age (Altman, 1969, 1972). This early peak in serum thyroxine is followed by a more gradual increase from 5 to 15–17 days (Samel, 1968; Clos, Crepel, Legrand, Legrand, Rabié, and Vigouroux, 1974), corresponding to the time course of cessation of cell proliferation (onset of neuronal differentiation) in the EGL (Fig. 5). Whether or not these temporal correlations are causally related remains to be determined.

Recently, the effects of altered thyroid states on the rate of cell proliferation in the EGL have been studied in this and other laboratories in an attempt to explain changes in the rate of cell acquisition observed in previous studies of cerebellar development in neonatal hypo- and hyperthyroidism. These investigations indicate that hypothyroidism does not

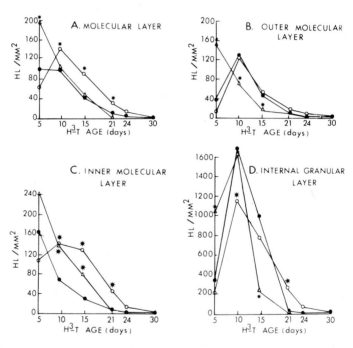

FIG. 5. Cell differentiation in the pyramis (sagittal plane). **A:** Density of heavily labeled cells in the whole molecular layer (basket and stellate cells). **B:** Density of heavily labeled cells in the outer half of the molecular layer (mainly stellate cells). **C:** Density of heavily labeled cells in the inner half of the molecular layer (mainly basket cells). **D:** Density of heavily labeled cells in the internal granular layer. [^{3}H]thymidine (10 μCi/g of body weight) injected on days indicated. Animals sacrificed at 60 days of age. Symbols as in Fig. 4. F-Test comparisons of treated animals and controls significant at $p < 0.01$ (Duncan's multiple range test). (Revised from Nicholson and Altman, 1972a.)

significantly change the length of the cell cycle in the EGL, as determined using the percent-labeled mitoses method (Lauder, 1976; Lewis, Patel, Johnson, and Balázs, 1976). However, there is evidence that some EGL cells may spend a prolonged time in mitosis, especially in anaphase-telophase, which could lead to a decreased rate of cell proliferation and acquisition in hypothyroidism (Lauder, 1976). An increased amount of cell death, which has been reported to occur in the internal granular layer at certain times during the postnatal period, probably also contributes to the lower rate of cell acquisition in the hypothyroid cerebellum as a whole (total DNA; Patel, Rabié, Lewis, and Balázs, 1976).

In the EGL excessive levels of thyroxine shorten the cell cycle, primarily by decreasing the length of the pre-DNA synthetic phase G_1 (Lauder, 1976). This could account for the apparent stimulation of cell proliferation at 5 days and for the early termination of proliferation at 10 days. Thyroid hormone could then act as a "time clock" in the developing cerebellum (Hamburgh et al., 1971), not by triggering differentiation in an all-or-none fashion, but by controlling the rate at which cells complete a fixed number of cell cycles. Alternatively, thyroid hormone might influence proliferative activities of cells that are rapidly dividing (e.g., synthesis or activation of thymidine kinase) or functions of differentiation in cells approaching their last cell cycle(s) (e.g., new protein synthesis). Answers to these questions, however, must await detailed examination of cell proliferation in the hypo- and hyperthyroid EGL. Studies of these models may help elucidate the mechanisms of normal EGL cell proliferation.

THE ONSET OF NEURONAL DIFFERENTIATION

After our initial studies of EGL cell proliferation in the hypo- and hyperthyroid rat (Nicholson and Altman, 1972a), we sought to determine whether altered thyroid states might influence the time when EGL cells stop dividing and begin to differentiate into neurons. We studied the onset of neuronal differentiation by using long-survival autoradiography, in which an animal is injected with [³H]thymidine on a given day of development and then allowed to survive for 1 to 2 months. During this time, those cells that continue to divide dilute their label in proportion to the number of divisions they undergo. The presence of heavily labeled cells in an adult cell population indicates that those cells stopped dividing (were "born" as neurons) on the day of isotope injection. Animals were injected with [³H]thymidine on the days indicated in Fig. 5 and allowed to survive until 60 days of age (Nicholson and Altman, 1972a). The times of origin of the cerebellar interneurons derived from the EGL (basket, stellate, and granule cells) were determined by this method (Fig. 5).

Hyperthyroidism increased the number of molecular layer cells differentiating on the peak day (Fig. 5A), whereas hypothyroidism prolonged the entire time course of differentiation. The peak of differentiation of cells in the outer half of the molecular layer (mainly stellate cells) was accelerated by 5 days in hyperthyroids, whereas the peak of differentiation of inner molecular layer cells (mainly basket cells) occurred on the same day as controls (Fig. 5B, C). Hypothyroidism, however, primarily affected cells in the inner molecular layer where the peak of cell differentiation was delayed by 5 days and was significantly prolonged. Granule cell differentiation (Fig. 5D) was also accelerated by hyperthyroidism and prolonged by hypothyroidism. Such data support the idea that thyroid hormone influences the time of onset of neuronal differentiation (termination of cell proliferation) in the cerebellar cortex.

CELL POPULATIONS

Since hypo- and hyperthyroidism were found to affect the time of onset of differentiation of basket, stellate, and granule cells, we explored the effects of such treatments on the final composition of these cell populations (Nicholson and Altman, 1972*a*). Counts were made in nonradioactive tissue of the total number of cells in the pyramis (identified as basket cells by their relatively light nuclei and darkly staining cytoplasm, large size compared with other cell types, and location in the inner half of the molecular layer). Granule cells were counted throughout the granular layer. The total number of granule cells per sagittal section was estimated by multiplying the number of granule cells per mm^2 by the area of the internal granular layer.

By 30 days, hyperthyroidism had reduced the number of cells in both populations, presumably as a result of the early termination of cell proliferation in the EGL. A similar effect on stellate cells might be expected, but these cells were not counted for technical reasons.

Hypothyroidism apparently exerted a differential effect on the number of basket and granule cells (Fig. 6), although further data are needed to confirm this finding. This treatment caused a slight reduction (statistically nonsignificant) in the number of basket cells by 30 days (Fig. 6B), whereas

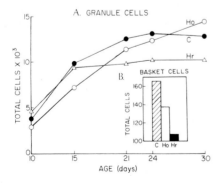

FIG. 6. Cell populations in the pyramis (sagittal plane). **A:** Developmental increase in granule cells. Statistical significance (Duncan's multiple range test): C-Ho, 15, 30 days, $p < 0.01$; 21 days, $p < 0.05$. C-Hr, 21–30 days, $p < 0.01$. **B:** Total basket cells at 30 days. Statistical significance: C-Hr, $p < 0.01$. C, controls; Ho, hypothyroids; Hr, hyperthyroids. (From Nicholson and Altman, 1972*a*.)

no such reduction in the number of granule cells (Fig. 6A) was found. Similar findings have been reported by Clos and Legrand (1973), who observed an apparent reduction in basket cells and approximately normal numbers of granule cells. They also reported a slight increase in the stellate cell population.

If these differential effects of hypothyroidism on the production of cerebellar interneurons can be confirmed by cell counts in semithin sections of plastic embedded tissue and electron microscopy, mechanisms controlling the formation of different cell types from the same precursor population may be found. This problem is of particular relevance to neurogenesis and its possible control by thyroid hormones.

Other interesting results were obtained with respect to the number of astroglia (mainly Bergmann glia) in the molecular layer (identified by their relatively large size, light nuclei, and cytoplasm) and the time course of local cell proliferation around Purkinje cell bodies, which may be the site of Bergmann glia production. Figure 7 illustrates these effects and provides

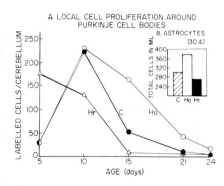

FIG. 7. A: Cell proliferation around Purkinje cell bodies in the pyramis. **B:** Total glia in the molecular layer of the pyramis at 30 days. Statistical significance (Duncan's multiple range test): C-Ho, $p < 0.01$; Ho-Hr, $p < 0.01$. C, controls; Ho, hypothyroids; Hr, hyperthyroids. (From Nicholson and Altman, 1972a.)

further evidence for the early termination of cell proliferation in hyperthyroidism and prolonged proliferation in hypothyroidism. A slight decrease in the number of these glial cells was observed in hyperthyroidism and a significant increase in hypothyroidism. The latter finding is supported by evidence of a larger amount of glial cytoplasm in the molecular layer of hypothyroid rat (Clos, Rebière, and Legrand, 1973).

NEUROPIL DEVELOPMENT AND SYNAPTOGENESIS

We studied the effects of altered thyroid states on the areal development of the molecular layer by using planimetric and linear methods of measurement on projected tracings of the sagittally sectioned vermis (Nicholson and Altman, 1972b,c). This study demonstrated a general retardation of neuropil development in hypothyroidism, with respect to total area, width, or vertical height of the molecular layer (Figs. 8 and 9). Hyperthyroidism, on the other

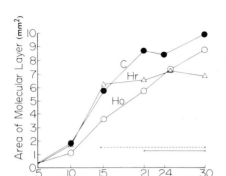

FIG. 8. Area of the molecular layer of the vermis (sagittal plane). C, controls; Ho, hypothyroids; Hr, hyperthyroids. Statistical significance at $p < 0.01$ (Duncan's multiple range test). C-Ho: (– – –), C-Hr: (———). (From Nicholson and Altman, 1972c.)

hand, produced a differential effect, sharply halting development of total area after 15 days (Fig. 8), while accelerating vertical growth of the molecular layer throughout development (Fig. 9). These two findings show that the areal deficit in hyperthyroidism consists of a deficit in the sagittal length of the molecular layer. Figure 10 demonstrates that this deficit reflects a decrease in the amount of cerebellar foliation of the cortical surface (Lauder, Altman, and Krebs, 1974).

The molecular layer is mainly composed of large numbers of parallel fibers (granule cell axons) and Purkinje cell dendritic trees which form characteristic synaptic connections, as well as lesser numbers of other axonal

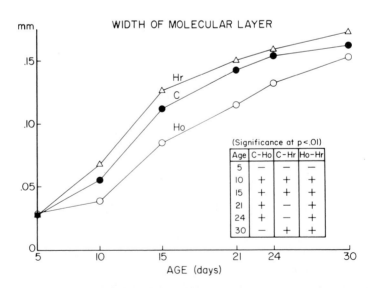

FIG. 9. Width of the molecular layer in the pyramis (sagittal plane). Statistical significance given in inset (Duncan's multiple range test). C, controls; Ho, hypothyroids; Hr, hyperthyroids. (From Nicholson and Altman, 1972b.)

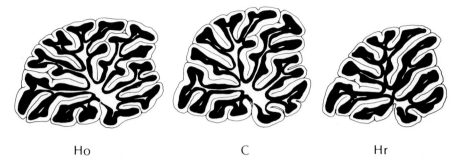

Ho   C   Hr

FIG. 10. Foliation of the cerebellar vermis (sagittal plane) at 30 days of age. **A:** Hypothyroid (Ho). Increased foliation appears to result from prolonged proliferation of the EGL and retarded growth of the rest of the cortex, producing a cerebellum which is more foliated but has shallower fissures. **B:** Control (C). **C:** Hyperthyroid (Hr). Decreased foliation seems to result from premature termination of cell proliferation in the EGL. (From Lauder, Altman, and Krebs, 1974.)

and dendritic processes and the cell bodies of basket, stellate, and glial cells. To examine the effects of hypo- and hyperthyroidism on synaptogenesis in this well-defined neuropil (Nicholson and Altman, 1972*b,c*), we used the ethanolic phosphotungstic acid method for the electron microscopic visualization of synaptic profiles (Bloom and Aghajanian, 1966). Hypothyroidism retarded the developmental increase in density of synapses in the molecular layer (Fig. 11) throughout the postnatal period, whereas hyperthyroidism caused a transient acceleration from days 10 to 21, but reached control values by 24 days. These results suggest that thyroid hor-

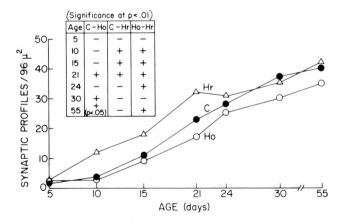

FIG. 11. Synaptogenesis. Density of synaptic profiles stained with ethanolic phosphotungstic acid (E-PTA) in the molecular layer of the pyramis (sagittal plane). Statistical significance given in inset (Duncan's multiple range test). C, controls; Ho, hypothyroids; Hr, hyperthyroids. (Revised from Nicholson and Altman, 1972*c*.)

mone may be important for the normal rate of synaptogenesis in the molecular layer.

To examine the effects of these treatments on the total number of synapses in the area of the sagittally sectioned molecular layer, we multiplied the density of synapses at each age by the area of the molecular layer (Fig. 12). These calculations led to the finding that hypothyroidism produced a general retardation of synaptogenesis, resulting in a deficit in the estimated total number of synapses at all ages examined. In hyperthyroidism, however, although the density of synapses reached control values by 24 days, the total number of synapses were drastically reduced after 15 days because of the deficit in area of the molecular layer. Both treatments produced a total synaptic deficit but for different reasons.

These results agree with other studies of the development of the Purkinje cell dendritic spines and synaptogenesis in the molecular layer (Rebière and Legrand, 1972a,b; Rabié and Legrand, 1973). Using the Golgi method, Rebière and Legrand (1972a) found a distinct retardation of Purkinje cell dendritic tree development as a result of hypothyroidism, which led to a significantly longer primary dendrite and a deficit in the density of dendritic spines. Hyperthyroidism, on the other hand, caused no change in the length of the primary dendritic trunk, but transiently accelerated development of spines. In another study, Rebière and Legrand (1972b) demonstrated a permanent retardation in the density of synapses in the hypothyroid molecular layer. Likewise, Rabié and Legrand (1973) reported a decreased concentration of synaptosomal protein, which was more pronounced than the deficits in total protein previously reported in hypothyroidism (Geel, Valcana, and Timiras, 1967; Balázs and Gaitonde, 1968; Dainat, Rebière, and Legrand, 1970; Geel and Timiras, 1970). Hyperthyroidism, however, produced a transient increase in the concentration of synaptosomal protein. Hajós, Patel, and Balázs (1973) found that somatic processes on Purkinje cells persist longer in hypothyroid animals, and suggested that the climbing fiber-somatic spine synapses that normally disappear with increasing maturity remain longer. This finding is supported by the work of Crepel

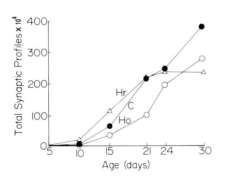

FIG. 12. Synaptogenesis. Estimated total E-PTA-stained synaptic profiles in the molecular layer of the vermis (sagittal plane). C, controls; Ho, hypothyroids; Hr, hyperthyroids. (Revised from Nicholson and Altman, 1972c.)

(1972, 1974) who reported that maturation of the mature climbing fiber response was delayed in hypothyroid animals.

PARALLEL FIBER DEVELOPMENT

To further specify the effects of altered thyroid states on neuropil development, the growth of axons in the molecular layer was studied during postnatal hypo- and hyperthyroidism by means of a method which allows the direct measurement of parallel fiber length (Brand, Dahl, and Mugnaini, 1976).

At various ages during the postnatal period, rats were lesioned in the sagittal plane of the vermis and allowed to survive for 1 to 2 days, depending on age. The cerebellum was then stained for degenerating axons and terminals with a silver-staining method (Fink and Heimer, 1967; DeOlmos and Ingram, 1971). We used the light microscope to measure the extent of degeneration on both sides of the lesion. The greatest distance measured was taken as the length of the longest parallel fibers lesioned. (For further details see Brand et al., 1976; Lauder, 1977.) Parallel fiber length was measured by this method in lobules II to VII at 10, 15, 21, 30, 60, and 90 days of age in controls and treated animals.

Parallel fibers grew rapidly between 10 and 30 days in controls, after which they increased more slowly through 90 days. In hypothyroidism, parallel fiber growth was retarded from the earliest age examined (15 days) through adulthood. At 90 days parallel fibers were still significantly shorter than in controls. Hyperthyroidism, on the other hand, accelerated parallel fiber growth and resulted in significantly longer parallel fibers at 60 and 90 days of age (Fig. 13). These data support the work of Crepel (1974, 1975).

Increased parallel fiber length in the hyperthyroid rat may have several functional consequences. First, because the efferent projections of the Purkinje cells in the vermis, paravermis, and hemispheres are considerably different (Bell and Dow, 1967; Palay and Chan-Palay, 1974), longer parallel fibers might excite more laterally placed Purkinje cells, possibly changing the efferent cerebellar output. Second, the accelerated growth of parallel fibers may be correlated with the accelerated development of Purkinje cell dendritic spines which has also been observed in hyperthyroidism (Rebière and Legrand, 1972*a*). It is impossible at present to ascertain whether dendritic spine and parallel fiber development are each directly accelerated by hyperthyroidism, or whether the accelerated growth of one may be the stimulus for the other. In any case, the increased rate of parallel fiber and Purkinje cell dendritic spine development appears to form the basis for the accelerated synaptogenesis seen in hyperthyroidism. The finding of longer parallel fibers in the adult rat made hyperthyroid from birth provides evidence that thyroid hormone influences not only the onset of neu-

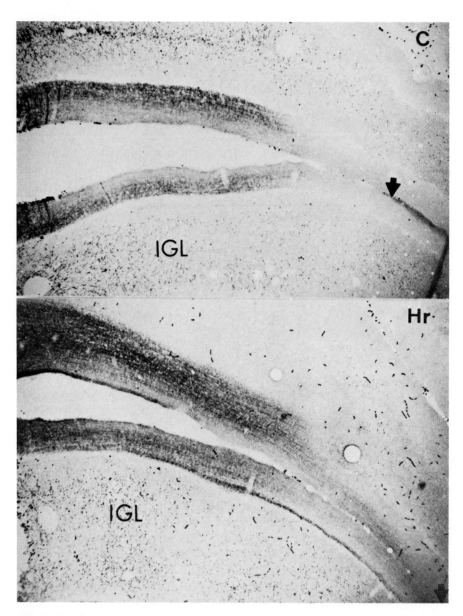

FIG. 13. Parallel fiber length at 90 days of age in lobules IV and V of the vermis (coronal plane, DeOlmos stain). *Arrows:* maximum length of parallel fiber degeneration. Note the increased length of the parallel fibers in hyperthyroidism (Hr) compared to controls (C). Magnification ×36.28. Internal granular layer, IGL. (From Lauder, 1977.)

ronal differentiation, but may regulate later aspects of differentiation such as axonal growth.

SYNAPTIC CAPACITY OF PARALLEL FIBERS

Because hyperthyroid rats have a normal density of synapses in the molecular layer at 30 days, but a greatly reduced number of granule cells contributing axons to this neuropil, it appeared likely that these axons must make more than the normal number of synapses to compensate for the cell deficit. In view of the known effects of hyperthyroidism on the development of the postsynaptic elements in this circuitry, it seemed important to understand how this was achieved.

To determine the average number of synaptic sites per parallel fiber in adult animals made hypo- or hyperthyroid from birth, we employed the rapid Golgi method to stain parallel fibers and their varicosities, which are the sites of the parallel fiber-Purkinje cell dendritic spine synapses (Palay and Chan-Palay, 1974). The number of varicosities per millimeter of parallel fiber length were counted at $1,000 \times$ magnification under oil immersion, with a sample size of 100 fiber lengths per animal (2 to 3 animals per treatment) at 60 days of age. In order to obtain an estimate of the average number of varicosities per parallel fiber, the number per unit length for each animal was multiplied by the average length of parallel fibers for that age and treatment (Lauder, 1977).

Hypothyroidism significantly reduced the average number of varicosities per unit length of parallel fiber. This reduction, combined with a decrease in the mean length of these axons, led to a marked reduction in the total number of varicosities per parallel fiber. In hyperthyroidism, no such reduction in varicosities per unit fiber length was observed, but longer parallel fibers produced a predicted increase in total varicosities (Nicholson and Altman, 1972b).

These data indicate that in hypothyroidism parallel fibers make fewer synapses as a result of both a decreased number of varicosities per unit fiber length and shorter parallel fibers. In hyperthyroidism, these axons contain more synaptic sites because the axons are longer, not because the number of sites per unit length are increased. This raises the possibility that thyroid hormone may affect synaptogenesis indirectly by stimulating axonal growth. This remains a tentative conclusion in the absence of more direct evidence.

CONCLUSIONS

The effects of neonatal hypo- and hyperthyroidism on cell proliferation, the onset of neuronal differentiation, axonal growth, and synaptogenesis in the rat cerebellar cortex have been studied by using quantitative light and electron microscopic methods. These studies indicate that proper levels of thyroid hormone are necessary for normal rates of many aspects of cell differentiation in the postnatally developing cerebellum, from the cessation of cell proliferation to the growth of axons and the formation of synaptic connections. Thyroid hormone also plays an important role in the timing, rate, and quantity of cell proliferation. By affecting these temporal processes thyroid hormone may coordinate the events of postnatal neurogenesis in the cerebellum.

ACKNOWLEDGMENTS

The author would like to thank Drs. Helmut Krebs and Enrico Mugnaini for critical reading of the manuscript. This work was partially supported by National Institutes of Health grant NS-09904. Several of these studies were carried out while Dr. Lauder (Nicholson) was the recipient of a National Institutes of Health predoctoral fellowship.

REFERENCES

Altman, J. (1969): Autoradiographic and histological studies of postnatal neurogenesis. III. Dating the time of production and onset of differentiation of cerebellar microneurons in rats. *J. Comp. Neurol.*, 136:269–294.

Altman, J. (1972): Postnatal development of the cerebellar cortex in the rat. I. The external germinal layer and the transitional molecular layer. *J. Comp. Neurol.*, 145:353–398.

Balázs, R., Cocks, W. A., Eayrs, J. T., and Kovacs, S. (1971*a*): Biochemical effects of thyroid hormones on the developing brain. In: *Hormones in Development,* edited by M. Hamburgh and E. J. W. Barrington, pp. 357–379. Appleton-Century-Crofts, New York.

Balázs, R., and Gaitonde, M. K. (1968): Factors affecting protein metabolism in the brain. *Biochem. J.,* 106:1–2p.

Balázs, R., Kovacs, S., Cocks, W. A., Johnson, A. L., and Eayrs, J. T. (1971*b*): Effect of thyroid hormone on the biochemical maturation of rat brain: Postnatal cell formation. *Brain Res.,* 25:555–570.

Balázs, R., Kovacs, S., Teichgräber, P., Cocks, W. A., and Eayrs, J. T. (1968): Biochemical effects of thyroid deficiency on the developing brain. *J. Neurochem.,* 15:1335–1349.

Bell, C., and Dow, R. S. (1967): Cerebellar circuitry. *Neurosci. Res. Prog. Bull.,* 5(2):177.

Bloom, F. E., and Aghajanian, G. K. (1966): Cytochemistry of synapses: A selective staining method for electron microscopy. *Science,* 154:1575–1577.

Brand, S., Dahl, A-L., and Mugnaini, E. (1975): The length of parallel fibers in the cat. An experimental light and electron microscopic study. (*In preparation.*)

Clos, J., Crepel, F., Legrand, C., Legrand, J., Rabié, A., and Vigouroux, E. (1974): Thyroid physiology during the postnatal period in the rat: A study of the development of thyroid function and of the morphogenetic effects of thyroxine with special reference to cerebellar maturation. *Gen. Comp. Endocrinol.,* 23:178–192.

Clos, J., and Legrand, J. (1973): Effects of thyroid deficiency on the different cell populations of the cerebellum in the young rat. *Brain Res.,* 63:450–455.

Clos, J., Rebière, A., and Legrand, J. (1973): Differential effects of hypothyroidism and undernutrition on the development of glia in the rat cerebellum. *Brain Res.,* 63:445–449.

Cocks, J. A., Balázs, R., Johnson, A. L., and Eayrs, J. T. (1970): Effect of thyroid hormone on the biochemical maturation of rat brain: Conversion of glucose-carbon into amino acids. *J. Neurochem.,* 17:1275–1285.

Cragg, B. G. (1970): Synapses and membranous bodies in experimental hypothyroidism. *Brain Res.,* 18:297–309.

Crepel, F. (1972): Maturation of cerebellar Purkinje cells. II. Hypothyroidism and ontogenesis of cerebellar Purkinje cells spontaneous firing. *Exp. Brain Res.*, 14:472–479.

Crepel, F. (1974): Excitatory and inhibitory processes acting upon cerebellar Purkinje cells during maturation in the rat: Influence of hypothyroidism. *Exp. Brain Res.*, 20:403–420.

Crepel, F. (1975): Consequences of hypothyroidism during infancy on the function of cerebellar neurons in the adult rat. *Brain Res.*, 85:157–160.

Dainat, J., Rebière, A., and Legrand, J. (1970): The effect of thyroid deficiency on the incorporation of L-[H³]-leucine into proteins of the cerebellum in the young rat. *J. Neurochem.*, 17:581–586.

DeOlmos, J. S., and Ingram, W. R. (1971): An improved cupric silver method for impregnation of axonal and terminal degeneration. *Brain Res.*, 33:523–529.

Eayrs, J. (1961): Protein anabolism as a factor ameliorating the effects of early thyroid deficiency. *Growth*, 25:175–189.

Eayrs, J., and Horn, G. (1955): The development of cerebral cortex in hypothyroid and starved rats. *Anat. Rec.*, 121:53–61.

Eayrs, J., and Taylor, S. H. (1951): The effect of thyroid deficiency induced by methylthiouracil on the maturation of the central nervous system. *J. Anat.*, 85:350–358.

Fink, R. P., and Heimer, L. (1967): Two methods for selective silver impregnation of degenerating axons and the synaptic endings in the central nervous system. *Brain Res.*, 4:369–374.

Geel, S. E., and Timiras, P. S. (1967): The influence of neonatal hypothyroidism and of thyroxine on the RNA and DNA concentration of rat cerebral cortex. *Brain Res.*, 4:135–142.

Geel, S. E., and Timiras, P. S. (1967): Influence of neonatal hypothyroidism and of thyroxine on the acetylcholinesterase and cholinesterase activities in the developing central nervous system of the rat. *Endocrinology*, 80:1069–1074.

Geel, S. E., and Timiras, P. S. (1970): The role of hormones in cerebral protein metabolism. In: *Protein Metabolism of the Nervous System*, edited by A. Lajtha, pp. 335–354. Plenum Press, New York.

Geel, S. E., and Timiras, P. S. (1971): The role of thyroid and growth hormones on RNA metabolism in the immature brain. In: *Hormones in Development*, edited by M. Hamburgh and E. J. W. Barrington, pp. 391–401. Appleton-Century-Crofts, New York.

Geel, S., Valcana, T., and Timiras, P. S. (1967): Effect of neonatal hypothyroidism and of thyroxine on L-[¹⁴C]-leucine incorporation in protein *in vivo* and the relationship to ionic levels in the developing brain of the rat. *Brain Res.*, 4:143–150.

Geloso, J. P., Hemon, P., Legrand, J., Legrand, C., and Jost, A. (1968): Some aspects of thyroid physiology during the perinatal period. *Gen. Comp. Endocrinol.*, 10:191–197.

Ghittoni, N. E., and Gómez, C. J. (1964): Respiration and aerobic glycolysis in rat cerebral cortex during postnatal maturation: Influence of hypothyroidism. *Life Sci.*, 3:979–986.

Gourdon, J., Clos, J., Coste, C., Dainat, J., and Legrand, J. (1973): Comparative effects of hypothyroidism, hyperthyroidism and undernutrition on the protein and nucleic acid contents of the cerebellum in the young rat. *J. Neurochem.*, 21:861–871.

Hajós, F., Patel, A. J., and Balázs, R. (1973): Effect of thyroid deficiencies on the synaptic organization of the rat cerebellar cortex. *Brain Res.*, 50:387–401.

Hamburgh, M., Mendoza, L. A., Burkart, J. F., and Weil, F. (1971): The thyroid as a time clock in the developing nervous system. In: *Cellular Aspects of Neural Growth and Differentiation*, edited by D. C. Pease, pp. 321–328. University of California Press, Berkeley.

Hamburgh, M., and Vicari, E. (1957): Effect of thyroid hormone on nervous system maturation. *Anat. Rec.*, 127:302.

Kerley, C. G. (1936): Childhood myxedema: observations through infancy, childhood and early life. *Endocrinology*, 20:611.

Krawiec, L., García Argiz, C. A., Gómez, C. J., and Pasquini, J. M. (1969): Hormonal regulation of brain development. III. Effects of triiodothyronine and growth hormone on the biochemical changes in the cerebral cortex and cerebellum of neonatally thyroidectomized rats. *Brain Res.*, 15:209–218.

Lauder, J. M. (1976): The effects of early hypo- and hyperthyroidism on the development of rat cerebellar cortex. III. Kinetics of cell proliferation in the external granular layer. *Brain Res. (In Press)*.

Lauder, J. M. (1977): Effects of early hypo- and hyperthyroidism on the development of rat cerebellar cortex. IV. The parallel fibers. *(In preparation.)*

Lauder, J. M., Altman, J., and Krebs, H. (1974): Some mechanisms of cerebellar foliation: Effects of early hypo- and hyperthyroidism. *Brain Res.,* 76:33–40.

Lefranc, G., George, Y., and Tusques, J. (1968): Etudes de l'activité acetylcholinesterasique du cortex cerebelleux du rat nouveau-né au cours de sa maturation sous l'action de la thyroxine. *C. R. Soc. Biol. (Paris),* 162:219–224.

Legrand, J. (1965): Influence de l'hypothyroidisme sur la maturation du cortex cerebelleux. *C. R. Acad. Sci. (Paris),* 261:544–547.

Legrand, J. (1967): Analyse de l'action morphogenetique des hormones thyroidiennes sur le cervelet du jeune rat. *Arch. Anat. Microsc. Morphol. Exp.,* 56:206–244.

Lewis, P. D., Patel, A. J., Johnson, A. L., and Balázs, R. (1976): Effect of thyroid deficiency on cell acquisition in the postnatal rat brain: A quantitative histological study. *Brain Res.,* 104:49–62.

Nicholson, J. L., and Altman, J. (1972a): The effects of early hypo- and hyperthyroidism on the development of rat cerebellar cortex. I. Cell proliferation and differentiation. *Brain Res.,* 44:13–23.

Nicholson, J. L., and Altman, J. (1972b): The effects of early hypo- and hyperthyroidism on the development of the rat cerebellar cortex. II. Synaptogenesis in the molecular layer. *Brain Res.,* 44:25–36.

Nicholson, J. L., and Altman, J. (1972c): Synaptogenesis in rat cerebellum: Effects of early hypo- and hyperthyroidism. *Science,* 176:530–532.

Palay, S. L., and Chan-Palay, V. (1974): *Cerebellar Cortex, Ctyology and Organization.* Springer-Verlag, New York, Heidelberg, Berlin.

Pasquini, J. M., Kaplún, B., García Argiz, C. A., and Gomez, C. J. (1967): Hormonal regulation of brain development. I. The effect of neonatal thyroidectomy upon nucleic acids, protein and two enzymes in developing cerebral cortex and cerebellum of the rat. *Brain Res.,* 6:621–634.

Patel, A. J., and Balázs, R. (1971): Effect of thyroid hormone on metabolic compartmentation in the developing rat brain. *Biochem. J.,* 121:469–481.

Patel, A. J., Rabie, A., Lewis, P. D., and Balázs, R. (1976): Effect of thyroid deficiency on postnatal cell formation in the rat brain: A biochemical study. *Brain Res.,* 104:33–48.

Rabié, A., and Legrand, J. (1973): Effects of thyroid hormone and undernourishment on the amount of synaptosomal fraction in the cerebellum of the young rat. *Brain Res.,* 61:267–278.

Rebière, A., and Legrand, J. (1972a): Comparative effects of underfeeding, hypothyroidism and hyperthyroidism on the histological maturation of the molecular layer of the cerebellar cortex of the young rat. *Arch. Anat. Microsc. Morphol. Exp.,* 61:105–126.

Rebière, A., and Legrand, J. (1972b). Données quantitatives sur la synaptogenese dans le cervelet du rat normal et rendu hypothyroïdien par le propylthiouracile. *C. R. Acad. Sci. (Paris),* 274:3581–3584.

Salmon, T. N. (1936): Effect of thyro-parathyroidectomy in newborn rats. *Proc. Soc. Exp. Biol. Med.,* 35:489–491.

Salmon, T. N. (1941): Effect of pituitary growth substance on the development of rats thyroidectomized at birth. *Endocrinology,* 29:291–296.

Samel, M. (1968): Thyroid function during postnatal development in the rat. *Gen. Comp. Endocrinol.,* 10:229–234.

Scow, R. O., and Simpson, M. E. (1945): Thyroidectomy in the newborn rat. *Anat. Rec.,* 91:209–226.

Weichsel, M. E., Jr. (1974): Effect of thyroxine on DNA synthesis and thymidine kinase activity during cerebellar development. *Brain Res.,* 78:455–465.

Zamenhof, S., van Marthens, E., and Bursztyn, H. (1971): The effects of hormones on DNA synthesis and cell number in the developing chick and rat brain. In: *Hormones in Development,* edited by M. Hamburgh and E. J. W. Barrington, pp. 101–119. Appleton-Century-Crofts, New York.

DISCUSSION

Balázs: I should like to venture to explain your observation that the numbers of varicosities per parallel fiber are abnormally great in the animals treated with thyroid hormone. Under these conditions, in comparison with controls, the number of

Purkinje cells is unaltered, but that of the granule cells is reduced. This situation will result in an increase in the number of synaptic contacts with Purkinje cells per parallel fiber.

Lauder: The longer parallel fibers in hyperthyroid animals may also have behavioral and electrophysiological consequences, because each parallel fiber may be contacting more Purkinje cells further laterally than they normally would, and may reach into the paravermal region. Since these laterally placed Purkinje cells have different projections from those in the vermis, this may be a testable consequence.

Valcana: What have you learned about afferent axons such as the mossy fibers? Are they altered in dysthyroid states?

Lauder: Since the mossy fibers grow postnatally they may be affected, especially if thyroid state affects the growth of all neuronal processes.

Valcana: I was not thinking of the direct effect of your treatment on the incoming fiber. I want to know the consequence of the reduction in numbers of granule cells to their presynaptic axons.

Lauder: There could be a number of consequences on the final synaptology in the glomeruli.

Valcana: I thought perhaps you and Dr. Altman would have examined these presynaptic elements in view of your previous work on irradiation, in which abnormalities developed in the mossy fiber.

Lauder: You have raised two different questions, since the mossy fibers may be directly influenced by the hormone, but irradiation presumably affects only the granule cells directly, and the mossy fibers secondarily.

Valcana: The questions are the same if we ask what controls synaptogenesis, and consider how closely pre- and postsynaptic development are related.

Lauder: At present I am studying 90-day-old animals to see if there are any altered synaptic relationships in the molecular layer and the glomeruli.

Gona: In the tadpole cerebellum the external granule cells appear as in mammals and migrate in the same fashion, but they do not show any proliferation while they are still in the external granular layer. Since even the mature frog cerebellum lacks foliation, one may say that it lacks foliation because the external granule cells do not proliferate.

Sokoloff: Dr. Lauder, you raised the question about how thyroid hormones might cause cellular differentiation and turn off proliferation. From a biochemical point of view, those do not have to be separate mechanisms because the same genome must be used as a template. If it is busy making RNA during differentiation, the template will not be available for replicating DNA which is required for proliferation, so the simple phenomenon of stimulating differentiation will turn off proliferation.

Kollros: I would like to comment on the lateral motor column system in the frog. If one keeps the tadpole hypothyroid by hypophysectomy, the initial population of cells which develops is increased by one-fifth or one-sixth. This is before any reduction appears in cell number brought about by an increased thyroid hormone content. If that is also done prematurely, e.g., before the usual cell population is there, which would be something like 50 cells/10-μm section, you could have a maximum of only 30 cells/10 μm because the destruction of cells has begun before the original maximum number has been formed. So you have genuine controls for cell number in both directions, depending on the thyroid state chosen for study.

Balázs: I should like to comment on your description of the abnormally long persistence of the external granular layer of the cerebellum in thyroid deficiency. It seems that a tendency toward the prolonged presence of this germinal zone is also observed in other conditions, such as undernutrition, after neonatal treatment with corticosteroids, and central deafferentation of the cerebellum. Thus, the response of the system to various insults is similar. However, in comparison with these conditions, the extent of mitotic activity beyond the age when active cell proliferation normally ceases, and the prolongation of the period when the external granular layer is present are much more pronounced in thyroid deficiency. These observations indicate that, concerning effects on active cellular proliferation, thyroid deficiency differs from other conditions quantitatively rather than qualitatively.

Bass: Even in euthyroidism the cerebellum seems to be very plastic in that differentiation continues for a long time. You carried out your experiments for many days, and parallel fibers kept getting longer. Does this continue throughout the life of the animal?

Lauder: I have pondered this question too. I am sure that the parallel fibers do not continue to grow forever, but an "adult" animal must be older than what we have thought. This is an important matter. If you are going to study adult rats, you should not consider rats younger than 90 days.

Bass: That teaches us a lesson about cutting developmental experiments short. We have learned about late myelinogenesis the hard way. Many events happen much later than expected.

There is much functional redundancy in the cerebellum; in many experiments you can ablate 75% of the cerebellum and still find no behavioral deficit in the animal. If you could increase the number of synapses or increase the length of axons throughout the life span of the animal, would not this indicate the immense scope of the plastic or regenerative capacity of the cerebellum?

Lauder: I feel that there must be an upper limit, but I do not think that 90 days is necessarily that limit. There may be slight increases in fiber length after that time. However, if you make a lesion in the adult cerebellum, you will not see regeneration of parallel fibers.

Bass: You may have the same problem that we had with the cortex when you say that a lesion is irreversible. If you had carried out your experiments another 100 days, you might have seen some recovery.

Ford: The rat is an unusual animal in that its nervous system continues to grow. I do not know if it grows forever, but it certainly grows for a prolonged period after apparent maturity. Thus, if one measures the volumes of ventral horn cells [the only cells on which I have data over a long period (Ford and Cohan, 1968)], one ends up with a curve which does not reach a plateau after 60 days. Gravimetric studies on a similar population of cells disclose that at 1 week of age a cell weighs about 8,000 pg, at 6 months up to 96,000 pg, and still gains thereafter.

Timiras: We have studied some aging processes in rats up to 3 years old, and we have found that total body growth never ceases, neither in weight nor in length.

Ford: In the rat CNS both glia and neurons continue to grow.

DISCUSSION REFERENCE

Ford, D. H., and Cohan, G. (1968): Changes in weight and volume of rat spinal cord motor neurons with increasing age. *Acta Anat.,* 71:311–319.

Thyroid Hormones and Brain Development,
edited by Gilman D. Grave. Raven Press,
New York, 1977.

Thyroid and Nutritional Influences on Electrocortical Activity Development

Manuel Salas, Sofia Diaz, and Leon Cintra*

During the course of our investigations on neural ontogenesis, we found that both neonatal administration of thyroxine (T_4) and early malnutrition delay the maturation of the CNS, as evidenced by spontaneous and evoked electrocortical events. We discuss these effects and their possible morphological correlates.

The genesis of cortical evoked potentials has been interpreted as: (1) due to activation of particular parts of the neuron (Vastola, 1966), (2) a response of neurons belonging to different cortical layers (von Euler and Ricci, 1958; Towe, 1966), (3) a result of a continuous interaction of cells of different cortical levels (Holubar, 1964), and (4) a result of activation of different afferent systems (Anokhin, 1964; Rose and Lindsley, 1968). Without rejecting any of these interpretations, we believe that the last hypothesis is best supported by experimental data.

The nerve impulses which produce the primary cortical responses are conducted through a fast pathway called the specific thalamic radiation. However, those impulses eliciting the secondary repetitive slow waves following primary responses are conducted centripetally by an extrathalamic nonspecific route (Fig. 1). Furthermore, positive and negative components of primary electrical potentials and secondary slow waves appear to have different anatomical substrates and seem to belong to two different systems of ascending cortical neurons (Purpura, 1962; Anokhin, 1964). The slow negative component develops earlier during ontogeny, whereas the fast positive component of evoked response appears much later in life (Purpura, 1962) (Fig. 2). The latter repetitive slow waves, so-called nonspecific responses with a latency of approximately 300 msec, are mediated by a nonspecific afferent pathway and are related to attentional and perceptual processes (Thompson and Shaw, 1965; Callaway, 1966; Wilkinson and Morlock, 1967). We present our observations concerning the development of the cortical evoked activity in response to sensory stimuli and its possible functional basis.

---

*Department of Physiology, Instituto de Investigaciones Biomédicas, Universidad Nacional Autónoma de México, México 20, D.F., México.

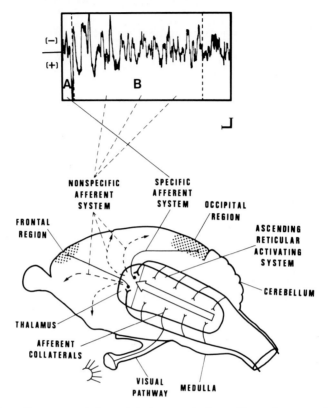

FIG. 1. Schematic representation of thalamocortical specific and nonspecific systems involved in the genesis of the cortical evoked potential. The short-latency primary response (A) is presumably related to the transmission of impulses through the specific afferent system. In contrast, the late repetitive responses following the primary potential (B) are presumably related to the transmission of impulses through the nonspecific system. Calibration: 100 msec and 50 μV.

METHODS

We used 132 male laboratory-bred Wistar rats between 12 and 45 days of age throughout the experiments. In all cases, split litters were used; half received the experimental treatment, and half served as controls. The procedure used to produce undernourished infant rats was as follows: Litter size was kept constant from birth at 8 pups/mother; when necessary, the litter was completed by pups taken from other litters. The control rats were freely nursed by the mother. Between days 2 to 23 postnatally, the undernourished animals were separated from mother and littermates for 12 hr/day and kept in an incubator at a temperature of 29°C. After 23 days, the rats were maintained on water and Purina food pellets *ad libitum*.

In 42 animals, Na$^+$-L-thyroxine (5 μg/g of body weight) was given

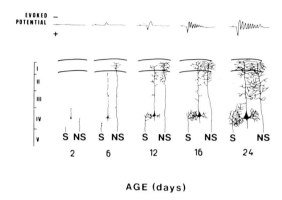

AGE (days)

FIG. 2. Schematic representation of the dendritic connective process between the large cortical pyramidal cells and the afferent thalamocortical systems, correlated with the evoked electrical activity during development. At 2 days of age, because the afferent systems are immature, no evoked activity is obtained. In the 6th postnatal day, because the nonspecific afferent system has attained the cortical surface, a long-latency negative component is obtained. At 12 days of age, because the specific afferent systems synapse with the basilar dendrites and cell bodies, a positive-negative biphasic evoked potential is recorded. Thereafter, the evoked potential is better organized, increases in amplitude, and is followed by a series of repetitive oscillatory waves. S, specific afferent system; NS, nonspecific afferent system. Cortical layers are indicated by roman numerals.

intraperitoneally on postnatal days 1 to 4. A similar control group received saline injections of equivalent volume (0.05 ml). Body weights are shown in Table 1.

Evoked responses were recorded from specific neocortical areas in paralyzed, artificially ventilated animals at 12, 16, 20, and 45 days of age. In the T_4-treated animals recording was additionally performed at day 30. Surgical procedures were performed under ether anesthesia. After animals had recovered from the anesthesia, electrical activity was recorded by the bipolar technique. Electrode resistance was measured during the course of acute experiments in order to ascertain small variations. The operative sites

TABLE 1. *Effects of excess thyroid hormone and malnutrition on body weight of rats during development*

Age (days)	Mean (±SE) body weight (g)		
	Control	Thyroxine (5 μg/g on days 1–4)	Malnutrition (starved 12 hr/day, days 2–23)
12	21.9 ± 0.840	18.9 ± 1.042	15.0 ± 1.087
16	22.8 ± 1.018	21.0 ± 2.223	17.0 ± 1.544
20	43.3 ± 1.559	26.7 ± 0.981	26.8 ± 1.330
30	66.9 ± 4.791	54.0 ± 6.636	
45	129.6 ± 8.286	98.8 ± 5.725	93.6 ± 7.379

were kept moist at all times with mineral oil, and the animal's body temperature was kept constant. The scalp, the incision sites, and the pressure points
were infiltrated with local anesthesia. Square pulses of 0.5 msec duration and
1 to 2 V intensity were used to stimulate the sciatic nerve. Brief flashes in a
darkened room from a photostimulator were used for visual stimulation.
Clicks of 0.2 msec duration and constant intensity from a speaker were used
as acoustic stimuli.

Evoked responses were amplified and recorded with standard neurophysiological equipment. The evoked response and the successive electrical
activity until 1,000 msec were analyzed by the following measurements: (1)
the mean peak latency of primary response, (2) the total duration of the
repetitive discharges from the stimulus presentation until the disappearance
of the oscillations, and (3) the amplitude between the highest and the lowest
peaks of evoked responses sampled at intervals of 100 msec (Fig. 3). In all
cases, 50 successive evoked potentials/animal and cortical area were
measured manually. These data were added to those obtained in animals of
the same age group and treatment. The differences between 300 samples
taken in 6 controls versus 6 experimental rats, at each developmental age
were graphed and analyzed by Student's t-test.

At 7, 12, 20, and 30 days of age, 3 brains of controls and 3 of T_4-treated
rats were chosen at random for morphological analysis. Vertical sections
(20 to 30 μm) from the frontal, parietal, and occipital specific cortical regions
were stained by a variant of the rapid Golgi technique (Globus and Scheibel,
1967). Slides were coded and blind counts were tabulated at ×675 magnification. Five cortical pyramidal neurons/cortical area were studied in each
animal. The number of spines counted included 2 apical, 2 terminal, 8
oblique, and 8 basilar dendrites in a 28.25-μm extent/count/cell. The experimental data were analyzed by the t-test to estimate the validity of the differences between means resulting from the experimental treatment.

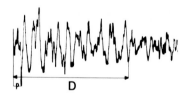

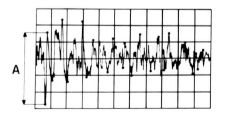

FIG. 3. Single cortical evoked potentials
indicate the procedure used to determine
the mean peak latency (P), the duration
of late afterdischarges (D), and the
amplitude of evoked cortical electrical
activity (A). Black spots in the lower
potential indicate the points between
which amplitude measurements were
done. Calibration: 100 msec and 50
μV.

RESULTS

Maturational Characteristics of Cortical Evoked Responses

At all ages the sensory cortex exhibited potential changes in response to afferent stimulation. This consisted of a large initial positive deflection, followed by a secondary negative component, in turn followed by a series of smaller waves regularly distributed in time. In the frontal region of the younger group of normally developed rats (12 days of age), the sciatic nerve stimulation gave rise to a conventional evoked potential. After an approximate latency of 45 msec, a short positive deflection of approximately 150 μV occurred followed by a secondary negative wave with a latency of approximately 100 msec. In the secondary wave, several repetitive oscillations could be distinguished, generally varying from 4 to 5 waves at intervals of about 90 to 100 msec. In the subsequent successive waves of repetitive discharges, each wave was generally smaller than the preceding one and the form was much broader than that of the primary response. With increasing age, the primary response latency became progressively reduced (Fig. 4) and the wave changed to a mature biphasic configuration until at 20 days, adult values were achieved (latency, 30 to 35 msec). The secondary negative

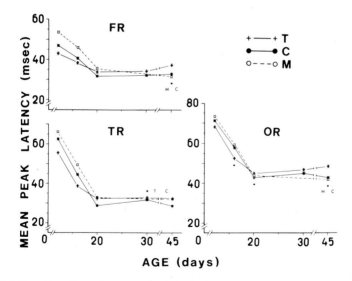

FIG. 4. Relationship of age to mean peak latencies of evoked potentials in the frontal (FR), temporal (TR), and occipital (OR) cortical regions. In general, before 20 days of age T_4 (T) decreased, and malnutrition (M) increased the latency of primary responses of the control rats (C). At 45 days of age T_4 prolonged the latency responses significantly in the temporal and occipital regions. Black squares indicate places where differences between malnutrition-control (M-C) and T_4-controls (T-C) were not statistically significant. Each point in the curve represents the mean of 300 responses.

component at the 20th postnatal day was set at about 85 msec of latency, with a duration of approximately 85 msec. The late repetitive discharges were increased from 7 to 8, and the separation among them was still at intervals of 90 to 100 msec.

Stimulation at 12 days of age evoked two types of responses to visual and auditory stimuli: (1) the conventionally evoked potential of short latency in the corresponding cortical projection areas (±75 msec for visual and ±60 msec for auditory responses); and (2) long-latency secondary response (±100 msec) of a large duration (±100 msec) followed by a series of repetitive waves similar to those seen in the frontal cortical region. With increasing age, the primary response progressively decreased in latency (Fig. 4), until at 20 days of age adult values were obtained (±45 and 30 msec for visual and auditory potentials, respectively). The secondary negative component at this age ranged from 90 to 110 msec in latency and ±100 msec duration. The general pattern of evoked response in the occipital and temporal cortical areas was less consistent than in the frontal region, presumably due to the more complex central pathways composing these sensory projecting systems. The repetitive secondary slow waves of evoked responses increased in number and were separated by intervals of 90 to 100 msec.

Neonatal T_4 treatment advanced the maturation of the evoked responses by approximately 2 to 3 days in all three cortical areas. Already at 12 days of age, consistent monophasic primary positive response and long-latency repetitive discharges were observed. From 12 to 16 days there was a better-organized configuration, shorter latency, and biphasic sensorial potentials compared with the controls (Fig. 4). These neocortical potentials assumed the adult appearance at this latter age, although significantly prolonged mean peak latencies were common at later ages. The number of repetitive discharges following primary response was significantly reduced compared with controls up to 20 days of age, after which they increased and assumed adult appearance.

Early malnutrition delayed the development of evoked potentials in all cortical areas. The malnourished animals exhibited a mean peak latency significantly longer than that of control rats; even at 20 days of age this effect was still present (Fig. 4). Moreover, the number of late repetitive discharges was increased compared to that shown by normally fed rats.

Figure 5 shows the development of the duration of somatesthetic-evoked repetitive afterdischarges in normal, malnourished, and hormonally treated rats. At 12 days of age, in normally developed rats, contralateral sciatic nerve stimulation elicited repetitive responses of a mean total duration of ±550 msec. This duration progressively increased in value until at 30 days of age the adult pattern (±950 msec) was achieved. At 12, 16, and 20 days of age the duration of repetitive afterdischarges of T_4-treated rats was shorter than that of normal subjects ($p < 0.001$). At 30 and 45 days of age, however, the duration was prolonged significantly compared with the controls

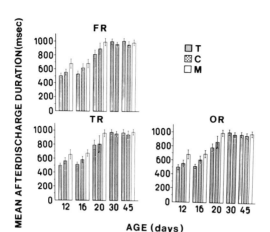

FIG. 5. Relationship of age to evoked afterdischarge duration in the frontal (FR), temporal (TR), and occipital (OR) cortical regions. At 12, 16, and 20 days of age T_4 (T) shortened and thereafter prolonged the duration of the afterdischarges (30 and 45 days of age). In contrast, malnutrition (M) prolonged the afterdischarge throughout experiments when compared with controls (C). Bars representing T_4-treated and starved rats differ from controls at a level of significance of $p < 0.001$. Each bar represents the mean of 300 samples.

$(p < 0.001)$. In the malnourished animals, the duration of late repetitive waves followed a similar sequence in development compared with controls; the duration of afterdischarges was, however, prolonged significantly $(p < 0.001)$ throughout the experiments.

In normally developing rats, the duration of visual and auditory cortical repetitive afterdischarges followed a sequence of development similar to somatesthetic responses (Fig. 5). In T_4-treated and early malnourished animals, the duration of the evoked repetitive afterdischarges to light and auditory cues followed a sequence of development similar to the frontal cortical area $(p < 0.001)$.

Figure 6 summarizes the variations in amplitude of cortically evoked responses in normal and experimental rats during development. The amplitude of the specific responses showed a considerable increment when compared with controls. At all ages, the frontal and temporal cortical areas of T_4-treated rats exhibited higher values than those of control and malnourished rats. In the occipital region, however, the hormonally treated rats tended to show greater evoked responses than control rats, although the values obtained often were low compared with malnourished animals.

Some Maturational Aspects of Cortical Dendritic Spines

Figure 7 shows the progressive dendritic spine development in both normal and hormonally treated rats. Compared with the controls, the T_4-

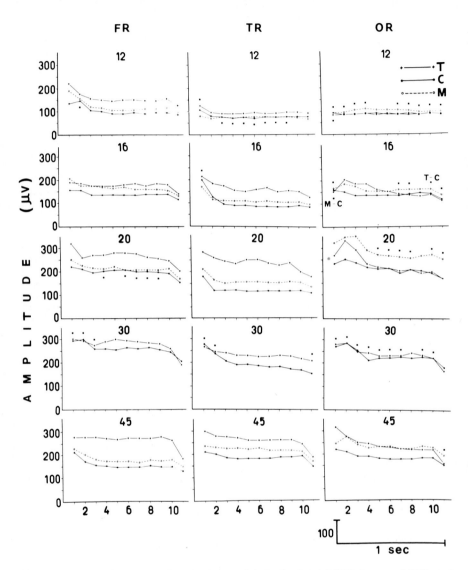

FIG. 6. Amplitude variations of evoked potentials in the frontal (FR), temporal (TR), and occipital (OR) cortical regions during development. In FR and TR, T_4 and malnutrition produce significantly higher amplitude variations compared with controls ($p < 0.05$). Hyperthyroid rats in most cases exhibit larger amplitude values than malnourished rats. Occipital cortical region shows less consistent variations in the evoked potentials during development. However, at 45 days of age the experimental treatments cause a clear increment in the amplitude of evoked responses. Points differ from control at a level of significance of at least $p < 0.05$. Black squares above and below the curves indicate places where the differences between T_4-control and malnutrition-control, respectively, were not statistically significant. Each point in the graphs represents the mean of 300 samples.

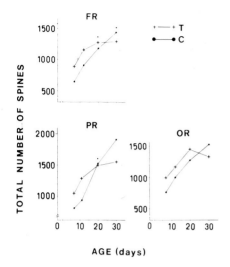

FIG. 7. Effect of neonatal T_4 treatment on dendritic spinal development of large cortical pyramidal cells. FR, frontal region; PR, parietal region; OR, occipital region. Points differ from control at a level of $p < 0.001$. Black squares indicate points where differences were not statistically significant. Each point in the curves represents the total number of spines obtained in the different dendritic prolongations of 5 neurons.

treated rats at 7 and 12 days of age showed an increased number of spines ($p < 0.001$) in all cortical-specific areas. However, at 20 days of age, these differences had disappeared in the parietal and frontal areas, whereas the occipital region still showed an increased number of spines ($p < 0.01$). After the 20th postnatal day, when the number of spines normally shows a rapidly accelerated growth, the T_4-treated rats showed only a small decrement in the frontal region and, in addition, a clear decrement in the number of spinal processes of the parietal and occipital cortical areas ($p < 0.05$). In these experiments, the variations in the number of spines took place without any change in the distribution of the various forms of spines on the dendritic tree.

The hormonally treated rats showed the behavioral signs of hyperthyroidism as manifested by hyperactivity, tremulousness, and exaggerated startle responses. Physical signs of accelerated ear and eye opening and maldevelopment of the pinna were also observed.

DISCUSSION

Our results show that an early excess of T_4 and food deprivation in the rat lead to pronounced deficits in cortical maturation as assessed by a number of electrophysiological and morphological parameters.

During the first 16 postnatal days, T_4-treated rats showed an accelerated maturation of primary evoked cortical potentials and of repetitive discharges following these potentials. These results agree with those of previous studies showing a precocious appearance of spontaneous cortical electrical activity (Schapiro and Norman, 1967) and advanced maturation of primary cortical evoked potentials in response to sensory stimulation (Salas and Schapiro, 1970). Furthermore, our data indicate that from the 20th postnatal day there is a subsequent retardation of the electrophysiological development, as evidenced by a prolonged mean peak latency of primary responses, persistence of an increased amplitude, and prolonged duration of the evoked repetitive discharges to sensory cues.

From previous studies of the development of the neocortex (Pappas and Purpura, 1961; Voeller, Pappas, and Purpura, 1963; Purpura, Shofer, and Scarff, 1965), it is clear that axodendritic synapses, which presumably underlie the excitatory electrical activity, mature relatively early and are numerous during this period. In contrast, the axosomatic and juxtasomatic synapses subserving inhibitory electrical activity (Eccles, 1964) are sparsely distributed and do not increase markedly until the second and third postnatal week (Purpura et al., 1965). The observed abnormalities in amplitude and duration of repetitive discharge during development were probably the result of two different maturational processes. During the first 20 days, treatment with T_4 increases: deposition of myelin (Myant and Cole, 1966; Schapiro, 1968), dendritic branching (Nicholson and Altman, 1972b); dendritic spinal processes (Schapiro, Vukovich, and Globus, 1973), and the number of afferent fibers in the cortex (which increase normally in proportion to the synaptic connections). After 20 days, T_4 causes premature cessation of dendritic proliferation, spinal reabsorption, and cell hypoplasia, which may lead to an ultimate reduction in total number of synapses.

The impairment of cerebral activity in the adult rat which was T_4-treated from birth represents the combined effect of two different actions. This assumption is supported not only by our work, but also by the observations of Hamburgh (1968) and Nicholson and Altman (1972a,b). T_4 causes an accelerated development of the cortical dendritic spines and enhances cortical cell differentiation followed by an ultimate reduction in the total number of synapses. The electrophysiological effects of an excess of T_4 correlate well with microchemical (Pelton and Bass, 1973) and behavioral (Eayrs, 1964; Schapiro, 1968; Davenport and González, 1973) findings, which show similar accelerated development and subsequent retardation.

Early malnutrition delays the maturation of evoked response by approximately 2 to 3 days in all three cortical areas. The undernourished animals show a prolonged primary mean peak latency compared with controls, until adult values are achieved at 20 days. They also show a larger amplitude and duration of primary and late repetitive discharges.

The data show that neonatal malnutrition affects the development of both specific and nonspecific afferent systems. These effects might be due to a delay in myelination (Davison and Dobbing, 1966; Bass, Netsky, and Young, 1970); reduced number of dendritic branches (Eayrs and Horn, 1955; Salas, Díaz, and Nieto, 1974); reduced number of dendritic spines and axon terminals (Salas et al., 1974; Cragg, 1972); retarded caliber growth and irreversible impairment in the perineural diffusion barrier of peripheral nerves (Sima and Sourander, 1973, 1974); as well as delayed biochemical maturation of the synaptic transmissions in the young rats (Bass et al., 1970; Cragg, 1972). Moreover, they agree with the findings that early malnutrition delays the latency of the first positive components and development of the mature waveform of visual, auditory, and somatosensory-evoked cortical potentials (Mourek, Himwich, Myslivecek, and Callison, 1967; Callison and Spencer, 1968; Salas and Cintra, 1973).

Our results in malnourished and hormonally treated adult rats not only emphasize changes in primary cortical potentials but also in the evoked late repetitive waves, closely related to the cortical activity triggered by the non-specific afferent impulses. The slowing of the development of powerful synaptic systems due to the reduction in number of spines and nerve terminals may have produced a differential retardation in the maturation of the cortical neurones. Cells responsible for excitatory and inhibitory processes mature at different ages; consequently, T_4 may disturb permanently the normal balance between excitatory and inhibitory actions.

According to Mungai (1967), the dendrites (site for excitatory synapses) occupy 96% of the total synaptic surface of the cortical pyramidal cells, whereas the cell body (site for inhibitory contacts) occupies only 4% of the surface. Similar findings have been reported by others (Eccles, 1964; Purpura et al., 1965; Uchizono, 1965; Colonnier, 1968). Because environmental conditions may interfere with the normal development, either accelerating (by T_4) or delaying (by malnutrition) demonstrates that the normal balance between the two antagonistic systems is easily upset, resulting in permanent impairment of functioning (Barnet and Lodge, 1967; Meisami, Valcana, and Timiras, 1970; Salas and Cintra, 1975).

Finally, the noxious effects of malnutrition or excess T_4 early in life upon cortical-subcortical structures connected with the nonspecific ascending system may be decisive for normal cerebral function in adulthood. This may be particularly important in view of the well-established roles the non-specific systems of the brainstem play in arousal, attention span and other basic cognitive processes (Lindsley, 1970).

ACKNOWLEDGMENTS

This work was supported in part by a grant from the Foundation's Fund for Research in Psychiatry.

The authors wish to express gratitude to Drs. P. Pacheco and K. Larsson for discussions and critical reading and writing during the preparation of the manuscript.

REFERENCES

Anokhin, P. K. (1964): The electroencephalogram as a resultant of ascending influences on the cells of cortex. *Electroencephalogr. Clin. Neurophysiol.*, 16:27–43.

Barnet, A. B., and Lodge, A. (1961): Click evoked EEG responses in normal and developmentally retarded infants. *Nature*, 214:252–255.

Bass, N. H., Netsky, M. G., and Young, E. (1970): Effect of neonatal malnutrition on developing cerebrum. I. Microchemical and histologic study of cellular differentiation in the rat. *Arch. Neurol.*, 23:289–302.

Callaway, E. (1966): Averaged evoked responses in psychiatry. *J. Nerv. Ment. Dis.*, 143:80–94.

Callison, D. A., and Spencer, J. W. (1968): Effect of chronic undernutrition and/or visual deprivation upon the visual evoked potential from the developing rat brain. *Dev. Psychobiol.*, 1:196–204.

Colonnier, M. (1968): Synaptic patterns on different cell types in the different laminae of the cat visual cortex. An electron microscope study. *Brain Res.*, 9:268–287.

Cragg, B. G. (1972): The development of cortical synapses during starvation in the rat. *Brain*, 95:143–150.

Davenport, J. W., and González, L. M. (1973): Neonatal thyroxine stimulation in rats: Accelerated behavioral maturation and subsequent learning deficit. *J. Comp. Physiol. Psychol.*, 85:397–408.

Davison, A. N., and Dobbing, J. (1966): Myelination as a vulnerable period in brain development. *Br. Med. Bull.*, 22:40–44.

Eayrs, J. T. (1964): Effect of neonatal hyperthyroidism on maturation and learning in the rat. *Anim. Behav.*, 12:195–199.

Eayrs, J. T., and Horn, G. (1955): The development of cerebral cortex in hypothyroid and starved rats. *Anat. Rec.*, 121:53–61.

Eccles, J. C. (1964): *The Physiology of Synapses*. Springer-Verlag, Berlin.

Globus, A., and Scheibel, A. B. (1967): Synaptic loci on visual cortical neurons of the rabbit: The specific afferent radiation. *Exp. Neurol.*, 18:116–131.

Hamburgh, M. (1968): An analysis of the action of thyroid hormone on development based on *in vivo* and *in vitro* studies. *Gen. Comp. Endocrinol.*, 10:198–213.

Holubar, J. (1964): Mechanisms of the primary cortical response (PCR) of the somatosensory area in rats. *Physiol. Bohemoslov.*, 13:385–396.

Lindsley, D. B. (1970): The role of nonspecific reticulothalamocortical system in emotion. In: *Physiological Correlates of Emotion*, edited by P. Black, pp. 147–188. Academic Press, New York and London.

Meisami, E., Valcana, T., and Timiras, P. S. (1970): Effects of neonatal hypothyroidism on the development of brain excitability in the rat. *Neuroendocrinology*, 6:160–167.

Mourek, J., Himwich, W. A., Myslivecek, J., and Callison, D. A. (1967): The role of nutrition in the development of evoked cortical responses in rat. *Brain Res.*, 6:241–251.

Mungai, J. M. (1967): Dendritic patterns in the somatic sensory cortex of the cat. *J. Anat.*, 101:403–418.

Myant, N. B., and Cole, L. A. (1966): Effect of thyroxine on the deposition of phospholipids in the brain *in vivo* and on synthesis of phospholipids by brain slices. *J. Neurochem.*, 13:1299–1307.

Nicholson, J. L., and Altman, J. (1972a): The effects of early hypo- and hyperthyroidism on the development of rat differentiation. *Brain Res.*, 44:13–23.

Nicholson, J. L., and Altman, J. (1972b): Synaptogenesis in the rat cerebellum: Effects of early hypo- and hyperthyroidism. *Science*, 176:530–532.

Pappas, G. D., and Purpura, D. P. (1961): Fine structure of dendrites in the superficial neocortical neuropil. *Exp. Neurol.*, 4:507–530.

Pelton, E. W., and Bass, N. H. (1973): Adverse effects of excess thyroid hormone on the maturation of rat cerebrum. *Arch. Neurol.*, 29:145–150.

Purpura, D. P. (1962): Synaptic organization of immature cerebral cortex. *World. Neurol.*, 3:275–293.

Pupura, D. P., Shofer, R. J., and Scarff, T. (1965): Properties of synaptic activities and spike potentials of neurons in immature neocortex. *J. Neurophysiol.*, 28:925–942.

Rose, G. H., and Lindsley, D. B. (1968): Development of visually evoked potentials in kittens: Specific and nonspecific responses. *J. Neurophysiol.*, 31:607–623.

Salas, M., and Cintra, L. (1973): Nutritional influences upon somatosensory evoked responses during development in the rat. *Physiol. Behav.*, 10:1019–1022.

Salas, M., and Cintra, L. (1975): Development of the electrocorticogram during starvation in the rat. *Physiol. Behav.*, 14:589–593.

Salas, M., Díaz, S., and Nieto, A. (1974): Effects of neonatal food deprivation on cortical spines and dendritic development of the rat. *Brain Res.,* 73:139–144.

Salas, M., and Schapiro, S. (1970): Hormonal influences upon the maturation of the rat brain's responsiveness to sensory stimuli. *Physiol. Behav.,* 5:7–11.

Schapiro, S. (1968): Some physiological, biochemical and behavioral consequences of neonatal hormone administration: Cortisol and thyroxine. *Gen. Comp. Endocrinol.,* 10:214–228.

Schapiro, S., and Norman R. J. (1967): Thyroxine: Effects of neonatal administration on maturation, development and behavior. *Science,* 155:1279–1281.

Schapiro, S., Vukovich, K., and Globus, A. (1973): Effects of neonatal thyroxine and hydrocortisone administration on the development of dendritic spines in the visual cortex of rats. *Exp. Neurol.,* 40:286–296.

Sima, A., and Sourander, P. (1973): The effect of perinatal undernutrition on perineurial diffusion barrier to exogenous protein. *Acta Neuropathol.,* 24:263–272.

Sima, A., and Sourander, P. (1974): The effect of early undernutrition on the calibre spectrum of the rat optic nerve. *Acta Neuropathol.,* 28:1–10.

Thompson, R. F., and Shaw, J. A. (1965): Behavioral correlates of evoked activity recorded from association areas of the cerebral cortex. *J. Comp. Physiol. Psychol.,* 60:329–339.

Towe, A. L. (1966): On the nature of the primary evoked response. *Exp. Neurol.,* 15:113–139.

Uchizono, K. (1965): Characteristics of excitatory and inhibitory synapses in the central nervous system of the cat. *Nature,* 207:642–643.

Vastola, E. F. (1966): Dependence between responses evoked in visual cortex. *Ann. N.Y. Acad. Sci.,* 3:914–920.

Voeller, K., Pappas, G. D., and Purpura, D. P. (1963): Electron microscope study of development of cat superficial neocortex. *Exp. Neurol.,* 7:107–130.

von Euler, C., and Ricci, O. F. (1958): Cortical evoked responses in auditory area and significance of apical dendrites. *J. Neurophysiol.,* 21:231–246.

Wilkinson, R. T., and Morlock, H. C. (1967): Auditory evoked response and reaction time. *Electroencephalogr. Clin. Neurophysiol.,* 23:50–56.

DISCUSSION

Lauder: The initial acceleration and subsequent retardation in growth of dendritic spines puzzles me. In the cerebellum this phenomenon presumably reflects a deficit in number of granule cells. But in the cerebral cortex that should not be the case.

Salas: We counted the number of dendritic spines of the large pyramidal cells in the Vth cortical layer of different areas. We found morphological changes in the cortical spines following early hyperthyroidism. We have not yet identified what parts of the cortical elements that make synaptic contacts with the large pyramidal cells are specifically affected by hyperthyroidism. We have analyzed only the postsynaptic elements, not spine resorption.

Lauder: I am talking about a developmental time course; I have not looked at dendritic spines and Purkinje cells. I assume that the dendritic spines increase along with the synapses. The ceiling in total number of synapses is not due to resorption of spines, but rather to the deficit in the total number of granule cells which make synapses.

Salas: We found a reduced number of synapses. We do not know if this means that the large pyramidal cells slow their growth process or that the number of interneurons and thalamocortical afferent fibers are reduced, or even if some spines are reabsorbed. You did not mention the possibility of reabsorption of the spines, but we have advanced this hypothesis to explain the electrophysiological effects.

Altman: Are you talking about the number of synapses per unit area, or *in toto?* If you have a growing system, you may not have a total reduction, but rather a reduction in density.

Lauder: There is no decrease in the density of synaptic profiles in hyperthyroid animals. There is an initial acceleration in density after which normal levels are reached.

Valcana: The number of synapses depends on the overall functional activity of the animal, or even on the environment in which it is kept. Could it be that the difference in your findings is the outcome of an initial acceleration followed by a return to normal, while the deficit may stem from a functional depression in the already established ones? They may regress because the animal is basically inactive.

Lauder: Cerebral cortex comprises a completely different system than cerebellum.

Bass: The correlation of evoked potential studies with cortical development seems to relate not so much to myelinogenesis but to synaptogenesis. The process of synaptogenesis in cortex is much different from that in cerebellum because the cortical microneurons are all in place at birth. Postnatally between 15 and 25 days of age, neuronal processes proliferate and form a synaptic hookup at the same time that the cortical evoked response exhibits its characteristic sequence of maturational changes. When a balance between inhibitory and excitatory synapses is achieved at 25 days of age, a mature electrical pattern and evoked potential response can be observed.

Interestingly, this all happens before myelinogenesis is finished in the thalamo-cortical connections. Without fully myelinated axons, Dr. Salas, you are still able to stimulate cortical responses through the eye and the ear. I do not know what part of the electrical profile reflects the speed of conduction of the stimulus to the cortex, but I would think that this electrical aspect might be severely affected in altered or delayed myelinogenesis. Based on our studies of hypothyroidism, the abnormality would occur between 20 and 50 days.

Salas: The latency of the evoked potential represents primarily the afferent conduction time in the axons of the sensorial pathways. So the process of myelination affects primarily the conduction of nerve impulses through myelinated pathways rather than the interaction of the neurons. The synaptic transmission of impulses happens quickly (0.6 msec); at the synaptic level myelin is not present.

Bass: The total maximal amplitude is the variable that would best correlate with myelinogenesis.

Salas: It would be difficult to explain any single part of the various components of the evoked potentials in terms of myelinogenesis, because the evoked response reflects the electrical interactions of cells in different cortical layers. Our attempts to establish structural and functional correlations may be criticized because other neuronal elements (such as fusiform cells and cortical interneurons) were not included in our experimental design. These elements participate in many of the synaptic events and mediate complex physiological processes such as memory (Altman, 1967). Our failure to establish a clear correlation between morphology and electrical activity could be due to the lack of adequate methods. Our idea is that T_4 in some way affects the physiological properties of the nonspecific system. This in turn may be reflected in the increased amplitude of cortically evoked activity and in the changes of the duration of the afterdischarge.

Valcana: Dr. Salas, you have shown us that some of the histological abnormalities are also manifested at the electrophysiological level. Have you done any intracellular recordings which might clarify the electrophysiological manifestations of the intracellular biochemical effects of T_4? For example, neuronal excitability may be affected by metabolic changes that accompany hypo- or hyperthyroidism.

Salas: We have not, but Meisami, Valcana, and Timiras (1970) and Woodbury, Hurley, Lewis, McArthur, Copeland, Kirschvink, and Goodman (1952) have shown that both neonatal hypo- and hyperthyroidism lower the threshold of the electroshock seizure. This change in excitability must be related to ionic or metabolic alterations of the nerve cells which might be detected by microchemical or micro-electrical techniques. However, at this time such correlations remain problematic.

Valcana: I wonder whether the depression in the activity of the sodium-potassium pump, for example, and the electrolyte changes that occur in the developing brain at the electrophysiological level, would be manifested as changes in resting potential or alterations in excitability properties.

Salas: While it might be interesting to analyze the problem by using this approach to correlate the physiological and electrical effects of T_4 on neurons, I am afraid that it would produce more inconclusive data.

Valcana: Would it be too difficult to utilize these techniques to show electro-physiological counterparts of the biochemical alterations that have been presented?

Salas: I am afraid so.

DISCUSSION REFERENCES

Altman, J. (1967): Postnatal growth and differentiation of the mammalian brain, with impli-cations for a morphological theory of memory. In: *The Neurosciences, A Study Program,* edited by G. C. Quarton, T. Melnechuk, and F. O. Schmitt, pp. 723–743. Rockefeller University Press, New York.

Meisami, E., Valcana, T., and Timiras, P. S. (1970): Effects of neonatal hypothyroidism on the development of brain excitability in the rat. *Neuroendocrinology,* 6:241–251.

Woodbury, D. M., Hurley, R. E., Lewis, N. G., McArthur, M. W., Copeland, W. W., Kirsch-vink, J. F., and Goodman, L. S. (1952): Effect of thyroxin, thyroidectomy and 6-N-propyl-2-thiouracil on brain function. *J. Pharmacol. Exp. Ther.,* 106:331–340.

Thyroid Hormones and Brain Development,
edited by Gilman D. Grave. Raven Press,
New York, 1977.

Effects of Neonatal Hypothyroidism on Protein Synthesis in the Developing Rat Brain: An Open Question

Theony Valcana* and Norman L. Eberhardt**

The rate of protein synthesis is increased by thyroid hormones in all tissues which respond to these hormones with an increased rate of oxygen consumption (Sokoloff, 1970). Although the adult brain is nonresponsive (in terms of protein synthesis and oxygen consumption), the developing brain is markedly impaired by lack of thyroid hormones in its overall growth, structural, functional, and biochemical development (Eayrs, 1966; Geel and Timiras, 1970; Balázs, 1971; Sokoloff and Kennedy, 1973). This impairment may be ascribed to changes in protein synthesis.

The rate of protein synthesis, as estimated by experiments *in vivo*, is depressed in the hypothyroid developing rat brain (Geel, Valcana, and Timiras, 1967; Balázs and Gaitonde, 1968; Dainat, Gourdon, and Legrand, 1970a; Dainat, Rebière, and Legrand, 1970b; Szijan, Kalbermann, and Gómez, 1971). Also, an early *in vitro* stimulatory effect of thyroxine (T$_4$), mediated through mitochondrial stimulation of the existing protein synthesizing machinery, has been described in the developing rat brain (Sokoloff, 1970).

Changes at the transcriptional (Szijan et al., 1971) and/or translational (Balázs, Kovacs, Teichgräber, Cocks, and Eayrs, 1968) levels have been suggested as the primary site of thyroid hormone interaction. We have proposed that the depressed protein synthesis in the developing hypothyroid brain may be related to alterations in the transport and/or metabolism of amino acids brought about either by changes of membrane permeability or by alterations of blood-brain exchange processes consequent to hypothyroidism (Geel et al., 1967). Regardless of this diversity of opinion, it is well accepted that the rate of protein synthesis is depressed in hypothyroidism. Some doubt has been introduced on the subject by the data of Andrews and Tata (1971) who, by employing a cell-free protein synthesizing system, showed that there was no depression in the protein synthetic capacity of hypothyroid brain. This discrepancy indicated that our sug-

---

* Chair of Human and Animal Physiology, School of Natural Sciences and Mathematics, University of Patras, Patras, Greece.
** Department of Biochemistry, University of California Medical School, San Francisco, California 94720.

gestion that T_4 plays a regulatory role in amino acid transport and metabolism [which would in turn influence protein synthesis (Geel et al., 1967)] warranted reexamination. The lack of agreement in the results obtained by experimentation *in vivo* by various groups (Geel et al., 1967; Dainat et al., 1970*a*; Szijan et al., 1971) and the results obtained by Andrews and Tata (1971) in cell-free systems could be explained by alterations in the amino acid transport and metabolism, processes which are not rate-limiting in the cell-free system.

Plasma amino acid levels are altered in hypo- and hyperthyroidism. For example, leucine and tyrosine are increased in hyperthyroidism and decreased in hypothyroidism (Ness, Takahashi, and Lee, 1969); in humans with thyrotoxicosis, blood tyrosine levels increase as much as 70% (Rivlin and Asper, 1966). In addition, other aspects of amino acid metabolism are altered in the brain of the adult (Rivlin and Kaufman, 1965; Kaplanskii and Akopyan, 1966; Mochizuki and Lee, 1970) and developing rat (Ramirez de Guglielmone and Gómez, 1966; Patel and Balázs, 1971). In hypothyroidism, the levels of free aspartic and glutamic acid concentrations are depressed (Ramirez de Guglielmone and Gómez, 1966) and the oxidation of leucine is increased (Patel and Balázs, 1971) in the developing brain. These findings are of considerable importance in interpreting *in vivo* experiments which use amino acids as precursors. In addition, leucine in the brain is oxidized 20 times faster than it is incorporated into protein (Diamond, *personal communication*). The above amino acid abnormalities, coupled with a depression of cerebral blood flow in hypothyroidism (Eayrs, 1954), make the *in vivo* experiments hard to interpret. The greatest difficulty in determining protein synthesis has been a lack of knowledge of the specific activity and size of the amino acid precursor pool and how these may be altered by hypothyroidism.

We decided, therefore, to circumvent some of the changes in plasma amino acids, alterations in cerebral blood flow, and their consequent differential equilibration in the brain amino acid pools by adopting the *in vitro* brain-slice system and examining aspects of amino acid transport and incorporation into protein. The adopted system is well defined *in vitro* as to requirements for protein synthesis, provides a simpler technical approach, and allows greater diversity in experimental design (Elliott, 1969). The main purpose of these experiments is to reexamine the question of whether neonatal hypothyroidism alters the rate of protein synthesis in the developing rat brain and whether such an alteration is the outcome of altered uptake and/or metabolism of amino acids.

MATERIALS AND METHODS

We used female Long-Evans rats born to mothers fed a low-iodide diet during the last week of gestation and for 4 days postnatally. Hypothyroidism was induced by intraperitoneal injections of ^{131}I (100 μCi/animal) at birth (Goldberg and Chaikoff, 1949). Littermate euthyroid animals served as controls. The developmental period in these studies covered days 13 to 42 postnatally.

Our initial experiments were designed to test the incorporation *in vitro* of amino acid into total brain protein and, more specifically, into proteins of subcellular components, particularly those of myelin, microsomes, and the soluble cytoplasmic fraction. It was thought that any depression in protein synthesis due to hypothyroidism would most likely be found in the synthesis of myelin membrane, a process known to be depressed in hypothyroidism (Walravens and Chase, 1969; Dalal, Valcana, Timiras, Einstein, 1971; Wysocki and Segal, 1972; Valcana, Einstein, Csejtey, Dalal, and Timiras, 1975).

For these experiments, the brain was excised and sliced into 0.5-mm coronal sections. To avoid topographically related differences in protein synthesis, slices from either the whole brain or half (bisected sagittally) were used. The ratio of tissue weight to medium volume was maintained at 100 mg/ml. The atmosphere was 95% O_2, 5% CO_2, and the incubation temperature 37°C. The incubation medium was Krebs-Ringer phosphate buffer pH 7.4 (122 mM NaCl, 3.1 mM KCl, 0.4 mM KH_2PO_4, 25 mM $NaHCO_3$, 1.2 mM Mg_2SO_4, 1.2 mM $CaCl_2$, 10 mM glucose). The amino acid precursors used were uniformly ^{14}C-labeled amino acids (Amersham Searle Company) and were used in trace amounts in the incubation medium (final concentrations: leucine 1.6 μM, 312 μCi/μM; tyrosine 12 μM, 460 μCi/μM; proline 1.0 μM, 260 μCi/μM). The uptake and incorporation of these amino acids into brain proteins were tested separately except in experiments in which both leucine and tyrosine, at the concentrations indicated, were present in the incubation medium. At the end of the incubation period, the tissue was removed from the solution by filtration and washed with cold 0.32 M sucrose. The tissue was homogenized in sucrose and samples of the homogenate were removed for determination of the levels of radioactivity and protein. The remainder of the homogenate was used to isolate the various subcellular fractions. Myelin was isolated from the crude mitochondrial fraction according to the method of Norton (1971). Microsomes and the cytoplasmic fraction were prepared by centrifuging the postmitochondrial fraction at 105,000 × g for 1 hr. The pellet obtained contained the microsomes and the supernatant material the cytoplasmic soluble fraction.

Because protein synthesis is depressed in the liver of hypothyroid animals (DuToit, 1952), in one experiment we determined the effects of neonatal hypothyroidism on the *in vitro* incorporation of amino acids into liver protein and compared it with that in brain of the same animals. The incubation conditions and the precursor concentrations were as described. In a parallel experiment we tested the effects of cycloheximide (40 mg/ml), a protein synthesis inhibitor, on the *in vitro* protein synthesis by brain slices.

Samples of brain and liver homogenate, as well as aliquots of subcellular fractions, were taken for determination of protein and radioactivity. The samples were precipitated with 10% trichloroacetic acid (TCA) and centrifuged at $3,000 \times g$ for 10 min. The supernatant fraction was removed, and the pellet was washed twice by resuspending it in 5% cold TCA and recentrifuging as above. The acid extracts were combined with the supernatant fraction of the first centrifugation and aliquots counted for activity of the acid-soluble component. The precipitate was washed consecutively with hot 5% TCA for 10 min at 90°C; ethanol containing 0.98% potassium acetate, and ethanol ether (3:1 v/v) at 74°C for 3 min. The ether-dried precipitate was dissolved in 1 N NaOH. An aliquot was used for determination of protein according to the procedure of Lowry, Rosebrough, Farr, and Randall (1951). Another aliquot was acidified and counted with Aquasol (New England Nuclear).

We planned a second series of experiments to clarify the results obtained from the above studies and to answer the original question. Specifically, we examined: (1) the uptake and incorporation into protein of additional amino acids by adding $[U-^{14}C]$-L-lysine and $[U-^{14}C]$-L-glutamic acid; (2) the effects of T_4 (10^{-8} M) in the incubation medium on the amino acid uptake and incorporation into protein by cerebral cortical slices obtained from control animals; (3) the concentration of free leucine, tyrosine, lysine, and glutamic acid in the cerebral cortex of control and hypothyroid animals. The incubation conditions were the same as described above, except that the tissue slices were obtained from the cerebral cortex only, and the ratio of tissue:medium was decreased to 30 to 50 mg/ml of incubation medium. Radioactivity also was determined as described above. The results are expressed as dpm or cpm/mg of wet tissue in the acid-soluble fraction; dpm or cpm/mg protein in the protein fraction; or as relative specific activity (RSA), which represents the ratio of the activity in the protein fraction/mg wet tissue:activity in the acid-soluble fraction/mg wet tissue. Free amino acids in the cerebral cortex were extracted in 75% ethanol and determined on a Beckman 120B amino acid analyzer.

RESULTS AND DISCUSSION

The amino acid incorporation into protein was higher in the brain slices obtained from hypothyroid animals than in those from controls. This was observed in protein of all subcellular compartments, at early (13 days) as well as at later (42 days) stages of hypothyroidism (Table 1). This effect was noted when leucine, tyrosine, or proline were used as precursors and even when the results were expressed in terms of RSA. These findings agree with results obtained by others *in vivo* in which both the activity incorporated

TABLE 1. *In vitro amino acid incorporation into protein of various subcellular fractions from control and hypothyroid rat brain*

Precursor Age (days)		Homogenate		Cytoplasm		Microsomes		Myelin	
		C	H	C	H	C	H	C	H
Leucine	13	8,561	10,528 (23%)	22,521	20,584	12,985	16,269 (25%)	9,143	13,306 (45%)
	43	1,102	1,347 (13%)	2,887	3,876 (34%)	6,740	7,460 (11%)	–	–
Tyrosine	13	4,609	6,064 (31%)	9,476	8,691	9,680	11,363 (17%)	4,705	5,553 (18%)
	43	1,108	3,465 (212%)	4,345	6,035 (39%)	8,080	11,580 (43%)	–	–
Proline	13	3,073	4,643 (51%)	6,183	7,597 (23%)	12,079	15,828 (31%)	4,409	8,287 (88%)
	43	399	1,890 (374%)	1,916	2,867 (49%)	10,000	11,720 (17%)	–	–

Brain tissue slices, 0.5 mm thick coronal sections, from whole brain of control (C) and hypothyroid (H) rats were incubated at 37°C for 2 hr in Krebs-Ringer medium (100 mg/ml). Final amino acid concentrations and specific activity in incubation medium were leucine: 1.6 μm, 312 μCi/μM; tyrosine: 12 μM, 460 μCi/μM; proline: 1.0 μM, 260 μCi/μM. Numbers represent means from 2 determinations, 4 animals per determination. Numbers in parentheses represent percent change from control values.

into cerebral protein and the activity of the acid-soluble fraction are higher in hypothyroid tissue. However, their findings disagree with respect to the RSA which they have found to be depressed *in vivo* by hypothyroidism (Geel et al., 1967; Balász and Gaitonde, 1968; Dainat et al., 1970a,b; Szijan et al., 1971).

In view of the overall hypoplasia that characterizes the developing hypothyroid brain and the depression of the rate of protein synthesis in the hypothyroid liver, we hypothesized that the observed rate of incorporation of amino acids into brain protein could not reflect a higher rate of protein synthesis but, rather, some other changes, such as a difference in transport or changes in the amino acid pool participating in protein synthesis. To substantiate this hypothesis, we conducted further experiments.

In one experiment, we employed cycloheximide in order to determine whether the higher activity in the acid soluble fraction (1) reflected protein synthesis, (2) was the outcome of depressed utilization of amino acids by other pathways, or (3) was indicative of enhanced transport. Cycloheximide depressed the incorporation of amino acid into both the protein and the acid soluble fraction in control tissue (Table 2). In tissue slices from hypothyroid animals, however, the incorporation into protein was depressed, but the incorporation into acid soluble fraction was enhanced. This indicated that the higher activity in this fraction in hypothyroidism in the absence of cyclo-

TABLE 2. *Effects of cycloheximide on the in vitro incorporation of amino acids into protein by control and hypothyroid brain tissue slices*

Precursor ± inhibitor	Specific activity (cpm/mg protein)		Acid soluble (cpm/mg wet tissue)	
	Control	Hypothyroid	Control	Hypothyroid
Leucine (−)	1,102	1,347	1,382	1,480
Leucine (+)	751 (32%)	174 (87%)	1,187	1,749
Proline (−)	399	1,890	2,144	1,711
Proline (+)	59 (85%)	153 (92%)	1,816	2,144
Leucine and tyrosine (−)	2,870	6,472	2,125	2,849
Leucine and tyrosine (+)	1,097 (62%)	1,490 (77%)	2,859	3,113

Whole brain from 35- to 42-day-old control (C) and hypothyroid (H) rats was sliced into 0.5-mm coronal sections and incubated (100 mg/ml) for 2 hr under the conditions described in Table 1. Numbers represent means of 2 to 4 determinations. Numbers in parentheses indicate the percent inhibition by cycloheximide (40 mg/ml).

heximide does not represent a response to higher rate of synthesis, but rather may reflect enhanced transport. Depression of other metabolic pathways was not considered in view of the fact that leucine oxidation is augmented in hypothyroidism (Patel and Balázs, 1971). Parallel experiments, which are not reported here in detail, show that the *in vitro* incorporation of leucine into the lipid fraction of myelin membrane is similarly enhanced as was its incorporation into protein.

The fact that cycloheximide inhibition of protein synthesis is more marked in hypothyroidism indicates that alterations in transport may also involve other substances including cycloheximide; i.e., the transport of this inhibitor may be enhanced in hypothyroidism. In addition, this experiment shows that the enhanced radioactivity of the protein fraction represents incorporation rather than sequestered radioactivity because the incorporation was depressed by an inhibitor of protein synthesis. No other factors peculiar to this group of animals or experimental procedures were suspected. In contrast to the situation in brain in which we observed an increased activity in both the protein and the acid soluble fraction, in liver slices from the same animal, we found the expected depression (DuToit, 1952) of amino acid incorporation into protein (Table 3).

Inasmuch as we originally examined the incorporation of amino acids during a 2-hr incubation, we thought that examination at shorter and more frequent intervals would help to elucidate these observations. Figure 1 summarizes the results of one such experiment after incubation of brain slices from 13-day-old control and hypothyroid rats for 5, 10, and 45 min. The activities in total homogenates and in the acid-soluble and protein fractions were higher in slices from hypothyroid animals at all time intervals. Al-

TABLE 3. *In vitro incorporation of amino acids into protein by liver slices from control and hypothyroid rats*

Precursor	Specific activity (cpm/mg protein)		Acid soluble (cpm/mg wet tissue)		RSA	
	C	H	C	H	C	H
Leucine	3,575	3,198	176	186	2.73	2.66
Tyrosine	1,212	820	142	141	1.39	0.89
Leucine and tyrosine	4,148	3,526	406	451	1.60	1.29

Liver slices from control (C) and hypothyroid (H) 37-day-old rats were incubated in Krebs-Ringer medium (100 mg/ml) for 2 hr at 37°C. Numbers are means of 2 determinations. The concentrations and specific activities of amino acids in medium are those indicated in Table 1. RSA = relative specific activity.

though the incorporation of amino acid into protein and the RSA in hypothyroid tissue are again higher than in the control tissue, the slopes of these lines indicate that the rate of incorporation is the same in both tissues. At the 5-min interval (which can be taken as a better index of influx of leucine into brain tissue), radioactivity is much higher in the TCA-soluble fraction of hypothyroid tissue than in control. This finding indicates an enhanced transport of leucine in this tissue.

Therefore, in the next series of experiments we tested whether T_4 at a physiological concentration would influence the uptake of amino acids by control tissue when added to the incubation medium. The 5- and 20-min uptake of leucine, tyrosine, lysine, and glutamic acid by cerebral cortical

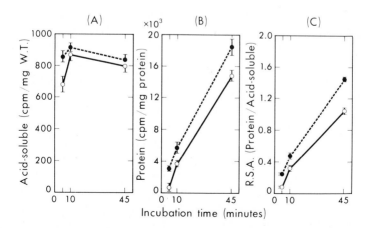

FIG. 1. *In vitro* incorporation of [U¹⁴C]-L-leucine into whole brain slices from control (——) and hypothyroid (----) 13-day-old rats. Incubation conditions and leucine concentration as in Table 1. In **(A)** radioactivity in the acid-soluble fraction, in **(B)** radioactivity in protein, and in **(C)** the relative specific activity (RSA).

slices was tested in the presence of 10^{-8} M T_4 in the incubation medium. There was no significant effect in the uptake of all amino acids except leucine, which was depressed in the acid-soluble fraction (Table 4). This finding is in agreement with the observations of Anthony Verity, Brown, Cheung, and Czer (1975) on the effects of T_4 on leucine uptake by synaptosomes *in vitro,* and of Adamson and Ingbar (1967) in embryonic bone tissue. These findings indicate that T_4 may influence the transport of certain amino acids into cerebral cortical tissue, particularly leucine, its transport being depressed in the presence of T_4 and increased in its absence.

TABLE 4. *In vitro effect of T_4 on leucine activity in the acid-soluble fraction of cerebral cortical tissue slices*

	Percent decrease	
Incubation period (min)	Exp. 1	Exp. 2
5	7	—
10	16	22
20	33	—
45	—	23

Cerebral cortical slices, 0.5 mm thick, from control 22-day-old animals (Exp. 1) and 14-day-old animals (Exp. 2) were incubated in medium and conditions described in Table 1, in the presence or absence of 10^{-8} M L-T_4. Numbers represent the percent decrease in radioactivity in acid-soluble fraction of tissues incubated in the presence and absence of T_4. The percent decrease at each time interval was determined in triplicate.

The higher incorporation of amino acid precursors into protein in hypothyroid tissues may reflect changes in the developmental pattern (Lajtha and Piccoli, 1971) of amino acid metabolism and transport that would lead to a depression of free amino acid content. Such changes are suggested by the work of Ramirez deGuglielmone and Gómez (1966), who have found that free glutamic and aspartic acid concentrations are depressed in the brain of neonatally thyroidectomized rats. We therefore chose to test the uptake and incorporation *in vitro* into protein in control and hypothyroid tissue of these same amino acids, as well as the uptake and incorporation of lysine, an amino acid with different transport properties and unchanged in concentration in neonatal hypothyroidism. The comparison of the kinetics of uptake and incorporation of these amino acids, together with the findings reported above, could help to elucidate whether the primary effect of hypothyroidism is due to changes in transport, to altered amino acid pool and/or both, and whether the higher incorporation of radioactivity into protein was caused by such changes.

The uptake into the acid-soluble fraction and the incorporation into protein of labeled glutamic acid and lysine by control and hypothyroid cerebral cortical slices are shown in Figs. 2 and 3, respectively. Unlike leucine, the uptake of both glutamic and lysine into the acid-soluble fraction is not significantly elevated by hypothyroidism, but their incorporation into protein and the RSA is significantly higher. It could be concluded that this higher incorporation of glutamic acid into protein arises from the known depression in the glutamic acid concentration with hypothyroidism. The lysine concentration, however, was not found to be changed by Ramirez deGuglielmone and Gómez (1966) and, inasmuch as no changes were found in the transport of lysine (Fig. 3A), we decided to investigate whether, under our experimental conditions, any change could be demonstrated in the free concentration of this amino acid as well as in tyrosine and leucine.

Hypothyroidism induced a marked depression in the free concentration of leucine, tyrosine, and lysine in the cerebral cortex of 29-day-old rats. Leucine was depressed by 65%, lysine by 50%, and tyrosine was not detectable in the hypothyroid cerebral cortical tissue. The free content of these amino acids in brain tissue is low relative to glutamic acid (Shaw and Heine, 1965), and the detection of changes may have been missed by previous investigators due to lack of sensitivity of the methods employed. On the other hand, the severity of hypothyroidism is probably higher in our animals, inasmuch as we had placed their mothers on a low-iodide diet during gesta-

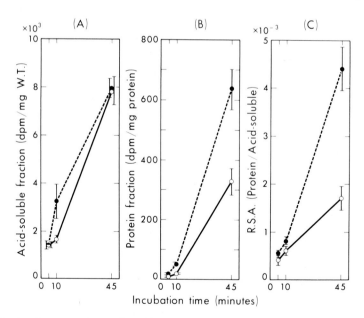

FIG. 2. *In vitro* incorporation of [U-¹⁴C]-L-glutamic acid into cerebral cortical tissue slices from control (————) and hypothyroid (- - - -) 21-day-old rats. Incubation medium and conditions as in Table 1. Glutamic acid concentration in medium 2.1 μM; 260μCi/μM. **(A), (B),** and **(C)** as defined in legend to Fig. 1.

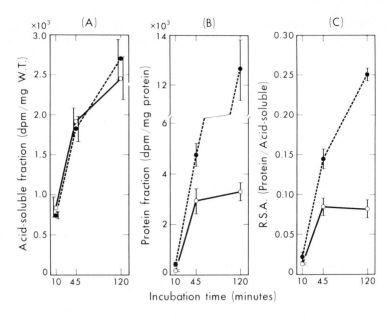

FIG. 3. *In vitro* incorporation of [U-¹⁴C]-L-lysine into cerebral cortical tissue slices from control (——) and hypothyroid (- - - -) 23-day-old rats. Incubation medium and conditions as in Table 1. Lysine concentration in medium 0.9 μM; 312μCi/μM. **(A)**, **(B)**, and **(C)** as defined in legend to Fig. 1.

tion and during the first 4 days postnatally. This procedure markedly influences the efficiency of hypothyroidism induced by ^{131}I injection at birth (Gorbman, 1950).

The decrease in the free amino acid concentration indicates that neither the *in vivo* nor *in vitro* determination of the specific activity of the acid-soluble pool represents the specific activity of the pool of amino acids from which the protein synthesizing system draws. In fact, in the hypothyroid state, the specific activity of the amino acid pool is markedly higher inasmuch as the amino acid concentration (at least for glutamic, aspartic, tyrosine, lysine, and leucine) is depressed by 50% or more. Therefore, the higher incorporation of amino acids into protein due to hypothyroidism, shown by these experiments and observed from *in vivo* experiments, is the result of a combination of changes in the amino acid concentration in the brain tissue as well as in transport of some amino acids.

The experimental approaches and results did not allow us to draw definite conclusions with respect to the rate of protein synthesis in hypothyroid brain tissue slices, although it can be concluded from the results presented in Fig. 1B and C that the rate of amino acid incorporation into protein is similar in control and hypothyroid tissue, in agreement with the conclusions of Andrews and Tata (1971). Dunlop, Van Elden, and Lajtha (1974) pointed out that determination of the rate of protein synthesis in brain tissue *in vivo* and *in vitro* is complicated by such factors as changes in amino acid pools, compartmentation, transport, and protein degradation. The present results indicate that such differences do exist between control and hypothyroid tissue. Therefore, the conclusions of Andrews and Tata (1971) regarding the rate of protein synthesis in the developing brain of hypothyroid animals may be more valid (inasmuch as no transport alterations or changes in specific activity in precursor pools would operate in their cell-free system) than the conclusions drawn from the brain-slice system and *in vivo* experiments. Even if the rate of protein synthesis determined *in vitro* in cell-free systems is not affected by hypothyroidism in the *in vivo* condition, particularly during the rapid growth phase of the brain, the reduction of free amino acid levels in hypothyroidism may limit the rate of protein synthesis and lead to the characteristic neuronal hypoplasia.

A better understanding of the overall hypoplasia may be provided by elucidation of catabolic processes in the brain and of turnover of cerebral proteins. In addition, changes in free amino acid pool *per se* in the brain may underlie many types of metabolic, neurological, and behavioral abnormalities that accompany hypothyroidism. Indeed, some of the free amino acids in brain serve as precursors in the synthesis of neurotransmitters, and others, such as glutamic acid and glycine, may participate directly in neurotransmission.

ACKNOWLEDGMENTS

This work was conducted in the laboratory of Prof. P. S. Timiras, whom we thank for interest, support, and critical review of the manuscript. We also thank Dr. D. B. Hudson for reviewing the manuscript and Ms. C. Miller and Mr. G. Bean for their technical assistance. This work was supported by National Institutes of Health grant HD-07340.

REFERENCES

Adamson, L. F., and Ingbar, S. H. (1967): Selective alteration by triiodothyronine of amino acid transport in embryonic bone. *Endocrinology*, 81:1362–1371.

Andrews, T. M., and Tata, J. R. (1971): Protein synthesis by membrane-bound and free ribosomes of the developing rat cerebral cortex. *Biochem. J.*, 124:883–889.

Anthony Verity, M., Brown, W. J., Cheung, M., and Czer, G. (1975): Paradoxical inhibition of synaptosomal protein synthesis by thyroid hormone. *Trans. Am. Soc. Neurochem.*, 6(1):279.

Balázs, R. (1971): Biochemical effects of thyroid hormones in the developing brain. In: *Cellular Aspects of Neural Growth and Differentiation*, edited by D. C. Pease, pp. 273–320. University of California Press, Los Angeles.

Balázs, R., and Gaitonde, M. K. (1968): Factors affecting protein metabolism in the brain. *Biochem. J.*, 106:1–2p.

Balázs, R., Kovacs, S., Teichgraber, P., Cocks, W. A., and Eayrs, J. T. (1968): Biochemical effects of thyroid deficiency on the developing brain. *J. Neurochem.*, 15:1335–1349.

Dainat, J., Gourdon, J., and Legrand, J. (1970*a*): Variations avec l'âge de l'incorporation de la leucine dans les proteines du cervelet après traitement par le propylthiouracile chez le rat. *C. R. Soc. Biol. (Paris),* 164:1550–1554.

Dainat, J., Rebière, A., and Legrand, J. (1970*b*): The effect of thyroid deficiency on the incorporation of L-(^{3}H) leucine into proteins of the cerebellum in the young rat. *J. Neurochem.,* 17:581–586.

Dalal, K. B., Valcana, T., Timiras, P. S., and Einstein, E. R. (1971): Regulatory role of thyroxine on myelinogenesis in the developing rat. *Neurobiology,* 1:211–224.

Dunlop, D. S., Van Elden, W., and Lajtha, A. (1974): Measurements of rates of protein synthesis in rat brain slices. *J. Neurochem.,* 22:821–830.

DuToit, C. H. (1952): The effects of thyroxine on phosphate metabolism. In: *Phosphorus Metabolism,* edited by W. D. McElroy and B. Glass, p. 597. Johns Hopkins Press, Baltimore.

Eayrs, J. T. (1954): The vascularity of the cerebral cortex in normal and cretinous rats. *J. Anat.,* 88:164–173.

Eayrs, J. T. (1966): Thyroid and central nervous development. In: *Scientific Basis of Medicine Annual Reviews,* edited by J. P. Ross, pp. 317–339. Athlone Press, London.

Elliott, K. A. C. (1969): The use of brain slices. In: *Handbook of Neurochemistry,* edited by A. Lajtha, Vol. 2, pp. 103–113. Plenum Press, New York.

Geel, S. E., and Timiras, P. S. (1970): The role of hormones in cerebral protein metabolism. In: *Protein Metabolism of the Nervous System,* edited by A. Lajtha, pp. 335–366. Plenum Press, New York.

Geel, S. E., Valcana, T., and Timiras, P. S. (1967): Effect of neonatal hypothyroidism and of thyroxine on L-(^{14}C) leucine incorporation in protein *in vivo* and the relationship to ionic levels in the developing brain of the rat. *Brain Res.,* 4:143–150.

Goldberg, R. C., and Chaikoff, I. L. (1949): A simplified procedure for thyroidectomy of the newborn rat without concomitant parathyroidectomy. *Endocrinology,* 45:64–70.

Gorbman, A. (1950): Functional and structural changes consequent to high dosages of radioactive iodine. *J. Clin. Endocrinol.,* 10:1177–1191.

Kaplanskii, S. Y., and Akopyan, Z. I. (1966): Phenylalanine and tyrosine metabolism and its regulation by thyroid hormones in the brain of albino rats. *Biochemistry (Biokhimiia),* 31:231–234.

Lajtha, A., and Piccoli, F. (1971): Alterations related to the cerebral free amino acid pool during development. In: *Cellular Aspects of Neural Growth and Differentiation,* edited by D. C. Pease, pp. 419–446. University of California Press, Los Angeles.

Lowry, O. H., Rosebrough, N. J., Farr, A. L., and Randall, K. J. (1951): Protein measurement with the folin phenol reagent. *J. Biol. Chem.,* 193:265–275.

Mochizuki, A., and Lee, Y. P. (1970): Effect of thyroid hormones on amino acid and protein metabolism. II. Glutamate concentration in rat tissues after thyroidectomy and thyroid hormone treatment. *Endocrinology,* 87:816–819.

Ness, G. C., Takahashi, T., and Lee, Y. P. (1969): Thyroid hormones on amino acid and protein metabolism. I. Concentration and composition of free amino acids in blood plasma of the rat. *Endocrinology,* 85:1166–1171.

Norton, W. T. (1971): Recent developments in the investigation of purified myelin. *Adv. Exp. Med. Biol.,* 13:327–337.

Patel, A. J., and Balázs, R. (1971): Effect of thyroid hormone on metabolic compartmentation in the developing rat brain. *Biochem. J.,* 121:469–481.

Ramirez de Guglielmone, A. E., and Gómez, C. J. (1966): Influence of neonatal hypothyroidism on amino acids in developing rat brain. *J. Neurochem.,* 13:1017–1025.

Rivlin, R. S., and Asper, S. P. (1966): Tyrosine and the thyroid hormones. *Am. J. Med.,* 40:823–827.

Rivlin, R. S., and Kaufman, S. (1965): Effects of altered thyroid function in rats upon the formation and distribution of tyrosine. *Endocrinology,* 77:295–307.

Shaw, R. K., and Heine, J. D. (1965): Ninhydrin positive substances present in different areas of normal rat brain. *J. Neurochem.,* 12:151–155.

Sokoloff, L. (1970): The mechanism of action of thyroid hormones on protein synthesis and its relationship to the differences in sensitivities of mature and immature brain. In: *Protein Metabolism of the Nervous System,* edited by A. Lajtha, pp. 367–382. Plenum Press, New York.

Sokoloff, L., and Kennedy, C. (1973): The action of thyroid hormones and their influence on brain development and function. In: *Biology of Brain Dysfunction,* edited by G. E. Gaull, Vol. 2, pp. 303–332. Plenum Press, New York.

Szijan, I., Kalbermann, L. E., and Gómez, C. J. (1971): Hormonal regulation of brain development. IV. Effect of neonatal thyroidectomy upon incorporation *in vivo* of L-(^{3}H) phenylalanine into proteins of developing rat cerebral tissues and pituitary gland. *Brain Res.,* 27:309–318.

Valcana, T., Einstein, E. R., Csejtey, J., Dalal, K. B., and Timiras, P. S. (1975): Influence of thyroid hormones on myelin proteins in the developing rat brain. *J. Neurol. Sci.,* 25:19–27.

Walravens, P., and Chase, H. P. (1969): Influence of thyroid on formation of myelin lipids. *J. Neurochem.,* 16:1477–1484.

Wysocki, S. J., and Segal, W. (1972): Influence of thyroid hormones on enzyme activities of myelinating rat central-nervous tissues. *Eur. J. Biochem.,* 28:183–189.

DISCUSSION

Sokoloff: Dr. Valcana raises an important point that has broad implications. The availability of radioisotopes has been a great boon to biochemistry, particularly in determining the direction and intermediates of biochemical pathways. When one uses radioisotopes to measure rates of reactions, especially those that are closely regulated, a number of precautions must be considered which too often are ignored, overlooked, or disregarded.

When one determines the rate of a chemical reaction by measuring radioactivity, one measures only the rate of the radioactive reaction, which may or may not reflect the true rate of the total biochemical reaction in the tissue. That depends also on the ratio of the concentration of the radioactive species of the precursor to that of the nonradioactive species.

Several years ago Dr. Patricia Middleton did some experiments in our laboratory. We had shown that T_4 would stimulate protein synthesis in the newborn rat brain in cell-free systems *in vitro.* We wanted to know whether the hyperthyroid state would also stimulate cerebral protein synthesis *in vivo.* We used three radioactive amino acids: [^{14}C]methionine, [^{14}C]lysine, and [^{14}C]leucine, and injected them individually. When we used methionine, we observed an apparent stimulation of protein synthesis by about 100%; lysine produced an apparent inhibition of protein synthesis by about 50%, and leucine resulted in a stimulation of about 5%. Obviously, if we were observing only protein synthesis, all three amino acids should have stimulated or inhibited by the same amount; i.e., the percentage effect should have been the same with each of them. Evidently hyperthyroidism had different effects on the uptake from the blood by the brain of the three amino acids or on the size or turnover rate of the tissue pools of the different amino acids.

By using matched animals and an amino acid analyzer we were able to separate each amino acid and measure the whole history of the specific activity of each amino acid in the precursor pool. We found that they all had different time courses.

When we corrected for the changes in specific activity of the precursor amino acid caused by the hyperthyroid state, all of the amino acids showed the same percentage stimulation of protein synthesis. When one measures a reaction by measuring a radioactive product, one must consider the entire history of the specific activity of the precursor.

Another problem has come up recently. You may have read a paper by Carter, Faas, and Wynn (1971) reporting that T_4 stimulates protein synthesis in cell-free systems from liver in the complete absence of mitochondria. They took our original system, left out the mitochondria, used the creatine phosphate system, and lowered the microsomal concentration (which lowered the rate of protein synthesis). To compensate for the reduced incorporation they used uniformly labeled amino acids, of the highest specific activity available. These were the changes that they made in our system. We examined each of the components that they altered (Sokoloff and Roberts, 1974), and we were able to repeat what they had reported. We were surprised to find, however, that when we left out the microsomes, we observed an even greater percent stimulation by T_4! We thought that we might have some ribosomal units contaminating our $100,000 \times g$ fraction, so we centrifuged at $300,000 \times g$ for 2 hr, but this made no difference. From a long series of experiments we were able to demonstrate that uniformly labeled amino acids of high specific activity are contaminated with small amounts of radioactive substances that are incorporated into protein by processes unrelated to protein synthesis. For instance, aldehydes can react with the amino groups on lysine residues and appear to be incorporated into proteins. This is not protein synthesis. That was one reason why when Kaufman and I first designed the system we were going to use, we specifically selected carboxyl-labeled amino acids, and specifically chose leucine. It can only get incorporated into protein or get transaminated and decarboxylated, in which case the radioactivity is lost, and there are no radioactive products. Because there is only one carbon labeled in carboxyl-labeled leucine, if it happens to decay in the solution, the product is not radioactive. With uniformly labeled amino acids, if one radioactive carbon decays (and it may sit and decay on the shelf for years), it becomes a nitrogen leaving a radioactive product that is no longer a natural amino acid. That product can then break up into other compounds, such as aldehydes. These radioactive amino acid decomposition products can sometimes be incorporated into protein or can take part in a number of contaminating reactions.

When you use radioisotopes to study chemical reactions, you must consider all of the factors that are peculiar to the use of radioisotopes. You cannot simply trace the label in the chemical reaction that you think you are measuring. An old biochemical principle demands that you always know and identify your precursor and your product.

I agree with you, Dr. Valcana, that different amino acids are transported differently. That is something that must be considered when you are studying protein synthesis *in vivo* in brain. You must be concerned about how that amino acid is getting into the pool in the brain and, in fact, whether you are dealing with the precursor pool for protein synthesis and not for some other reaction.

Valcana: I am familiar with the problems of contaminants, and the paper that describes this phenomenon. I have trusted the New England Nuclear Corporation's assay of the amino acids used in our study, but I have not done all of what you suggested. However, I find it difficult to believe that T_4 would stimulate the uptake of this specific decay product or contaminant of the amino acid, and not the amino acid itself. If true, the differences in radioactivity that we observe could reflect differences in breakdown products of amino acids in each case.

Sokoloff: First of all, you can trust New England Nuclear Corporation. They say that their radioactive compounds are better than 99% radioactively pure. But in your reaction you are incorporating 0.01% or less of your added radioactivity, so that 1% impurity contains more than enough counts to account for all of those that you incorporated. And if you chromatograph New England Nuclear Corporation's preparations, you will find that 99% of the radioactivity falls under the amino acid peak, but many other radioactive compounds comprise the remaining 1%.

Krawiec: Dr. Valcana, what is the meaning of the higher quantity of radioactivity being incorporated into protein by the hypothyroid brain as compared with the normal one?

Valcana: At this point, we do not know; we can only speculate. Perhaps we should look at permeability changes as well as catabolic processes before we conclude that protein synthesis is increased in the hypothyroid brain. As you have also suggested, these differences may simply reflect delays in the maturational decline in protein synthesis.

Ford: What occurs after you have injected labeled material into your organism, particularly tyrosine and leucine? What you are measuring afterwards is probably no longer all tyrosine or leucine. Only 45 or 50% of the label may continue to be associated with the original amino acid residue.

Valcana: With respect to leucine, you are absolutely right; it is quickly metabolized by brain tissue *in vitro*. Within the same time interval of 2 hr and in the same *in vitro* system, if tyrosine is substituted for leucine, 97% of the radioactivity in the acid-soluble pool remains tyrosine.

Ford: In an *in vivo* study, within an hour we found that at least 60% of the radioactivity was no longer associated with tyrosine but instead with virtually all the possible compounds to which tyrosine might contribute.

Valcana: That may be a discrepancy between systems *in vivo* and *in vitro*.

Ford: Might there be a decrease in turnover rate instead of an increase in the rate of the protein synthesis? In that case, nonlabeled amino acids in the precursor pool would not be exchanged as rapidly, and the label would then be maintained in the protein longer.

Balázs: Drs. Valcana and Timiras were the first to show that there is a depression in rate of cerebral protein synthesis in thyroid deficiency. Nevertheless, there are alternative explanations of their present results, and one has to keep an open mind until the various hypotheses have been tested.

I should like to raise a few questions. Everybody with some experience in the field will appreciate the difficulties in obtaining a valid estimate of the rate of protein synthesis, especially in the brain. Lajtha's group (Lajtha and Dunlop, 1974) has developed a neat technique for the estimation of rates of protein synthesis in the brain which seems to overcome one of the most formidable problems related to amino acid compartmentation. It is possible to determine the specific radioactivity of the free amino acids in the acid-soluble fraction, but this is not necessarily identical with the specific radioactivity of the particular pools that are involved in protein synthesis. That is why the new technique is promising: it involves the flooding of the amino acid pools with a large amount of the precursor amino acid. Consequently the specific radioactivity of the amino acid in each compartment approaches a uniform value. I would suggest that you check your results by using this method.

I would not place the same reliance on the results obtained in experiments *in vitro* and *in vivo*. It is not possible to compare the rates of protein synthesis *in vivo* and *in vitro* during the age period when your experiments were done (approximately the first 3 postnatal weeks), since the rate in slices decreases dramatically from day 1, whereas this is not the case *in vivo*. The precipitous fall in the rate with age is characteristic of the *in vitro* preparations, suggesting that certain factors are not under control.

Valcana: But those results were observed in a circumscribed time interval of a few days postnatally. In this study, we have a time interval of 13 to 42 days; within this period, there is a decline in protein synthesis in the *in vivo* system, too.

Balázs: But there is a great difference in degree. The results are expressed as a percentage of the rate of amino acid incorporation into protein at birth; they are less than 10% by the end of the third week, and the sharp fall occurs in the first 10 postnatal days.

Another question is the relevance of amino acid exchange *in vivo* in thyroid deficiency. In comparison with controls, the utilization of the precursor amino acid is reduced in the hypothyroid animal, primarily because of depressed rate of protein synthesis throughout the body. As a result, the concentration of the radioactive precursor amino acid in the blood is elevated, and the clearance of the amino acid from the blood is prolonged. It follows that the availability of the radioactive precursor to the brain is also elevated, and consequently the cerebral acid-soluble fraction will contain more radioactivity (mediated through exchange and/or net uptake) than that of the controls. The increased acid-soluble radioactivity in thyroid deficiency, therefore, is a consequence of the reduced utilization of the precursor in the body as a whole, rather than a reflection of a change in the rate of amino acid exchange between blood and brain.

Valcana: If the higher specific activity is a function of the depressed utilization in other parts of the body, then you should be able to compensate for this by examining results shortly after injection, in terms of the specific activity of the acid-soluble fraction, or else by using a system *in vitro* as we have done.

Balázs: The results may be explained by mechanisms other than exchange, such as differences between treated and untreated animals in the utilization of amino acids by the rest of the body.

You said that the rate of incorporation of labeled leucine into protein is slow relative to that of leucine oxidation. There must be some mistake, since 10 min after the injection of [U-^{14}C]leucine, about 50% of the total radioactivity has already been incorporated into protein, and only 15 to 30% is converted into intermediates of leucine catabolism (Patel and Balázs, 1975). Thus, the situation is just the opposite: the rate of leucine incorporation into protein is very fast, whereas that of leucine oxidation is relatively slow.

Valcana: I referred to the work of Dr. Ivan Diamond (*personal communication*).

Sokoloff: Dr. Diamond reported his work at the 5th Annual Meeting of the American Society of Neurochemistry. He was measuring leucine metabolism in adult brains. His observations do not apply to the brains of newborn animals.

DISCUSSION REFERENCES

Carter, W. J., Fass, F. H., and Wynn, J. (1971): Thyroxine stimulation of protein synthesis *in vitro* in the absence of mitochondria. *J. Biol. Chem.*, 246:4973–4977.

Lajtha, A., and Dunlop, D. (1974): Alterations of protein metabolism during development of the brain. In: *Drugs and the Developing Brain*, edited by A. Vernadakis and N. Weiner, pp. 215–229. Plenum, New York.

Patel, A. J., and Balazs, R. (1970): Manifestation of metabolic compartmentation during the maturation of the rat brain. *J. Neurochem.*, 17:955–971.

Sokoloff, L., and Roberts, P. A. (1974): Artifacts in studies of protein synthesis with radioactive amino acids. *J. Biol. Chem.*, 249:5520–5526.

Thyroid Hormones and Brain Development,
edited by Gilman D. Grave. Raven Press,
New York, 1977.

Effect of Thyroid Hormone and Undernutrition on Cell Acquisition in the Rat Brain

Robert Balázs*

This chapter considers the influence of thyroid deficiency on cell proliferation in the rat brain. Certain comparisons are also made with the effects of undernutrition which may complicate thyroid deficiency. Finally, we generalize on the mechanisms which may contribute to impaired functional brain development following exposure to metabolic insults during early life.

THYROID DEFICIENCY AND ITS EFFECTS ON POSTNATAL CELL ACQUISITION IN THE RAT BRAIN

Thyroid deficiency has a rather selective effect on postnatal cell acquisition in the cerebellum (Balázs, Kovács, Teichgräber, Cocks, and Eayrs, 1968). We have found that the postnatal rise in cell numbers in the forebrain was not affected significantly in comparison with controls, whereas in the cerebellum it was depressed, especially during the second week after birth; cell numbers were normal in the first week and again by day 35. In these experiments rats were thyroidectomized by a relatively high dose of radioiodine (^{131}I, 150 μCi) at birth. In order to minimize the possibility that the effects resulted from radiation damage to the brain, the experiments were repeated by inducing thyroid deficiency in the young by treating the mother rats with propylthiouracil from the 18th day of gestation throughout the experimental period. The new results confirmed our previous observations (Patel, Rabié, Lewis, and Balázs, 1976): the age course of DNA acquisition was significantly affected by thyroid deficiency in the cerebellum (Fig. 1a), although it was normal in the forebrain. In addition, the DNA content also was apparently irreversibly depressed in the olfactory bulbs of the hypothyroid animals.

These results are of interest because of certain peculiarities of postnatal cell formation in the brain. As a percentage of final cell numbers, cell acquisition after birth accounts for about 50% in the forebrain, 80% in the olfactory bulbs, and 97% in the cerebellum (Patel et al., 1976). Also, there is an important qualitative difference among these brain parts; most of

---

* MRC Developmental Neurobiology Unit, Medical Research Council Laboratories, Woodmansterne Road, Carshalton, Surrey SM5 4EF, England

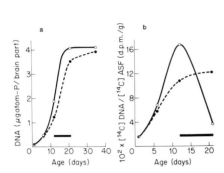

FIG. 1. Effect of thyroid deficiency on **(a)** the content of DNA-P per cerebellum, and **(b)** the incorporation of ^{14}C into total cerebellar DNA 30 min after the subcutaneous injection of $[2\text{-}^{14}C]$thymidine (15 μCi/100 g body wt); the values in **(b)** were corrected on the basis of the concentration of acid-soluble ^{14}C ($[^{14}C]$ASF). Thyroid deficiency in the young was induced by feeding daily 50 mg of propylthiouracil to mother rats by stomach tube from the 18th day of gestation throughout the suckling period. Four controls and four hypothyroid animals were studied at each age. Analysis of variance indicated that the age curves for the thyroid-deficient animals differed significantly from controls in both **(a)** and **(b)** ($p < 0.05$); the horizontal bars show the periods when the differences were significant. O———O, control; ●----●, hypothyroid animals. (From Patel et al., 1975.)

the cells formed during the postnatal period are glial cells in the forebrain (an important exception is the fascia dentata in the hippocampus), whereas neurogenesis is significant in the olfactory bulbs and the cerebellum (Altman, 1969). These findings, therefore, are consistent with the hypothesis that thyroid hormone is selectively required by the CNS for the genesis and/or maintenance of nerve cells.

We determined as an index of mitotic activity (Patel, Balázs, and Johnson, 1973), the labeling of DNA at 0.5 hr after subcutaneous administration of $[2\text{-}^{14}C]$thymidine. In comparison with controls, mitotic activity was significantly lower in the hypothyroid cerebellum at day 12, whereas it was 3 to 4 times higher at day 21. This sustained high mitotic activity (at a time when in controls active cell proliferation is just about to cease) accounts for the restoration in the thyroid-deficient cerebellum of normal cell numbers by 35 days of age.

The biochemical observations agree with the morphological findings of Legrand (1967), Hamburgh (1968), and Nicholson and Altman (1972), who have shown that the external granular layer (which is the major germinal site in the cerebellum) persists for a longer time than in controls. Concurrent observations in our laboratory show that the external granular layer is multicellular until about day 32 in treated animals, and is reduced only by day 35 to the same thickness as in 21-day-old controls (Lewis, Patel, Johnson, and Balázs, 1976).

We next analyzed the depressed rate of cell acquisition observed in the hypothyroid cerebellum from 7 to 21 days after birth (Fig. 1a). At day 12, when the total ^{14}C combined in DNA was less than in controls (Fig. 1b), the specific radioactivity of DNA was normal (corrected on the basis of the acid-soluble ^{14}C concentration). At this stage we investigated whether the conversion of [^{14}C]thymidine into thymidine nucleotides was impaired in the thyroid-deficient cerebellum (Patel et al., 1976).

Figure 2 shows that as a function of time, the concentration of acid-soluble ^{14}C at 2 hr and 4 hr fell to about 10% and 4%, respectively, of the value at 15 min after injection. Although these estimates were significantly elevated in the cerebellum of thyroid-deficient animals, the overall trend of decay was similar to that in controls. Further analysis indicated that the difference between the treated and untreated animals was mainly due to abnormally high [^{14}C]thymidine concentrations in the hypothyroid cerebellum (by 4 hr the difference was nearly threefold).

These changes are mainly attributable to increased and prolonged availability of [^{14}C]thymidine to the brain, resulting from a slower utilization of thymidine for DNA synthesis in the whole body in hypothyroid rats. In the brain, [^{14}C]thymidine metabolism was affected only slightly. At 15 min, in comparison with controls the concentration of [^{14}C]thymidine nucleotides was about 80%; later, it was similar or slightly elevated. Thus, although the initial decrease in [^{14}C]thymidine nucleotides suggests a slight

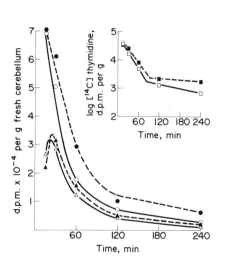

FIG. 2. Effect of thyroid deficiency on the kinetics of [^{14}C]thymidine metabolism in the cerebellum. We gave 14-day-old control and hypothyroid rats a subcutaneous injection of [2-^{14}C]thymidine and killed them by immersion into Freon at $-150°C$ at the times indicated in Fig. 2. Thymidine and thymidine nucleotides were separated by paper chromatography using the upper phase of ethyl acetate-formic acid-water (15:2:8 by vol) mixture as the solvent system.

The results are the mean of 2 to 3 animals at each time point; analysis of variance indicated that all curves for the hypothyroid rats differed significantly from controls ($p < 0.01$). The inset is a semilogarithmic plot of the decay curves of [^{14}C]thymidine in the cerebellum. The half-life ($t_{1/2}$) of the fast component calculated from the slope of the regression line was 15 min in controls and 22 min in thyroid deficiency ($p < 0.002$). Controls: concentration of acid-soluble ^{14}C, ○, and [^{14}C]thymidine nucleotides, △; logarithm of concentration of [^{14}C]thymidine, □. Hypothyroid animals: concentration of acid-soluble ^{14}C, ●----●, and [^{14}C]thymidine nucleotides, ▲----▲, and logarithm of concentration of [^{14}C]thymidine, ■----■. (From Patel et al., 1976.)

retardation in the rate of thymidine conversion, the whole time course—in agreement with the observations of Yamagami, Kiriike, and Kawakita (1973)—did not indicate a marked impairment in the supply of the proper precursor for DNA synthesis in the hypothyroid brain.

The depression in the rate of cell acquisition and of [^{14}C]DNA formation may result from a reduced rate of cell replication in the external granular layer, as proposed by Nicholson and Altman (1972). This hypothesis can be tested by constructing a "percentage labeled mitosis" (PLM) curve which, after proper analysis, provides estimates of cell cycle variables (reviewed by Cleaver, 1967). The assumption in this method is that the tissue is exposed to a pulse of the radioactive precursor. This, however, is never achieved *in vivo*, and the protracted availability of the labeled precursor results in distortions in the PLM curve leading to errors in the estimates of cell cycle variables. These limitations also apply to our present experiments. However, important information can be extracted from kinetic observations on [^{14}C]thymidine metabolism, with respect to the validity of the comparison of two experimental conditions, in terms of cell cycle variables based on the PLM method. The semilogarithmic plot of the concentration of [^{14}C]thymidine against time (Fig. 2) indicates that the decay has a fast and a slow component. The fast decay characterized approximately the first 80- and 95-min periods in controls and hypothyroid animals, respectively. It is important that the rise in the [^{14}C]DNA content of the cerebellum occurred only during this period. [^{14}C]DNA synthesis was rapid in controls in the first 30 min after [^{14}C]thymidine injection, but slowed considerably later. Although in the hypothyroid animals the rapid phase of [^{14}C]DNA synthesis lasted about 15 min longer than in controls, the [^{14}C]DNA content of the cerebellum in both treated and untreated rats reached a constant value by 60 min. Thus, although [^{14}C]thymidine was detectable beyond 1 hr, its ^{14}C concentration was too low to cause appreciable changes in the [^{14}C]DNA estimates. In order to compare the two experimental situations, the characteristics of the rapid decay of [^{14}C]-thymidine must be considered primarily: the half-life was increased only from 15 min in controls to 22 min in thyroid-deficient animals. Considering the time course of the concentration of [^{14}C]thymidine, [^{14}C]thymidine nucleotides, and [^{14}C]DNA, thyroid deficiency caused a displacement to the right on the time axis by about 15 min. Because the cell cycle time and the length of the DNA synthesis phase in the external granular layer are about 1,200 and 600 min, respectively, it is unlikely that the slight prolongation in the availability of [^{14}C]thymidine to the thyroid-deficient brain could introduce significant errors in comparison with controls in the estimation of cell cycle variables by the autoradiographic technique.

Investigation of the generation cycle of dividing cells in the external granular layer showed that thyroid deficiency had no significant effect on either the length of the cell cycle or on the duration of the DNA synthesis phase. However, there was a tendency for a slight, but not significant, prolongation of the doubling time of cells in the germinal zone because of a reduction of the labeling index (estimated 1 hr after [³H]thymidine injection; Lewis et al., 1976).

Thus far the results did not provide a lead concerning the mechanisms involved in the impairment of cell acquisition in the hypothyroid cerebellum in the second week after birth. Further studies, however, helped to elucidate such mechanisms (Lewis et al., 1976). An approximate comparison of numbers of replicating cells in the cerebellum of thyroid-deficient and control rats was made by estimating the cross-sectional area of the external granular layer and the packing density of cells in this layer. At day 12, the number of cells in the hypothyroid external granular layer was only two-thirds that in controls (Lewis et al., 1976). A similar reduction in the proliferative zone of the external granular layer has been observed by Nicholson and Altman (1972), whose results also indicated that the deficit in replicating external granule cells is confined to the second postnatal week in thyroid deficiency.

Certain reassuring agreements between the biochemical and morphological findings were observed. Although in comparison with controls, the area of the external granular layer was reduced in the 12-day-old hypothyroid rats, it constituted a similar proportion of the total cross-sectional area of the cerebellum. These observations are consistent with the biochemical findings: at day 12, the amount of [¹⁴C]DNA per cerebellum, i.e., the total number of replicating cells, was less than in controls, but the specific radioactivity of DNA, i.e., the proportion of cells in replication, was normal (Lewis et al., 1975*b*; Patel et al., 1975). It is not yet known how the deficit in replicating cells becomes established in thyroid deficiency. However, it is evident that a decrease in the number of proliferating cells results in a reduction in overall cell production, in spite of a normal rate of cell replication.

Another important factor in the decreased rate of cell acquisition is the effect of thyroid deficiency on the maintenance of cells in the cerebellum. The postnatal increase in cell numbers in the cerebellum relates to both the formation and the loss of cells. Experiments concerning the effect of thyroid deficiency on cell formation were extended to determine cell loss by estimating the proportion of degenerating cells (pyknotic index). The major effect was a transient and remarkable increase in cell degeneration in the internal granular layer; at 12 days of age the pyknotic index increased from a control value of about 0.1% to over 1.2%. The most abundant cells in this layer are the granule cells, which are formed in the external granular layer and migrate through the molecular layer to their final position below the Purkinje cells. In terms of differentiation, these cells are already irrevocably committed on arrival to the internal granular layer. Because the pyknotic indices were normal in both the external granular layer and the molecular layer at day 12, thyroid deficiency did not seem to affect adversely the replicating and migrating cells. It follows that certain conditions in thyroid deficiency are unfavorable for the survival of a specific fraction of differentiated cells.

The key to the understanding of the nature of such adverse conditions seems to be the influence of thyroid deficiency on the structural development of the cerebellar cortex. Significantly, the maturation of the Purkinje cells is severely retarded. At day 12, the dendritic arborization of these cells is less than half that of controls (Legrand, 1967). The axons of the granule cells, the parallel fibers, establish their most abundant synaptic contacts with the tertiary dendritic spines on the Purkinje cells (Eccles, Ito, and Szentágothai, 1967; Palay and Chan-Palay, 1974). The availability of synaptic sites for the parallel fibers is further reduced in thyroid deficiency by the marked decrease in the number of basket cells (Nicholson and Altman, 1972; Clos and Legrand, 1973). In accordance with the redundancy hypothesis of Hamburger and Levi-Montalcini (1949), it is proposed that death of a fraction of the granule cells is a consequence of a severe deficit in available postsynaptic sites for the termination of their axons. A similar mechanism has been suggested to operate in the developing cerebellum of "staggerer" mutant mice (Sotelo and Changeux, 1974).

We simulated the age curve of cerebellar DNA content in thyroid deficiency by assuming that the two factors, i.e., reduced number of germinal cells and enhanced loss of granule cells, are exclusively responsible for the decrease in cell number in the second week of life. The calculated shortfall in cell number was about 17% in the 14-day-old hypothyroid rat, which is somewhat less than the 25% deficit observed. Thus, other factors such as depressed output rates from the hypothyroid external granular layer may also be involved in the transient retardation in cell acquisition.

UNDERNUTRITION AND POSTNATAL CELL FORMATION

Another condition which causes retardation in the rate of postnatal cell acquisition in the brain is undernutrition during early life (Winick and Noble, 1966). Because this may color the symptoms of neonatal thyroid deficiency, we investigated its influence on cell formation in the rat brain (Patel et al., 1973; Lewis, Balázs, Patel, and Johnson, 1975).

We underfed mother rats, by giving them 50% of their usual feed from the 6th day of pregnancy throughout lactation (Chow and Lee, 1964). This resulted in reproducible growth retardation in the young, as in the studies of Altman, Das, Sudarshan, and Anderson (1971), who compared different techniques of undernutrition. We observed that the nutritional deprivation during gestation had no significant effect on brain growth, although the newborns were slightly smaller than controls. On the other hand, undernutrition during the suckling period resulted in a severe retardation in growth, also affecting the brain, although to a much smaller extent. Our results showed that by weaning there was about a 15% deficit in cell numbers in the brain, which seemed to persist (Dobbing and Smart, 1974).

We also found that, in contrast to this relatively small deficit, undernutrition had a powerful influence on the *in vivo* rate of DNA synthesis. Depending on age, this was depressed in comparison with controls, e.g., in the cerebellum by up to 70% (Table 1) (Patel et al., 1973). These results were surprising, because it would have been expected that the two estimates, both reflecting cell acquisition rates, should be influenced similarly. We have proposed three alternative mechanisms which may account for the apparent discrepancy (Balázs and Patel, 1973).

TABLE 1. *Effect of undernutrition on postnatal cell formation in the rat cerebellum*

Age (days)	(a) DNA content	(b) [^{14}C]DNA formation[a]	(c) Generation time	S-phase	G_1-phase
1	100	91	105	152	8
6	98	30	104	143	5
10 (12[b])	67	39	129	179	3
21	87	73	125	129	129

[a] Labeling of DNA per cerebellum was determined at 30 min after subcutaneous injection of 20 μCi of [2-^{14}C]thymidine.

[b] Cell cycle variables were estimated in 12-day-old rats.

Results are expressed as percent of control values: in (a) and (b) they refer to the mean of 4 undernourished and normal rats at each age (Patel et al., 1973) and in (c) to the median values derived from computer-generated curves (Steel and Hanes, 1971; we are indebted to Dr. Steel for these analyses) fitted to the percent labeled mitosis data from 16 treated and untreated animals at each age (Lewis et al., 1975). The results were analyzed by analysis of variance; significance of difference between the age curves of experimental and control groups (p) was <0.01 in (a) and (b). In (c) the data for the cerebellum and cerebrum were combined because the main effect of the "brain region" was not significant in any of the analyses: significance of difference between undernourished and corresponding control ($p < 0.05$) was observed at day 12 for generation time and at days 1, 6, and 12 for the length of both the S- and the G_1-phases of the cell cycle.

1. A compensation for the reduced mitotic activity may be provided by a decrease in the normal degree of cell loss. However, the proportion of degenerating cells was not lower than in controls, either in the germinal sites of the forebrain and the cerebellum (in fact, the pyknotic index was higher at 12 days of age; Lewis, 1975) or in sites containing differentiated cells, such as the internal granular layer in the cerebellum (Lewis, *unpublished observation*).

2. The *in vivo* rate of DNA synthesis is determined by the labeling of DNA after the administration of [^{14}C]thymidine. A depression in the rate of conversion of [^{14}C]thymidine into [^{14}C]thymidine nucleotides would result in a decrease in DNA labeling not necessarily paralleled by a decrease in cell

acquisition. Therefore, we studied the effect of undernutrition on the time course of [^{14}C]thymidine nucleotide synthesis at day 12 when a marked depression of DNA labeling is found (Patel et al., 1973). The results (*unpublished observations* by Patel, Balázs, and Lewis) indicated that the rate is slightly slower, because the peak incorporation of ^{14}C into thymidine nucleotides occurs 15 to 30 min later. However the supply of [^{14}C]thymidine nucleotides is high in the undernourished brain. Therefore, it seems unlikely that the slowing of the DNA labeling is a consequence of impaired [^{14}C]-thymidine nucleotide formation.

3. The rate of cell acquisition in an asynchronously replicating cell population is related to the cell cycle time or the doubling time of proliferating cells, whereas the rate of DNA synthesis is primarily a function of the length of the S-phase. The observed discrepancy between the effect of undernutrition on the rate of cell acquisition and the rate of DNA synthesis may be accounted for by a disproportionately greater prolongation of the S-phase than of the cell cycle time. The results support this hypothesis (Table 1; Lewis et al., 1975). In undernutrition, cell cycle time was affected only slightly, in contrast to the pronounced lengthening of the S-phase, which at day 12 was almost twice the normal value.

The relatively small effect of the treatment on cell cycle time, in spite of the pronounced prolongation of the DNA synthesis phase, resulted from a severe curtailment of the length of the G_1-phase. The latter effect may be of great importance. Certain processes which occur during a limited period in the G_1-phase have been claimed to be critical in terms of the final differentiation of some cells (Vonderhaar and Topper, 1974). It is possible, therefore, that the virtual elimination of the G_1-phase may affect the progeny of the dividing cells in the brain adversely.

COMPARISON OF THE EFFECTS OF UNDERNUTRITION AND THYROID DEFICIENCY

These two conditions evidently have distinct influences on cell acquisition in the brain during the postnatal period. The major differences are as follows:

1. In undernutrition, the rate of cell acquisition is depressed throughout the brain and during the whole postnatal period of treatment. On the other hand, the effects of thyroid deficiency seem to be confined to those parts of the brain where neurogenesis is significant after birth.

2. The rate of [^{14}C]DNA synthesis is markedly slowed throughout the brain in undernutrition during most of the postnatal period. In thyroid deficiency, [^{14}C]DNA formation is mainly reduced in the cerebellum and only in the second week after birth.

3. The most prominent difference between these two conditions lies in their effect on the generation cycle of the dividing cells. Undernutrition results in a marked prolongation of the S-phase of the cell cycle, whereas

the G_1-phase is curtailed drastically. In contrast, the generation cycle of replicating cells in thyroid deficiency is more or less normal. However, in both conditions, the total number of germinal cells, at least in the cerebellum in the second week of life, is less than in controls.

4. In thyroid deficiency, the shortfall in cell number in the cerebellum at the end of the normal period of active cell proliferation is compensated by high mitotic activity at day 21 which exceeds that at day 12 when, in untreated rats, cell replication is maximal (Fig. 1b). Furthermore, relatively pronounced cell multiplication proceeds for nearly 2 weeks longer in the external granular layer of hypothyroid rats than in controls. Similar changes are slight and short-lived in the undernourished brain (Lewis et al., 1975).

5. Finally, cell death in the major germinal sites in the external granular and the subependymal layers may account for about 3% of the newly formed cells in controls, and up to 8% in undernourished animals at day 12 (Lewis, 1975). The pyknotic indices for the hypothyroid animal, however, are normal. On the other hand, thyroid deficiency rather than undernutrition seems to be associated with cell degeneration in the internal granular layer, and accounts for the loss of about 1% of the total cerebellar cell population in 24 hr. Nevertheless, there are indications that differentiated cells in certain parts of the CNS are also lost in undernutrition (Dobbing, Hopewell, and Lynch, 1971).

There are also other differences between these two conditions in terms of both the biochemical and morphological manifestations of brain maturation. These have been reviewed by Patel and Balázs (1975) and Balázs, Lewis, and Patel (1975); some important aspects are also considered by other contributors in this volume.

POSSIBLE FUNCTIONAL CONSEQUENCES

Permanent changes in brain function may result from metabolic imbalance during the period of active brain development (Eayrs, 1964; Dobbing and Smart, 1974; Tizard, 1974). Although here we have emphasized interference with cell acquisition, this is only one factor that contributes to behavioral anomalies that may develop after various insults in early life. Effects on neuronal differentiation and the development of neuronal circuits are also important. Both undernutrition and thyroid deficiency influence these processes adversely (reviewed by Balázs, 1974; Balázs et al., 1975).

The functional effects of insults may depend, in part, on the time of interference with cell formation which, in turn, determines the cell types affected (Balázs, 1972a; Barnes and Altman, 1973). The rat cerebellum is a good model to indicate certain critical aspects of this hypothesis, because knowledge is relatively advanced concerning the timing of neurogenesis (Altman, 1969) and the role of the various nerve cells in the cerebellar circuits (Eccles et al., 1967; Palay and Chan-Palay, 1974). The Purkinje cells are the only efferent cells in the cerebellar cortex and are formed prenatally. The functioning of both the input and output systems is modulated by internal circuits in which the cerebellar interneurons play an important role. There is a strict chronological order in the formation of nerve cells in the CNS, and this also applies to the interneurons in the cerebellum (Altman, 1969). Among the inhibitory interneurons, the Golgi cells are formed first (perinatal period), followed by the basket cells (by the end of the first postnatal week), and finally the stellate cells are generated (in a rather sharp burst about the end of the second week). The only excitatory nerve cell, the granule cell, is the most abundant cell type in the cerebellar cortex; 50% of these cells are formed. The balance of the excitatory and inhibitory intracerebellar influences on the Purkinje cells is affected differently depending on whether the interference with cell formation occurs during the first 2 postnatal weeks (thus affecting the inhibitory interneurons) or in the third week (when the excitatory interneurons only would be affected). Furthermore, the localization of the synapses on the postsynaptic cell affects the efficiency of polarization of the cell by presynaptic stimulation (Rall, 1970). Thus an insult in the first postnatal week would lead to more drastic consequences than one in the second week, since the terminals of the basket cells are strategically localized on the lower part of the cell bodies and on the initial segments of the axons of Purkinje cells, whereas the synaptic sites of the stellate cells are on the dendrites of the Purkinje cells.

Powerful compensatory mechanisms operate in the developing brain to balance the adverse effects of the various insults. For example, in the hypothyroid cerebellum, although the rate of cell acquisition is retarded, normal cell number is ultimately reached because the period of extensive cell proliferation is prolonged. However, a compensation in cell numbers does not necessarily mean normal cell composition. In thyroid deficiency the number of basket cells is persistently reduced, whereas that of glial cells (especially Bergmann glia) is increased (Nicholson and Altman, 1972; Clos and Legrand, 1973). The results with respect to the basket cells are unexpected. In thyroid deficiency, the interference with cell acquisition is detected only after the first week of life, i.e., after the basket cells are usually formed. Balázs (1972b) and Nicholson and Altman (1972) have suggested that the "ontogenetic clock" is slower in the hypothyroid animal, and thus the formation and differentiation of the basket cells may occur after the first week. A contributing factor to basket cell deficit may be the retardation of the maturation of the Purkinje cells in thyroid deficiency, in terms of the longer persistence of the transitory climbing fiber synaptic contact on the soma of the Purkinje cells (Hajós, Patel, and Balázs, 1973). This may reflect changes in the properties of the Purkinje cell membrane. Thus, a fraction of the basket cells may be lost because of failure to make proper synaptic contact with the Purkinje cells.

Another example of the compensatory faculty of the developing CNS is observed in undernutrition when the lengthening of the S-phase is balanced partly by a severe curtailment of the G_1-phase of the cell cycle. However, it is not yet known if the virtual elimination of the G_1-phase in cells, which are at or near to their final division, will ultimately impair the expression of some of their differentiated functions.

Finally, there are powerful safety factors built into the structural design of the CNS as a result of convergence and divergence of neuronal interconnections and the abundant reiteration of neuronal circuits of the same function.

ACKNOWLEDGMENTS

I am happy to acknowledge the important contributions of Drs. P. D. Lewis (Royal Postgraduate Medical School, Hammersmith Hospital) and A. J. Patel (from our unit) to the reported work. I am also indebted to Dr. A. L. Johnson (MRC Statistical Research and Services Unit, University College, London) for his help in the statistical analysis of the results and to Dr. A. Rabié (Laboratoire de Physiologie Comparé, Montpelier) for his collaboration in a part of these studies and appreciate their permission to refer to unpublished results.

REFERENCES

Altman, J. (1969): DNA metabolism and cell proliferation. In: *Handbook of Neurochemistry*, edited by A. Lajtha, Vol. 2, pp. 137–182. Plenum, New York.

Altman, J., Das, G. D., Sudarshan, K., and Anderson, J. B. (1971): The influence of nutrition on neural and behavioural development. II. Growth of body and brain in infant rats using different techniques of undernutrition. *Dev. Psychobiol.*, 4:55–70.

Balázs, R. (1972a): Hormonal aspects of brain development. In: *The Brain in Unclassified Mental Retardation*, I.R.M.R. Study Group No. 3, edited by J. B. Cavanagh, pp. 61–72. Churchill, London.

Balázs, R. (1972b): Effects of hormones and nutrition on brain development. In: *Human Development and the Thyroid Gland—Relation to Endemic Cretinism*, Advances in Experimental Medicine and Biology, Vol. 30, edited by J. B. Stanbury and R. L. Kroc, pp. 385–415. Plenum, New York.

Balázs, R. (1974): Influence of metabolic factors on brain development. *Br. Med. Bull.*, 30:126–134.

Balázs, R., Kovács, S., Teichgräber, P., Cocks, W. A., and Eayrs, J. T. (1968): Biochemical effects of thyroid deficiency on the developing brain. *J. Neurochem.*, 15:1335–1379.

Balázs, R., Lewis, P. D., and Patel, A. J. (1975): Effects of metabolic factors on brain development. In: *Growth and Development of the Brain*, edited by M. A. B. Brazier, pp. 83–115. Raven Press, New York.

Balázs, R., and Patel, A. J. (1973): Factors affecting the biochemical maturation of the brain. Effect of undernutrition during early life. In: *Neurobiological Aspects of Maturation and Aging, Progress in Brain Research*, Vol. 40, edited by D. H. Ford, pp. 115–128. Elsevier, Amsterdam.

Barnes, D., and Altman, J. (1973): Effects of different schedules of early undernutrition on the preweaning growth of the rat cerebellum. *Exp. Neurol.*, 38:406–419.

Chow, B. F., and Lee, C. U. (1964): Effect of dietary restriction of pregnant rats on body weight gain of the offspring. *J. Nutr.*, 82:10–18.

Cleaver, J. E. (1967): *Thymidine Metabolism and Cell Kinetics.* North Holland, Amsterdam.

Clos, J., and Legrand, J. (1973): Effects of thyroid deficiency on the different cell populations of the cerebellum in the young rat. *Brain Res.,* 63:450–455.

Dobbing, J., Hopewell, J. W., and Lynch, A. (1971): Vulnerability of developing brain. VII. Permanent deficit of neurons in cerebral and cerebellar cortex following early mild undernutrition. *Exp. Neurol.,* 32:439–447.

Dobbing, J., and Smart, J. L. (1974): Vulnerability of developing brain and behaviour. *Br. Med. Bull.,* 30:164–168.

Eayrs, J. T. (1964): Effect of thyroid hormones on brain differentiation. In: *Brain-Thyroid Relationships,* CIBA Foundation Study Group No. 18, edited by M. P. Cameron and M. O'Connor, pp. 60–71. Churchill, London.

Eccles, J. C., Ito, M., and Szentágothai, J. (1967): *The Cerebellum as a Neuronal Machine,* Springer-Verlag, Berlin.

Hajós, F., Patel, A. J., and Balázs, R. (1973): Effect of thyroid deficiency on the synaptic organization of the rat cerebellar cortex. *Brain Res.,* 50:387–401.

Hamburger, V., and Levi-Montalcini, R. (1949): Proliferation, differentiation and degeneration in the spinal ganglia of the chick embryo under normal and experimental conditions. *J. Exp. Zool.,* 111:457–500.

Hamburgh, M. (1968): An analysis of the action of thyroid hormone on development based on *in vivo* and *in vitro* studies. *Gen. Comp. Endocrinol.,* 10:198–213.

Legrand, J. (1967): Analyse de l'action morphogénétique des hormones thyroïdiennes sur le cervelet du jeune rat. *Arch. Anat. Microsc. Morphol. Exp.,* 56:205–244.

Lewis, P. D. (1975): Cell death in the germinal layers of the postnatal rat brain. *Neuropathol. Appl. Neurobiol.,* 1:21–29.

Lewis, P. D., Balázs, R., Patel, A. J., and Johnson, A. L. (1975): The effect of undernutrition in early life on cell generation in the rat brain. *Brain Res.,* 83:235–247.

Lewis, P. D., Patel, A. J., Johnson, A. L., and Balázs, R. (1976): Effect of thyroid deficiency on cell acquisition in the postnatal rat brain: A quantitative histological study. *Brain Res.,* 104:49–62.

Nicholson, J. L., and Altman, J. (1972): The effects of early hypo- and hyperthyroidism on the development of rat cerebellar cortex. I. Cell proliferation and differentiation. *Brain Res.,* 44:12–23.

Palay, S. L., and Chan-Palay, V. (1974): *Cerebellar Cortex, Cytology and Organization.* Springer-Verlag, Berlin.

Patel, A. J., and Balázs, R. (1975): Factors affecting the development of metabolic compartmentation in the brain. In: *Metabolic Compartmentation and Neurotransmission,* edited by S. Berl, D. D. Clarke, and D. Schneider, pp. 363–383. Plenum, New York.

Patel, A. J., Balázs, R., and Johnson, A. L. (1973): Effect of undernutrition on cell formation in the rat brain. *J. Neurochem.,* 20:1151–1165.

Patel, A. J., Rabié, A., Lewis, P. D., and Balázs, R. (1976): Effect of thyroid deficiency on postnatal cell formation in the rat brain: A biochemical investigation. *Brain Res.,* 104:33–48.

Rall, W. (1970): Cable properties of dendrites and effects on synaptic location. In: *Excitatory Synaptic Mechanisms,* edited by K. S. Jansen, pp. 175–187. Universitetsforlaget, Oslo.

Sotelo, C., and Changeux, J.-P. (1974): Transsynaptic degeneration "en cascade" in the cerebellar cortex of staggerer mutant mice. *Brain Res.,* 67:519–526.

Tizard, J. (1974): Early malnutrition, growth and mental development in man. *Br. Med. Bull.,* 30:169–174.

Vonderhaar, B. K., and Topper, Y. J. (1974): A role of the cell cycle in hormone-dependent differentiation. *J. Cell Biol.,* 63:707–712.

Winick, M., and Noble, A. (1966): Cellular response in rats during malnutrition at various ages. *J. Nutr.,* 89:300–306.

Yamagami, S., Kiriike, N., and Kawakita, Y. (1973): Effect of neonatal thyroidectomy on thymidine metabolism and deoxyribonucleic acid synthesis in the developing cerebellum. *4th International Meeting of the International Society for Neurochemistry* (Tokyo), p. 430.

DISCUSSION

Lauder: At what ages did you determine the total number of proliferating cells in your animals?

Balázs: We usually did them at 6, 12, 14, and 21 days of age. The comparison of the number of proliferating cells between treated and untreated animals was done at 12 days of age, when the depression in cell acquisition rate seemed to be maximal.

Lauder: I would have expected, depending on the age, an increase in the number of proliferating cells, because they are sitting in the external granular layer (EGL) and proliferating.

Balázs: If you consider the age curve representing mitotic activity in terms of the rate of [^{14}C]thymidine incorporation into DNA (see Fig. 1b), at day 12 the activity in hypothyroid cerebellum is lower than in controls. However, after that age the rate falls precipitously in the controls, whereas it remains high in thyroid deficiency. Thus, the two age curves cross each other. By the end of the second and the beginning of the third weeks, in comparison with controls, the mitotic activities in the treated animals are similar, whereas later they are elevated.

Lauder: At 12 days in our hypothyroid animals the area of the proliferative zone of the EGL and the total number of proliferating cells in the EGL are also less than controls due to the retarded increase in the number of cells in this area (see Lauder, Fig. 4). I would like to compliment you for your very enlightening work on the cell cycle.

Timiras: I am surprised to find that, in speaking of the morphology of the cerebellum, no mention is made of the respective differences in the number of cells. In some species, there is one Purkinje cell per 1,400 granule cells.

Balázs: The ratio of granule cells to Purkinje cells in the adult rat cerebellar cortex is approximately 250:1 (Smolyaninov, 1971).

Timiras: Despite that large ratio, the granule cells might be destroyed or become pyknotic because they do not attach properly. I do not know the functional implication in view of the high ratio of granule to Purkinje cells. The second consideration is based on the case of the weaver or stagger mice, in which the granule layer is not present. By a special arrangement, the mossy fibers bypass the granule cell which is missing, synapse directly on the Purkinje cell, and provide the excitatory input directly to these cells.

Dr. Balázs, at a recent neurochemical meeting Dr. Bloom spoke of animals from your laboratory in which the granule layer had been completely destroyed by neonatal irradiation and in which the Purkinje cell looked as it does in the hypothyroid animal. When measured electrophysiologically, the Purkinje cell responded normally to various drugs. We concluded that even though the cell had lost its normal connections and was morphologically abnormal, it seemed to act normally at least in terms of electrophysiological and neurochemical responses. All of these considerations must be weighed when we interpret the functional consequences of morphologic alterations.

Balázs: I am glad that you raised the question of relationship between physical alterations in the brain and functional changes. I have proposed certain neurological mechanisms which may be instrumental in the impaired brain function which frequently develops after insults in early life: the emphasis being on *possible* mechanisms. Furthermore, there is an important quantitative aspect of this problem. How badly must the system be damaged in order to overtax the compensating faculties? Finally, functional deficiencies are usually the result of multiple defects in the system. Evidently, it is a formidable task to unravel the valid relationships. We are still far from fulfilling this aim, but at least we are able to identify certain biological mechanisms which *may* contribute to behavioral impairment. An important caveat is that the physical alterations which are observed, for example in thyroid deficiency, are not completely irreversible. We have experienced great difficulties in studying spontaneous reversibility, since our hypothyroid animals die relatively young. However, Eayrs (1971) has found that, although the behavioral deficit is persistent in the cretinous animal even when treated with thyroid hormone after weaning, some morphological alterations indicate a certain degree of reversibility. This discrepancy raises the question of identifying the valid correlations between physical variables and behavior.

Concerning your other comment, Dr. Timiras, Crepel (1974 and 1975) studied the electrophysiology of the cerebellar cortex in thyroid deficiency. The results indicate a delay in the maturation of the climbing fiber-Purkinje cell circuit. This correlates well with the longer persistence of the climbing fiber synapses on the soma of the Purkinje cells (Hajós, Patel, and Balázs, 1973). Crepel also observed that, in comparison with the climbing fiber-Purkinje cell circuit, the functional maturation of the mossy fiber-granule cell-Purkinje cell circuit is much more severely retarded, and this finding is also consistent with the relevant morphologic changes in thyroid deficiency. However, when rats were rendered hypothyroid in the first month after birth and made euthyroid for 4 months, restoration of the electrophysiological responses of the Purkinje cells was virtually complete. We do not know yet whether the reversal of the electrophysiological changes is accompanied by normalization of the ultrastructure of the cerebellar glomeruli.

Hamburgh: Dr. Balázs, you said that a large proportion of granule cells die out because they cannot make a synaptic connection with the Purkinje cells. However, other workers have evidence that it may be the other way around. It may be that the granule cells induce synaptic connections in the Purkinje cells. This system seems to be one of the least well ensured in development, because there are so many genetic mutants that affect granule cell migration and Purkinje cell arborization. Lack of granule cells in some mutants is accompanied by Purkinje cell abnormalities.

Altman: Dr. Balázs, you postulated that there is an interaction between parallel fibers and Purkinje cells at 12 days, but that might only represent the beginning of parallel fiber synaptogenesis.

Balázs: We were concerned with this problem and studied pyknotic indices in two parts of the cerebellum, in the nodule (which is part of the archicerebellum and develops earlier than the other part) and the paramedian lobule (part of the neocerebellum): The effect of thyroid deficiency on cell degeneration was similar in the two parts.

The puzzling observations in thyroid deficiency were that in the second postnatal week, the rate of cell acquisition was depressed in the cerebellum. Concomitantly, mitotic activity in terms of [^{14}C]DNA synthesis per cerebellum was also less than in controls. However, cell proliferation in terms of the variables of the cell cycle was normal.

We identified two factors involved in the impairment of cell acquisition in the hypothyroid cerebellum. (1) In the second postnatal week the total number of proliferating cells in the external granular layer was less than in controls. Thus, although cells replicated at the same rate, the overall increase in cell numbers was reduced, since the total number of replicating cells was less. (2) At the same time, the loss of granule cells was abnormally high in the thyroid deficient animal.

Lauder: You stated that the rate of cell proliferation, the length of the cell cycle, and the doubling time were not significantly different in the hypothyroid animals, yet the rate of cell acquisition was slower than controls. Could you explain this seemingly paradoxical situation?

Balázs: I can summarize briefly the different approaches we used to understand the retardation in cell acquisition rates in the cerebellum of hypothyroid animals in the second postnatal week. (1) The estimation of DNA content showed that cell number in the whole cerebellum was less than in controls. (2) At the age of 12 days we determined (as an index of mitotic activity) the labeling of DNA 30 min after a subcutaneous injection of [^{14}C]thymidine. The [^{14}C]DNA content per cerebellum was significantly depressed. This was a transient phenomenon, since at day 21 the [^{14}C]DNA content was about threefold higher than in controls as a result of the persistence of active cell proliferation in the cerebellum. (3) We established that the supply of [^{14}C]thymidine nucleotides in the cerebellum was not inadequate in thyroid deficiency. Furthermore, the availability of [^{14}C]thymidine to the brain was slightly increased because of the depression of mitotic activity in the whole body. In general, the changes in the kinetics of [^{14}C]thymidine metabolism were too small to affect significantly the estimation of the cell cycle variables by the auto-radiographic methods. (4) Cell cycle variables were estimated by determining the percentage of radioactively labeled mitoses (the PLM technique). The results showed no significant differences in either the cell cycle time or the length of the S-phase. This applied not only to the 12-day-old animals, but also to 6- and 21-day-old rats. (5) Labeling indices in the external granular layer were determined at 1 hr after [^{3}H]thymidine injection. The values were lower than in controls at all the ages studied (6, 12, and 21 days of age), but the differences were *not* significant. The doubling time was calculated on the basis of the formula, doubling time $= 100 \times$ length of S-phase/labeling index. The results indicated a prolongation of the doubling time. However, since this calculation was based on the labeling indices, which were not significantly different from controls, we cannot accept the prolongation in doubling time as significant. A much more extensive study would be required to establish whether this indication is valid.

Valcana: I would like to return to our previous discussion of whether the differential uptake of amino acids, as well as nucleotides by control and hypothyroid tissue, is due to changes in cell density as you propose or to differences in uptake of these substances *per se*. Changes in cell density are not responsible for the differential uptake of these substances. This is based on my finding that control tissue incubated in the presence of T_4 showed decreased uptake, whereas tissue from hypothyroid animals showed increased uptake of leucine.

Bass: What is the endogenous thymidine pool? We have a problem with pools that is important and can lead us to misinterpret the results.

Balázs: The time course of labeled thymidine metabolism did not indicate severe abnormalities in thyroid deficiency, and the concentration of thymidine nucleotides is normal according to the observations of Yamagami, Kiriike, and Kawakita (1973). Thus I feel that the evidence is sufficient and that there is no compelling reason to do further work to substantiate the claim that the reduction in cell acquisition rate in the second postnatal week is not the result of derangement of thymidine metabolism in the cerebellum.

Hamburgh: One question as to the relevance or the significance: You mentioned Eayrs' old paper where he reversed all the histological effects of hypothyroid brain but did not get any improvement in functional deficit. This was reported for the somatic sensory cortex. Are these morphologic changes irrelevant to the higher function in the cortex?

Altman: An answer to this may be that the chronology is important. You can get almost complete recovery in a number of granule cells if you stop irradiation early enough. Nevertheless, the animal's behavior will be markedly affected; the reason is that the interaction is now different because of abnormal time course.

And if you say that there are no physiological deficits, you have not yet used the right physiological measures, because the animal behaves abnormally.

Balázs: In the experiments of Eayrs (1971), the demonstration of recovery of brain structure by neurohistological techniques was not complete after treating neonatally thyroidectomized rats with thyroid hormone from day 24 or 70. There was a tendency for recovery, since the neurohistological methods indicated that, after replacement therapy, the brain was nearer to normal than without treatment; nevertheless, the probability of axo-dendritic interaction was still abnormal.

Hamburgh: You have to be very sophisticated to see any differences.

Balázs: We must be very cautious when proposing correlations between physical and behavioral effects.

DISCUSSION REFERENCES

Crepel, F. (1974): Excitatory and inhibitory processes acting upon cerebellar Purkinje cells during maturation in the rat: Influence of hypothyroidism. *Exp. Brain Res.,* 20:403–420.

Crepel, F. (1975): Hypothyroidism and cerebellum. *Brain Res.,* 85:157–160.

Eayrs, J. T. (1971): Thyroid and developing brain: Anatomical and behavioural effects. In: *Hormones in Development,* edited by M. Hamburgh and E. J. W. Barrington, pp. 345–355. Appleton-Century-Crofts, New York.

Hajós, F., Patel, A. J., and Balázs, R. (1973): Effect of thyroid deficiency on the synaptic organization of the rat cerebellar cortex. *Brain Res.,* 50:387–401.

Hámori, J. (1969): Development of synaptic organization in the partially agranular and in the transneuronally atrophied cerebellar cortex. In: *Neurobiology of Cerebellar Evolution and Development,* edited by R. Llinás, pp. 845–858. American Medical Association, Chicago.

Smolyaninov, V. V. (1971): Some special features of the organization of the cerebellar cortex. In: *Models of the Structural-Functional Organization of Certain Biological Systems,* edited by I. M. Gelfand, V. S. Garfinkel, S. V. Fomin, and M. L. Tsetlin, pp. 250–423. MIT Press, Cambridge, Mass.

Yamagami, S., Kiriike, N., and Kawakita, Y. (1973): Effect of neonatal thyroidectomy on thymidine metabolism and deoxyribonucleic acid synthesis in the developing rat cerebellum. 4th International Meeting, ISN, Tokyo, p. 543.

Thyroid Hormones and Brain Development,
edited by Gilman D. Grave. Raven Press,
New York, 1977.

Accelerated Appearance Of Cerebral D(−)-β-Hydroxybutyric Dehydrogenase in Hyperthyroidism

Gilman D. Grave*

D(−)-β-hydroxybutyric dehydrogenase (HO-BDH) is a ubiquitous NAD-dependent oxidative enzyme which is tightly bound to intramitochondrial membranes. It acquired a recent fascination when it became clear that the presence of this enzyme in brain tissue has enabled the human race to survive periods of famine by allowing the brain to derive energy by oxidizing stores of fat accumulated during periods of plenty.

The enzyme's substrate, β-hydroxybutyric acid, is an organic acid typically found, among other places, in rancid butter; it contains four carbon atoms, one of which is asymmetric (Fig. 1). The compound therefore exists as a pair of stereoisomers; although D(−)-β-hydroxybutyric acid belongs to Fisher's D series, the compound rotates light to the left (indicated by the minus (−) sign). Both stereoisomers exist in the mammalian body, but each is acted upon only by its stereospecific enzymes.

For the past several years we have studied the effects of L-thyroxine on HO-BDH of rat brain *in vivo* and *in vitro*. The presence of HO-BDH has been known in liver since Dakin (1910) described its action, and its presence in brain has been known since Quastel (1939) observed the oxidation of D(−)-β-hydroxybutyrate by slices of rat brain *in vitro*. But its crucial importance to brain metabolism in states of ketosis was not suspected until recently when George Cahill and his group (Owen, Morgan, Kemp, Sullivan, Herrera, and Cahill, 1967) starved three grossly obese patients for 40 days on the metabolic ward of the Peter Bent Brigham Hospital.

Because the human body's glucose reserves are only 300 g, barely enough to supply the energy requirements of the brain for 2 days, Dr. Cahill rightly suspected that ketone bodies were being metabolized by human brain tissue. As their enormous quantities of fat stores were catabolized, these patients became ketotic; their arterial levels of acetoacetate and D(−)-β-hydroxybutyrate rose from normal values of 0.04 and 0.08 mM to values of 1.2 and 6.6 mM, respectively. The mean arteriovenous difference of acetoacetate across the brain was found to be 0.06 mM, and that of D(−)-β-hydroxy-

---

* Developmental Biology and Nutrition Branch, National Institute of Child Health and Human Development, Bethesda, Maryland 20014.

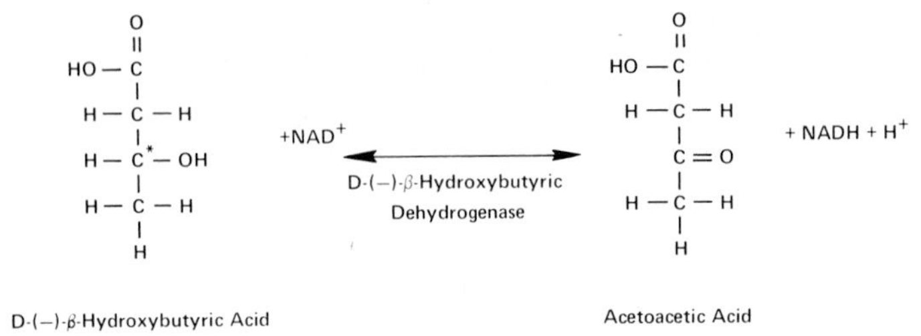

FIG. 1. Reversible reaction catalyzed by D(−)-β-hydroxybutyric dehydrogenase (EC 1.1.1.30). * = asymmetric carbon atom of β-hydroxybutyric acid.

butyrate 0.34 mM. In these ketotic, starved patients more than half of the brain's energy was being supplied by D(−)-β-hydroxybutyrate. This discovery astounded workers in the field of cerebral metabolism; until then it had been thought that the only significant energy-yielding substrate capable of being consumed by the brain was glucose (Kety, 1957; Sokoloff, 1960; Reinmuth, Scheinberg, and Bourne, 1965).

In the nine years that have elapsed since this discovery by Cahill and his group, the metabolism of the ketone bodies has been well documented by Sokoloff and his group in this country (Klee and Sokoloff, 1967; Sokoloff, 1972, 1973) and by Krebs and his group in England (Hawkins, Williamson, and Krebs, 1971; Page, Krebs, and Williamson, 1971; Page and Williamson, 1971).

These groups have demonstrated that in states of ketosis, acetoacetate and β-hydroxybutyrate are produced by the liver, released into the bloodstream, and utilized by the brain as well as by other peripheral tissues. HO-BDH enables the brain to oxidize the relatively large quantities of D(−)-β-hydroxybutyrate that are presented to the brain in ketosis. Several workers have now shown that the ketone bodies are utilized by the brain in direct proportion to their concentration in arterial blood (Hawkins et al., 1971; Krebs, Williamson, Bates, Page, and Hawkins, 1971; Spitzer and Weng, 1972; Persson, Settergren, and Dahlquist, 1972).

The brain utilizes these substrates as they become available, and the higher the concentration of the ketone bodies in arterial blood, the more they are catabolized by the brain.

The presence of HO-BDH in brain enables mammals to rely on D(−)-β-hydroxybutyrate as the major source of cerebral energy during starvation ketosis. When fat stores are catabolized, the equilibrium of the reversible reaction catalyzed by HO-BDH (Fig. 1) is shifted to the left, and D(−)-β-hydroxybutyrate appears in arterial blood at six times the concentration of acetoacetate, instead of twice the concentration normally found.

At the same time that Dr. Cahill was starving his 3 patients in Boston, Drs. Louis Sokoloff and Claude Klee at NIH were discovering that a homogenate of adult rat brain was not an adequate ATP-generating system for protein synthesis *in vitro* when β-hydroxybutyrate was used as a substrate, although succinate or α-ketoglutarate were more than adequate (Klee and Sokoloff, 1967). Subsequently, they found that homogenates of brain of younger rats (about 25 days old) were able to oxidize β-hydroxybutyrate three times faster than those of adult rats, and that immature rat brain could serve as an adequate ATP-generating system even when β-hydroxybutyrate was used as the substrate. This observation led to their working out the unique age curve of the activity of this enzyme, which rises sixfold from a low level at birth to a peak at weaning and then gradually drops off in adulthood to about one-third its peak activity (Fig. 2).

Fazekas, Graves, and Alman (1951) showed that thyroxine (T_4) augments oxidative metabolism in immature mouse brain, and Hamburgh and Flexner (1957) found that succinic dehydrogenase activity is low in immature hypothyroid rats but can be brought to normal levels by thyroid replacement during the critical first 3 weeks of life. In view of these demonstrations of the effect of T_4 on oxidative metabolism and oxidative enzymes in young brain, we sought to discover if T_4 accelerated the development of the unique maturational pattern of cerebral D(−)-β-hydroxybutyric dehydrogenase.

METHODS

Detailed methodologies concerning use of chemicals and animals, preparation of brain homogenates, assay of HO-BDH activity, and chemical determinations of brain DNA, RNA, and proteolipid protein have been reported elsewhere (Grave, Kennedy, and Sokoloff, 1972; Grave, Satterthwaite, Kennedy, and Sokoloff, 1973). Three separate series of experiments were performed, each with a different dosage of Na$^+$-L-T$_4$. In the first series of experiments (I), each of three litters of Sprague-Dawley newborn rat pups were divided randomly into control and experimental animals. The

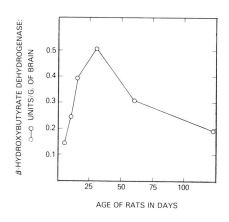

FIG. 2. Characteristic maturational curve of activity of D(−)-β-hydroxybutyric dehydrogenase in brain of rats. (Adapted with permission from Klee and Sokoloff, 1967, Fig. 1.)

latter received 10 μg of T_4 subcutaneously every 48 hr. Pairs of control and experimental rat pups were selected at 3, 6, 9, 13, 17, and 20 days of post-natal age for assay of brain HO-BDH activity. These experimental animals become thyrotoxic from the high dose of T_4 employed, and both their body and their brain growth lagged behind those of the controls (Fig. 3). Similar effects were observed by Balázs, Kovacs, Cocks, Johnson, and Eayrs (1971) with comparable doses of triiodo-L-thyronine.

A second series of experiments (II) was performed in which a lower dosage of T_4 was used, one less likely to exhibit the catabolic actions of the hormone. These experimental animals received 10 μg of Na^+-L-T_4 sub-cutaneously every 72 hr. This dosage schedule still accelerated eye-opening, righting, startle, and placing reflexes, but did not affect body or brain weights (Fig. 3). At twelve different ages between birth and 70 days, two pairs of control and experimental animals were removed for biochemical studies of their brains.

A third series of experiments (III) was carried out in order to compare two procedures (see below) for assaying the activity of HO-BDH in the

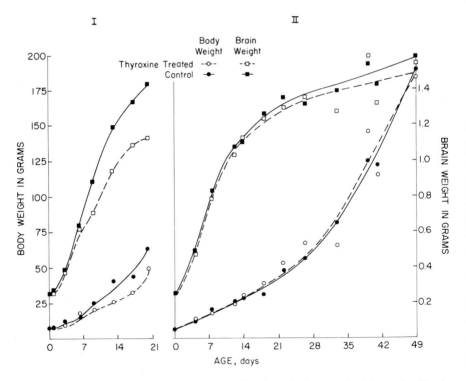

FIG. 3. Effects of exogenously administered L-T_4 (thyroxine) on postnatal growth of body and brain of rat in two different experiments (I and II) with different dosage schedules of L-T_4. (Reproduced with permission from Grave et al., 1973, Fig. 1.)

same brain preparations from both control and hyperthyroid rats across the age span. In this third series the experimental animals received 10 μg of T_4 every 48 hr for the first 6 days and every 72 hr thereafter. Pairs of control and hyperthyroid animals were removed at six different ages between 8 and 66 days for assay of brain HO-BDH activity.

Activity of HO-BDH was assayed by oxidation of D($-$)-β-hydroxybutyrate (Fig. 1); the acetoacetate produced was measured by an adaptation (Wadkins and Lehninger, 1963) of the method introduced by Walker (1954). This method is elegant and highly specific; it takes advantage of a reaction discovered nearly a century ago by Victor Meyer in which a reactive methylene group situated between two keto groups couples with aromatic diazo compounds to form intensely yellow compounds called formazans (Fig. 4). The reaction proceeds to completion at room temperature in the presence of minute quantities (as little as 10 nmoles) of acetoacetate. The only other common organic compounds that have such reactive methylene groups are oxaloacetic and malonic acids.

In Series I and II, the enzyme assay reaction mixture consisted of 0.11 M sucrose; 0.044 mM EDTA; 0.015 M potassium phosphate buffer, pH 7.4; 5.9 mM $MgCl_2$; 0.029 M sodium DL-β-hydroxybutyrate; and 0.75 ml of fresh whole brain homogenate containing 4.5 to 9.0 mg of protein (depending on the age of rat) in a total volume of 1.7 ml. The oxidation reaction was started by adding the DL-β-hydroxybutyrate and was halted by adding 1.7 ml of 5% (w/v) trichloroacetic acid. Incubations were done in 25-ml Erlenmeyer flasks shaken at 92 oscillations/min in a water bath maintained at 37°C.

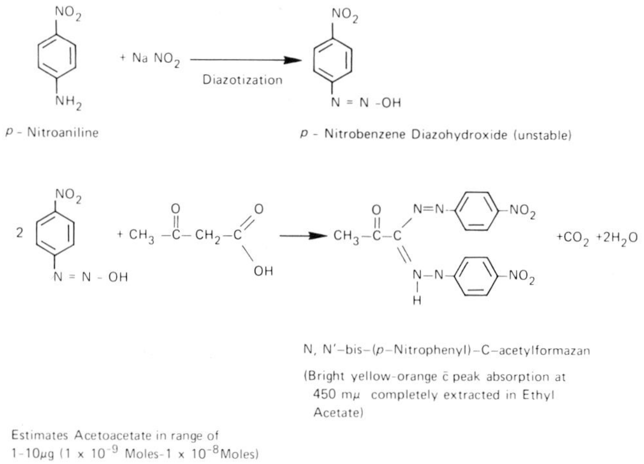

FIG. 4. Reaction of acetoacetate with p-nitrobenzene diazohydroxide which produces N,N'-bis-(p-nitrophenyl)-C-acetylformazan. This reaction is assayed by absorption spectrophotometry.

The time of the incubation was 10 min, well within the linear range of the reaction.

During the course of the experiments in Series I and II, we learned that considerable latent enzyme activity could be released from the fresh homogenates by freezing and thawing (Pull and McIlwain, 1971); after this treatment, however, the reaction exhibited an absolute dependence on added NAD^+. The experiments in Series III were done with an assay system modified to incorporate these findings. In the new assay, 0.25 ml of frozen-thawed homogenate (containing 1.5 to 3.0 mg of protein) at a saturating level of NAD^+ (2.0 mM) were used in the reaction mixture detailed above.

Each brain homogenate in Series III was assayed in parallel flasks with the earlier assay for comparison. Enzyme activity of the same brain preparations in the new assay system was a mean of 1.8 times that of the earlier assay. This ratio was not affected by the age of the rat nor by treatment with T_4. The results of the enzyme assays in Series I and II were then normalized to those of Series III by multiplying them by this experimentally determined factor of 1.8.

RESULTS

All three schedules of T_4 administration produced signs of hyperthyroidism within 48 hr of the second injection. The experimental animals became tremulous and hyperactive, and their rate of maturation accelerated dramatically. Eye opening occurred in every T_4-treated rat by day 12 instead of the usual 14 to 17 days required by untreated rat pups. Advancement of the appearance of eye opening in hyperthyroid rat pups has been described previously (Morton and Fahn, 1955) and has been shown to exhibit a classic log-dose response (Khamsi and Eayrs, 1966).

The high dose of T_4 used in Series I caused a marked retardation of body and brain growth (Fig. 3-I), which became increasingly apparent with advancing age. T_4, however, caused a more rapid rise in level of activity of HO-BDH in the brain tissue with increasing age (Fig. 5-I).

In Series II the lower dose of T_4 caused no significant effects on body or brain growth (Fig. 3-II). Nor were there any detectable effects on the DNA, RNA, and total protein contents of the brain, although a significantly more rapid accumulation of proteolipid protein was found in the T_4-treated animals [$p < 0.01$ (Grave et al., 1973)]. The effects on the age-dependent activity of HO-BDH were nearly identical to those found in Series I (Figs. 5-I and 5-II). T_4 hastened the entire pattern of postnatal development of activity of this unique mitochondrial oxidative enzyme in the brain. T_4 accelerated both the rise in HO-BDH activity to its peak in the suckling rat and the decline from the peak following weaning. In Series III the effects of hyperthyroidism on the activity of HO-BDH in the brain were the same as those noted in Series II (Figs. 5-II and 5-III).

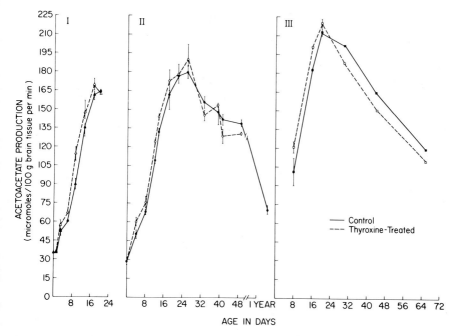

FIG. 5. Effects of administration of L-thyroxine (T_4) from birth on the postnatal development of D(−)-β-hydroxybutyric dehydrogenase activity in the rat brain in I, II, III (I and II refer to animals in Series I and II of Fig. 3). In all three series, acceleration of the rise of enzyme activity by T_4 was statistically significant on the basis of multivariate profile analysis. The f and p values for Series I, II, and III were, respectively, $f = 148.1$, $p < 0.001$; $f = 21.3$, $p < 0.005$; $f = 27.1$, $p < 0.05$. The effect of T_4 on the descending phase was statistically insignificant in Series II ($f = 2.24$, $p > 0.05$). Because the number of animals was insufficient for multivariate profile analysis in the descending phase of Series III, Student's t-test was employed, which indicated significantly lower values for enzyme activities in the T_4-treated animals ($t = 7.15$; $p < 0.02$). (Reproduced with permission from Fig. 2, Grave et al., 1973).

DISCUSSION

These studies reconfirm that neurophysiologic precocity can be induced by hyperthyroidism in the immediate postnatal period. Eye opening, appearance of righting, placing, and startle reflexes, and attainment of neuromuscular agility are all advanced by administration of T_4. In all three series of experiments the dosage of T_4 employed shifted the unique maturational pattern of cerebral HO-BDH activity to the left by 2 days, thus providing another biochemical correlate of the dramatic acceleration of neurological precocity produced by a hyperthyroid state during postnatal development of the mammalian brain.

In order to ascertain if the effect of T_4 on cerebral HO-BDH was truly maturational and not simply a direct enhancement of enzyme activity, we experimented with the effects of a range of T_4 concentrations on brain homogenates and cerebral mitochondrial preparations *in vitro*. Not only was no enhancement of enzyme activity noted, but instead a pronounced inhibition of oxidation of β-hydroxybutyrate was observed in the flasks containing T_4, even at saturating levels of substrate and coenzyme. The degree of inhibition did not vary across the age span, and the effect was clearly concentration-dependent on T_4. The inhibitory effect responded to T_4 in a log-dose manner over a range of concentrations of the hormone from 6.5×10^{-9} M to 6.5×10^{-5} M. The properties and mechanism of this inhibitory effect are presently under study, and preliminary results have been recently reported (Grave, Fitzgerald, and Sokoloff, 1975). Wolff and Wolff (1957) observed a similar inhibitory effect of T_4 on five other NAD^+-linked dehydrogenases. β-Hydroxybutyric dehydrogenase bears a striking similarity to malic dehydrogenase in its enzymatic behavior in the presence of T_4.

In view of the direct inhibition of HO-BDH *in vitro*, we may conclude that the effect on this cerebral enzyme produced *in vivo* by exogenous T_4 is truly maturational; i.e., during the first 25 days of postnatal life the activity of the HO-BDH of the hyperthyroid animals is specifically augmented 2 days earlier than normal and, moreover, that the activity of the enzyme is specifically decreased earlier than usual after weaning. The fact that the acceleration of the maturational pattern of the activity of HO-BDH by T_4 was documented under conditions in which no changes in total brain protein were observed indicates a high degree of specificity for the effects of the hormone on this enzyme. The site of action of T_4 in producing this maturational effect is unknown, but it would appear that T_4 enhances specifically the production of this oxidative enzyme in growing mammalian brain.

In summary, T_4 appears to have two different and independent effects on cerebral HO-BDH. On the one hand, it accelerates the maturational pattern of the enzyme; but at the same time it seems to exert a distinct control on its activity. These apparently contradictory actions enhance the appeal and the mystery of this protean hormone.

REFERENCES

Balázs, R., Kovacs, S., Cocks, W. A., Johnson, A. L., and Eayrs, J. T. (1971): Effect of thyroid hormone on the biochemical maturation of rat brain: Postnatal cell formation. *Brain Res.,* 25:555–570.

Dakin, H. D. (1910): The formation in the animal body of *l*-β-oxybutyric acid by the reduction of aceto-acetic acid. *J. Biol. Chem.,* 8:97–104.

Fazekas, J. F., Graves, F. B., and Alman, R. W. (1951): The influence of the thyroid on cerebral metabolism. *Endocrinology,* 48:169–174.

Grave, G. D., Kennedy, C., and Sokoloff, L. (1972): Impairment of growth and development of the rat brain by hyperoxia at atmospheric pressure. *J. Neurochem.,* 19:187–194.

Grave, G. D., Satterthwaite, H. S., Kennedy, C., and Sokoloff, L. (1973): Accelerated postnatal development of D(−)β-hydroxybutyric dehydrogenase activity in the brain in hyperthyroidism. *J. Neurochem.,* 20:495–502.

Grave, G. D., Fitzgerald, G., and Sokoloff, L. (1975): Inhibition of activity of rat brain D(−)β-hydroxybutyric dehydrogenase by thyroid hormones *in vitro. Trans. Am. Soc. Neurochem.,* 6:203 (abstract).

Hamburgh, M., and Flexner, L. B. (1957): Physiological differentiation during morphogenesis, XXI. Effect of hypothyroidism and hormone therapy on enzyme activities of the developing cerebral cortex of the rat. *J. Neurochem.*, 1:279–288.

Hawkins, R. A., Williamson, D. H., and Krebs, H. A. (1971): Ketone-body utilization by adult and suckling rat brain *in vivo. Biochem. J.*, 122:13–18.

Kety, S. S. (1956): The general metabolism of the brain *in vivo*. In: *The Metabolism of the Nervous System*, edited by D. Richter, p. 221. Pergamon Press, London.

Khamsi, F., and Eayrs, J. T. (1966): A study of the effects of thyroid hormones on growth and development. *Growth*, 30:143–156.

Klee, C. B., and Sokoloff, L. (1967): Changes in D(−)β-hydroxybutyric dehydrogenase activity during brain maturation in the rat. *J. Biol. Chem.*, 242:3880–3883.

Krebs, H. A., Williamson, D. H., Bates, M. W., Page, M. A., and Hawkins, R. A. (1971): The role of ketone bodies in caloric homeostasis. *Adv. Enzyme Regul.*, 9:387–409.

Morton, D. L., and Fahn, S. (1955): Acceleration of maturation of newborn rats by thyroxine. *Anat. Rec.*, 121:410 (abstract).

Owen, O. E., Morgan, A. P., Kemp, H. G., Sullivan, J. M., Herrera, M. G., and Cahill, G. F., Jr. (1967): Brain metabolism during fasting. *J. Clin. Invest.*, 46:1589–1595.

Page, M. A., Krebs, H. A., and Williamson, D. H. (1971): Activities of enzymes of ketone-body utilization in brain and other tissues of suckling rats. *Biochem. J.*, 121:49–53.

Page, M. A., and Williamson, D. H. (1971): Enzymes of ketone-body utilization in human brain. *Lancet*, 2:66–68.

Persson, B., Settergren, G., and Dahlquist, G. (1972): Cerebral arteriovenous difference of acetoacetate and D-β-hydroxybutyrate in children. *Acta Paediatr. Scand.*, 61:273–278.

Pull, I., and McIlwain, H. (1971): 3-Hydroxybutyrate dehydrogenase of rat brain on dietary change and during maturation. *J. Neurochem.*, 18:1163–1165.

Quastel, J. H. (1939): Respiration in the central nervous system. *Physiol. Rev.*, 19:135–183.

Reinmuth, O. M., Scheinberg, P., and Bourne, B. (1965): Total cerebral blood flow and metabolism. *Arch. Neurol.*, 12:49–66.

Sokoloff, L. (1960): Metabolism of the central nervous system *in vivo*. In: *Handbook of Physiology, Section 1, Neurophysiology*, p. 843. Waverly Press, Baltimore.

Sokoloff, L. (1972): Circulation and energy metabolism of the brain. In: *Basic Neurochemistry*, edited by R. W. Alberts, B. Agranoff, R. Katzman, and G. J. Seigel, pp. 299–325. Little, Brown, Boston.

Sokoloff, L. (1973): Metabolism of ketone bodies by the brain. *Ann. Rev. Med.*, 24:271–280.

Spitzer, J. J., and Weng, J. J. (1972): Removal and utilization of ketone bodies by the brain of newborn puppies. *J. Neurochem.*, 19:2169–2173.

Wadkins, C. L., and Lehninger, A. L. (1963): In: *Methods in Enzymology*, edited by S. P. Colowick and N. O. Kaplan, Vol. III, p. 265. Academic Press, New York.

Walker, P. G. (1954): A colorimetric method for the estimation of acetoacetate. *Biochem. J.*, 58:699–704.

Wolff, J., and Wolff, E. C. (1957): The effect of thyroxine on isolated dehydrogenases. *Biochim. Biophys. Acta*, 26:387–396.

DISCUSSION

Valcana: In the early stages of development, is the acceleration an induction phenomenon or some other indirect effect of T_4 on the enzyme?

Grave: T_4 in excessive concentrations makes animals ketotic. An early hypothesis was that the ketosis might induce the enzyme or perhaps preserve it, but this hypothesis was shown to be incorrect by Grave et al. (1973).

Sokoloff: We do not know the mechanism of the induction, but T_4 appears to inhibit HO-BDH directly as well as to accelerate the appearance of increased enzymatic activity in the brain during the maturational period. It may be more than fortuitous that this double effect takes place. As Dr. Baláuzs mentioned, the utilization of ketone bodies by brain is important during the immediate postnatal period. When the animal is first born, it has low levels of the enzymes which metabolize ketone bodies. As soon as the rat (which has been studied most extensively) starts to nurse, it becomes ketotic because its maternal milk is ketogenic. It also becomes hypoglycemic, so it depends on ketone bodies as its substrate for energy metabolism. If thyroid hormone (which is high in the animal at that time) inhibits this enzyme, it would inhibit a major source of energy production. Thus, it is fortunate that the tissue makes more enzyme, possibly to compensate for the partial inhibition of the enzyme that is present. Peak enzyme activity occurs at 22 days of age, at weaning. When the young rats are weaned onto a nonketogenic diet, the ketosis disappears and the brain begins to use glucose as its major substrate. It no longer depends on the utilization of ketone bodies, and activity and/or the amount of HO-BDH declines. In some way, nature has coordinated the dietary changes that occur in this animal and the enzyme levels in the brain that use these substrates.

Valcana: Does the metabolism of ketone bodies by the brain depend only on the circulating levels of ketone bodies and not on production of ketone bodies by brain?

Sokoloff: That is right. They are made mainly in liver.

Valcana: Is it established that there is no ketone body formation by brain?

Sokoloff: It would be a trivial amount compared to that produced by the liver.

Grave: Most of the ketone bodies are produced in the liver, which cannot metabolize them, and are released into the blood. The liver lacks acetyl Co-A succinyl transferase that the brain has in abundance.

Kollros: What would happen if the rat were weaned to a different diet. Does the level of HO-BDH depend on what the rat eats?

Sokoloff: If you wean animals at 22 days of age onto an artificial diet that simulates maternal milk, then the level of HO-BDH also falls, but not nearly as fast as normally. If you wean the animals prematurely at about 10 days of age onto a synthetic maternal milk diet, the enzyme level stays high. If you wean them at 10 days of age to a diet high in carbohydrate, then the enzyme level falls prematurely. There is some relationship between the dietary intake, the level of ketone bodies in the blood, and the enzyme level, at least during this part of the animal's life.

We have been interested in discovering the mechanism that regulates the level of the enzyme in the brain. Is it a matter of change in the rate of synthesis or degradation of the enzyme? One really should study this by pulse-labeling of the enzyme and using specific antibodies to study whether it is being synthesized or degraded.

Dr. Fitzgerald has been trying to purify the enzyme enough to get specific antibodies. She managed to purify the enzyme partially, but has not purified it enough to produce highly specific antibodies. I would like to know the molecular mechanisms of this regulation by diet and T_4.

Timiras: As I recall, the fetus is relatively hypoglycemic. Should we expect the enzyme activity to be so low at birth?

Grave: It is indeed low at birth, and it rises sixfold within the first 3 weeks of life.

Hamburgh: Is the rise linear from birth, or is there a long lag period?

Grave: There is no lag at all. It rises linearly throughout the first 3 weeks of postnatal life.

Hamburgh: Was there no lag period between the first dose of T_4 and the increase in enzyme activity?

Grave: The first T_4 effect was sampled at 3 days, and at this time we observed a significant effect. We would have had to sample within those first 3 days to find a lag.

Hamburgh: Would you not think that this increase in HO-BDH activity is just another expression of a general effect on protein synthesis?

Grave: I think that more molecules of HO-BDH are produced in neonatal hyperthyroidism; other cerebral enzymes probably experience a similar rise in concentration and activity. In order to achieve the augmented activity in the face of the inhibition engendered by T_4 more enzyme must be made.

Bass: The concentrations of T_4 used in order to inhibit the enzyme *in vitro* were fairly high. Would you equate it to the situation *in vivo?*

Grave: I measured an inhibition of activity by 3% *in vitro* at a T_4 concentration of 6.5×10^{-9} M at saturating levels (2.94×10^{-3} M) of NAD. *In vivo* there is 1,000 times less NAD available. Therefore, we would predict much greater inhibition *in vivo* because the inhibition is inversely related to the NAD concentration.

Valcana: This inhibition by T_4 on enzymatic activity *in vitro* is not necessarily found only in dehydrogenases. Opposite effects *in vivo* and *in vitro* have also been demonstrated with other enzymes. When ATPase is assayed *in vitro* in the presence of T_4 at the doses you have used, we also observe inhibition of enzymatic activity.

Grave: What happens when you use concentrations of 10^{-8} M or 10^{-9} M?

Valcana: Nothing; at 10^{-6} M one sees some inhibition, and at 10^{-5} M and above, inhibition is quite detectable.

Grave: Do you ever observe increased activity at !ow levels of T_4?

Valcana: No, not *in vitro,* but *in vivo* we do.

Sokoloff: We had the same experience with the ion-stimulated ATPase: *in vitro* inhibition, but *in vivo* augmentation.

DISCUSSION REFERENCE

Grave, G. D., Satterthwaite, H. S., Kennedy, C., and Sokoloff, L. (1973): Accelerated post-natal development of D(−)β-hydroxybutyric dehydrogenase activity in the brain in hyperthyroidism. *J. Neurochem.,* 20:495.

Thyroid Hormones and Brain Development,
edited by Gilman D. Grave. Raven Press,
New York, 1977.

Influence of Neonatal Hypothyroidism
on Brain RNA Synthesis

Leon Krawiec,* Carlos A. Montalbano,*,** Beatriz H.
Duvilanski,* Alicia E. R. de Guglielmone,* and
Carlos J. Gómez*

During the normal maturation of the rat brain there are important changes
in the levels of DNA, RNA, and structural proteins, with concomitant
variations in the activity of different enzymes. These modifications are
mediated, at least partially, by normal thyroid function, because thyroidectomy immediately after birth prevents normal development of the brain
(Pasquini, Kaplun, Garcia Argiz, and Gomez, 1967; Garcia Argiz, Pasquini,
Kaplun, and Gomez, 1967; Krawiec, Garcia Argiz, Gomez, and Pasquini,
1969).

Furthermore, Faryna de Raveglia, Gomez, and Ghittoni (1972) observed
a decrease in the lipid content of the cerebral cortex in this condition and a
transitory decrease of cephalin and lecithin. In view of the importance of
lipids as myelin components, their diminished synthesis could explain the
deficient myelination of the thyroidectomized rat.

These alterations appear about the second week of postnatal life, showing
that there is a critical period during which the thyroid hormone is important
for the normal maturation of the brain (Krawiec et al., 1969). The principal
effect of thyroid function on enzymatic activity represents a hormonal
induction of *de novo* synthesis of protein rather than a simple activation of
the enzymes. The hormone is also active in the formation of structural
components of the membranes. This increase in protein synthesis reflects
an action of thyroid hormone on either transcription or translation.

SYNTHESIS OF RNA IN VIVO

The earliest effect of neonatal thyroid deficiency is an alteration in the
cerebral metabolism of RNA (Gomez, Duvilanski, Soto, and Guglielmone,
1972). In brains of normal 10-day-old rats, the incorporation *in vivo* of
labeled precursor into nuclear RNA increases almost linearly during the
first hour after the injection of the isotope and then levels off (Table 1).

* Departamento de Química Biológica, Facultad de Farmacia y Bioquímica, Universidad de
Buenos Aires, Junín 956, Buenos Aires, Argentina.
** Fellowship from the Consejo Nacional de Investigaciones Científicas y Técnicas, Argen-
tina.

TABLE 1. *Effect of neonatal thyroidectomy on the incorporation of labeled precursor into nuclear RNA*

Time after injection (hr)	Nuclear RNA (RSR)		
	Normal		Hypothyroid
0.33	71.4 ± 2.1	$p < 0.001$	43.2 ± 3.7
1	162.9 ± 5.4	$p < 0.001$	103.7 ± 9.6
2	182.8 ± 10.8		175.3 ± 10.7
4	172.5 ± 9.9		179.9 ± 9.3
24	214.5 ± 18.7	$p < 0.005$	440.2 ± 37.1

The results were obtained after the subarachnoidal injection of 2 μCi of [^{3}H]orotic acid in 10-day-old normal and neonatally hypothyroid rats. Each value represents the mean ±SEM of 5 experiments. Results from normal and hypothyroid rats were compared by Student's *t*-test, and the *p* value is included only when the difference is significant. RNA = ribonucleic acid; RSR = relative specific radioactivity. RNA extraction and purification from subcellular fractions carried out as described by Gomez et al. (1972).

Because the total radioactivity of the initial homogenate depends on the amount of the injected precursor, the incorporation of the isotope into the RNA of subcellular fractions is related in each experiment to the total radioactivity of the initial homogenate. Thus, the results are expressed as relative specific radioactivity (RSR), the ratio between the specific radioactivity of RNA in each fraction (disintegrations/min/mg of RNA) and that of the initial homogenate (disintegrations/min/mg of wet tissue).

During the first 60 min, the RSR of nuclear RNA in hypothyroid brain is about 40% lower than that of the RNA in normal brain, and after 2 and 4 hr the values are the same in both groups of animals. Twenty-four hours after the injection, the RSR of nuclear RNA from hypothyroid brain is twice as high as that of the normal brain.

In both normal and hypothyroid rats, the incorporation of the labeled precursor, [^{3}H]orotic acid, into brain microsomal RNA is almost linear throughout the period studied (Table 2).

During the first 4 hr, the incorporation is significantly lower (35 to 45%) in hypothyroid than in normal brain RNA, and this difference disappears 24 hr after the injection of the labeled precursor. The differences obtained during the first hour suggest that neonatal thyroidectomy markedly decreases the synthesis of "rapidly labeled" RNA, and the results in longer periods suggest an altered transport of newly formed RNA from the nucleus to the microsomes. This is further supported by comparing the changes of the incorporation ratio between nuclear and microsomal RNA. During the first hour after the injection, this ratio is not significantly different in normal and hypothyroid rats (Table 3), but it is markedly higher in hypothyroid rats at longer times.

TABLE 2. *Effect of neonatal thyroidectomy on the incorporation of labeled precursor into microsomal RNA*

Time after injection (hr)	Microsomal RNA (RSR)		
	Normal		Hypothyroid
0.33	2.00 ± 0.12	$p < 0.005$	1.09 ± 0.14
1	7.50 ± 0.24	$p < 0.001$	4.89 ± 0.34
2	11.80 ± 0.71	$p < 0.01$	7.07 ± 0.18
4	25.5 ± 1.4	$p < 0.02$	17.2 ± 1.8
24	122.1 ± 11.3		113.4 ± 10.7

Each value represents the mean ±SEM of 5 experiments. Experimental conditions and statistical comparison as in Table 1.

The gradient analysis of the nuclear RNA in normal brains shows that the highest RSR in the heaviest region of the gradient (which involves a large DNA-like RNA) was reached during the first hour; then the radioactivity decreased rapidly and linearly. In hypothyroid brain, both the rates of synthesis and degradation of this RNA are delayed. These differences indicate at least two alterations: one during transcription and the other in posttranscriptional processes.

Although these experiments demonstrate an alteration in the synthesis of "rapidly labeled" RNA and in the posttranscriptional regulatory mechanisms, it is difficult to establish the type of RNA which is affected, as well as the reversibility of this process. In looking for an answer to these questions, we studied the effects of neonatal thyroidectomy on the incorporation *in vivo* of tritiated orotic acid into acid-soluble uridine nucleotides, nuclear RNA, and microsomal RNA of the rat brain at 10 and 30 days of age.

At 10 days of age (Fig. 1) the ^3H content of the acid-soluble uridine nucleotides is almost the same in both the normal and hypothyroid cerebrum.

TABLE 3. *Ratio of relative specific radioactivity of nuclear RNA to microsomal RNA at different intervals after injection of [^3H]orotic acid*

Time after injection (hr)	Normal	Hypothyroid	p value
0.33	35.7 ± 3.0	39.6 ± 3.3	N.S.
1	21.7 ± 0.9	21.2 ± 0.9	N.S.
2	15.6 ± 1.0	24.3 ± 0.8	<0.001
4	6.78 ± 0.33	10.54 ± 0.97	<0.01
24	1.79 ± 0.15	3.90 ± 0.41	<0.01

Each value represents the mean ±SEM of 5 experiments. Experimental conditions and statistical comparison as in Table 1.

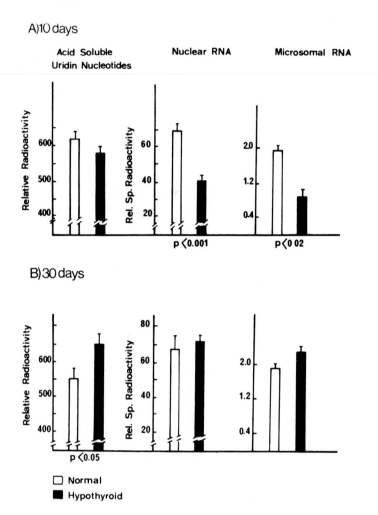

FIG. 1. Labeling of acid-soluble metabolites and of nuclear and microsomal RNA in 10- and 30-day-old rat brain. Acid-soluble uridine nucleotides were obtained from the total homogenate as described by Ramirez de Guglielmone and Duvilanski (1972). Other technical details as described by Gomez et al. (1972).

In normal rats, at 30 days after birth the cerebral metabolism of orotate is similar to that observed at 10 days.

In hypothyroid 30-day-old rats there is a slight increase in the content of soluble pyrimidines with respect to normal animals of the same age. On the 10th postnatal day the incorporation of [³H]orotic acid into nuclear and microsomal RNA is about 40% lower in hypothyroid than in normal rats, thus confirming previous results. However, on the 30th day, the rate of synthesis of nuclear and microsomal RNA is the same in the cerebrum of normal and hypothyroid rats.

Thus, thyroid deficiency affects only transiently RNA synthesis in developing brain, and suggests that the alteration observed at day 10 is a consequence of a transcriptional defect. This view is supported by the fact that alterations in RNA metabolism occur with only minor changes in the formation of labeled uridine nucleotides. Others (Balázs, Kovacs, Teichgräber, Cocks, and Eayrs, 1968; Geel and Valcana, 1971) have shown that the lack of thyroid function does not affect the pool size of cerebral uridine nucleotides.

SYNTHESIS OF RNA IN VITRO

Different molecular species of RNA polymerases exist in the cell nuclei of mammals. Those species show differences in the requirements for divalent cations, in their nuclear localization, and in the type of RNA they synthesize (Pogo, 1969; Roeder and Rutter, 1970). RNA polymerase type I is a magnesium-dependent enzyme. It has a nucleolar localization and promotes the transcription of a GC-type RNA or ribosomal RNA. RNA polymerase type II depends on the presence of manganese. It has a nucleoplasmic localization and promotes the synthesis of an AU-type RNA, presumably messenger RNA. We studied the activity of these two RNA polymerases in isolated nuclei from the brain of normal and neonatally thyroidectomized rats in order to establish which type of RNA is affected, and to confirm the transitory character of the alteration in RNA synthesis. Assays were done in a medium of relatively low ionic strength, which preserves the morphological integrity of the nuclei, using magnesium or manganese as divalent cations. In this way, the different functions are preserved, which represent different stages of interactions with a multimolecular complex involving all chromosomal and nucleolar components (Sirlin, 1972). This enabled us to study changes in priming efficiency. In another condition, the ionic strength was increased in the presence of the two divalent cations, thus producing nuclear lysis and disrupting the multimolecular structure, leading to the loss of the probable regulatory mechanisms.

The reaction does not require an ATP-generating system and shows the typical characteristics of a DNA-primed RNA synthesis, in that it is dependent on the presence of the four ribonucleoside triphosphates and is strongly inhibited by DNase and pyrophosphate. The acid-insoluble product of the reaction is hydrolized by RNase but not by DNase. The presence of 50 mm NaCl in the low-ionic-strength medium enhances the precursor incorporation and improves the UMP/GMP ratio of the product, confirming previous studies made by Pogo (1969) and Gomez et al. (1971). When the assays are done at low ionic strength and at 37°C, the nucleotide incorporation is linear for only 2 min and levels off at 10 min. This is in agreement with the observations of Glasser, Chytil, and Spelsberg (1972), who ascribe this fact to the action of nucleases present in the nuclei.

Taking into consideration the observations of Chambon, Ramuz, Mandel, and Doly (1968), who demonstrated the negligible nuclease activity at 15°C, we tested the enzyme activity at this temperature under the three conditions described (Fig. 2). The incorporation was linear for at least 30 min. For this reason we incubated for 15 min at 15°C and found that the nucleotide incorporation is proportional to the amount of nuclei added to the incubation mixture up to 100 μg of DNA (Fig. 3). Fifty to 80 μg of DNA per assay were used in all the experiments.

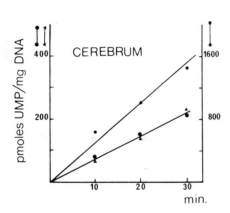

FIG. 2. Kinetics of [³H]UMP incorporation in RNA of isolated cell nuclei of rat brain. The nuclei were isolated by a modification of the method of Glasser et al. (1972). The incubation mixture contained with a final volume of 0.25 ml: 40 mM Tris-HCl, pH 8.0; 1.6 mM 2-mercaptoethanol; 0.6 mM of each unlabeled nucleotide, and 0.1 mM of the labeled nucleotide, corresponding to 1 μCi of [³H]UTP or [³H] GTP. 0.050 ml of nuclear suspension containing 50 to 80 μg of DNA was added to the incubation mixture. When polymerase I was measured, the low-ionic-strength medium also contained 5 mM MgCl₂ and 50 mM NaCl; for the assay of polymerase II, 1.6 mM MnCl₂ was used instead of MgCl₂. The high-ionic-strength medium contained the basic constituents and 2 mM MgCl₂, 1.6 mM MnCl₂, 8 mM KCl, and 0.24 M (NH₄)₂SO₄. Other technical details as described by Gomez et al. (1971). ● = low ionic strength, Mg²⁺; ▲ = low ionic strength, Mn²⁺; ★ = high ionic strength.

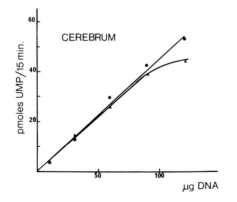

FIG. 3. Effect of nuclear concentration on the [³H]UMP incorporation in RNA. Technical details are the same as in Fig. 2. ● = low ionic strength, Mg²⁺; ▲ = low ionic strength, Mn²⁺.

CHARACTERIZATION OF THE NEWLY SYNTHESIZED RNA

We studied the influence of different media on newly formed RNA by assaying the same nuclear preparation under different ionic conditions. We measured the relative incorporation of radioactive uridine and guanosine monophosphate (UMP and GMP) in the presence of the other three unlabeled nucleotides (Pogo, 1969). At low ionic strength and in the presence of magnesium, the U/G ratio of 0.5 to 0.7 suggested the formation of a product resembling ribosomal RNA. When manganese was used instead of magnesium, there was an upward shift of the U/G ratio reaching a value of 1.0 to 1.2, which corresponds to a DNA-like product.

At a high ionic strength, with the addition of ammonium sulfate, magnesium, and manganese together in the same incubation mixture, the pre-

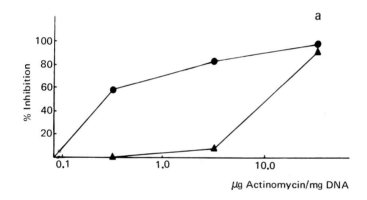

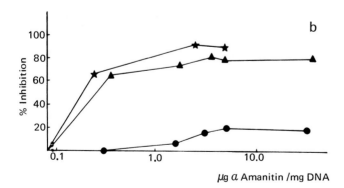

FIG. 4. Effect of different concentrations of actinomycin D **(a)** and α-amanitin **(b)** on RNA synthesis in isolated cell nuclei of rat brain. [³H]GMP incorporation was measured at low ionic strength and in the presence of Mg^{2+} (●) whereas [³H]UMP was measured in the presence of Mn^{2+} (▲) or at high ionic strength (★). Other details as in Fig. 2.

cursor incorporation into RNA increased two to three times, and the U/G ratio was greater than 1.0.

In order to confirm that the RNA formed was of the GC or AU type, we studied the *in vitro* effects of α-amanitin and actinomycin D. In the magnesium-low ionic strength medium with 3 μg/mg of DNA of actinomycin D (at this concentration a selective inhibitor of the ribosomal RNA synthesis), the nucleotide incorporation decreased by 80% (Fig. 4). Under the same conditions, if manganese is used instead of magnesium, there is no inhibition.

α-Amanitin, 1.8 μg/mg of DNA (a specific inhibitor of RNA polymerase II), decreased the incorporation at low ionic strength in the presence of manganese by 70% and 90% with ammonium sulphate. On the other hand, there was little effect of α-amanitin on the enzyme activity in a magnesium-low ionic strength medium.

From these results we can infer that when the isolated nuclei are tested in an isosmotic condition, it is possible to measure the endogenous activity of both polymerases I or II with a template in which most of the regulatory mechanisms are maintained. But when the nuclei are exposed to high concentrations of ammonium sulfate, most of the nuclear DNA becomes available for transcription; however, in these conditions, the incorporation does not indicate the template efficiency of the intact nuclei.

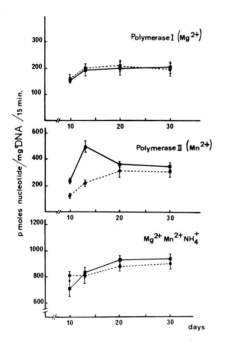

FIG. 5. Changes in RNA synthesis in isolated cell nuclei in normal and hypothyroid rat brain. Methods were as in Fig. 2. Each value represents the mean ±SEM of 5 to 7 experiments. Results from normal and hypothyroid rats were compared by Student's *t*-test. When the differences were significant, the *p* value was lower than 0.005. ■———■ normal; ●---● hypothyroid.

EFFECTS OF THE NEONATAL THYROID DEPRIVATION ON THE RNA POLYMERASES ACTIVITIES IN ISOLATED CELL NUCLEI OF RAT BRAIN

The transcription capacity for the GC-type RNA increases slightly during the normal development of the rat brain, reaching a plateau at 13 days after birth (Fig. 5). These changes are not affected by thyroid deprivation. On the other hand, the ability of nuclei to transcribe an AU-rich RNA increases at an early stage of normal maturation, attaining its maximum at 13 days and declining thereafter.

Between 10 and 13 days of postnatal life we detected an important decrease in the activity of RNA polymerase II (45 to 50%) produced by the lack of thyroid hormone. When assays were done in high-ionic-strength medium, the enzyme activity increased during the first 20 days after birth and was not affected by the absence of thyroid function.

In all cases, the U/G ratio characteristics of each incubation condition were the same for normal and hypothyroid rats (Table 4).

TABLE 4. *U/G ratio of incorporation in isolated cell nuclei of normal and hypothyroid rat brain*

Enzyme	Age (days)	Normal	Hypothyroid
Polymerase I	10	0.58 ± 0.07	0.60 ± 0.08
	13	0.61 ± 0.07	0.64 ± 0.06
	20	0.62 ± 0.11	0.65 ± 0.10
	30	0.63 ± 0.09	0.67 ± 0.12
Polymerase II	10	1.00 ± 0.08	1.07 ± 0.10
	13	1.10 ± 0.13	1.05 ± 0.09
	20	1.11 ± 0.12	1.17 ± 0.13
	30	1.16 ± 0.13	0.98 ± 0.12
Mg^{2+}-Mn^{2+}-$(NH_4)_2SO_4$	10	0.92 ± 0.11	1.21 ± 0.10
	13	1.06 ± 0.13	1.01 ± 0.12
	20	1.29 ± 0.11	1.16 ± 0.14
	30	1.16 ± 0.10	1.05 ± 0.09

Each value represents the mean $\pm$SEM of 5 to 7 experiments. Results were compared by Student's *t*-test, and the differences were not significant. U = uridine monophosphate; G = guanosine monophosphate.

CONCLUSIONS

The only alteration observed in RNA synthesis *in vitro* by brain cell nuclei of hypothyroid rats is a marked depression in the transcription of a DNA-like RNA. This decrease is only transient. This effect agrees with the results obtained *in vivo* with neonatally thyroidectomized rats, in which the synthesis of the rapidly labeled RNA is depressed at 10 but not at 30 days of age.

We conclude that one of the effects of thyroid hormone on the maturation of the brain is stimulation of the synthesis of a messenger-type RNA during a critical period of brain development.

ACKNOWLEDGMENT

This work was supported by grants from the Consejo Nacional de Investigaciones Científicas y Técnicas (1003d) and the Instituto Nacional de Farmacología y Bromatología (Argentina).

REFERENCES

Balázs, R., Kovacs, S., Teichgräber, P., Cocks, W. A., and Eayrs, J. T. (1968): Biochemical effects of thyroid deficiency on the developing brain. *J. Neurochem.*, 15:1335–1349.

Chambon, P., Ramuz, M., Mandel, P., and Doly, J. (1968): The influence of ionic strength and a polyanion on transcription *in vitro*. I. Stimulation of the aggregate RNA polymerase from rat-liver nuclei. *Biochim. Biophys. Acta*, 157:504–519.

Faryna de Raveglia, I., Gomez, C. J., and Ghittoni, N. E. (1972): Hormonal regulation of brain development. V. Effect of neonatal thyroidectomy on lipid changes in cerebral cortex and cerebellum of developing rats. *Brain Res.*, 43:181–195.

Garcia Argiz, C. A., Pasquini, J. M., Kaplun, B., and Gomez, C. J. (1967): Hormonal regulation of brain development. II. Effect of neonatal thyroidectomy on succinate dehydrogenase and other enzymes in developing cerebral cortex and cerebellum of the rat. *Brain Res.*, 6:635–646.

Geel, S. E., and Valcana, T. (1971): Cerebral RNA metabolism and thyroid function in early life. In: *Influence of Hormones on the Nervous System*, edited by D. H. Ford, pp. 165–173. S. Karger, Basel.

Glasser, S. R., Chytil, F., and Spelsberg, T. C. (1972): Early effects of oestradiol-17β on the chromatin and activity of the deoxyribonucleic acid-dependent ribonucleic acid polymerases (I and II) of the rat uterus. *Biochem. J.*, 130:947–957.

Gomez, C. J., Duvilanski, B. H., Soto, A. M., and Guglielmone, A. E. R. (1972): Hormonal regulation of brain development. VI. Kinetic studies on the incorporation *in vivo* of (^{3}H) orotic acid into RNA of brain subcellular fractions of 10-day-old normal and hypothyroid rats. *Brain Res.*, 44:231–243.

Gomez, C. J., Garcia Argiz, C. A., Franzoni, L., and Krawiec, L. (1971): Ribonucleic acid synthesis in isolated cell nuclei of developing rat brain. *Neurobiology*, 1:129–143.

Krawiec, L., Garcia Argiz, C. A., Gomez, C. J., and Pasquini, J. M. (1969): Hormonal regulation of brain development. III. Effects of triiodothyronine and growth hormone on the biochemical changes in the cerebral cortex and cerebellum of neonatally thyroidectomized rats. *Brain Res.*, 15:209–218.

Pasquini, J. M., Kaplun, B., Garcia Argiz, C. A., and Gomez, C. J. (1967): Hormonal regulation of brain development. I. The effect of neonatal thyroidectomy upon nucleic acids, protein and two enzymes in developing cerebral cortex and cerebellum of the rat. *Brain Res.*, 6:621–634.

Pogo, A. O. (1969): Modification of ribonucleic acid synthesis in isolated rat liver nuclei by low salt concentration and specific divalent cations. *Biochim. Biophys. Acta*, 182:57–65.

Ramirez de Guglielmone, A. E., and Duvilanski, B. (1972): RNA metabolism in brain of suckling normal and hypothyroid rats. *Experientia*, 28:1101–1103.

Roeder, R. G., and Rutter, W. J. (1970): Specific nucleolar and nucleoplasmic RNA polymerases. *Proc. Natl. Acad. Sci. (USA)*, 65:675–682.

Sirlin, J. L. (1972): In: *Biology of RNA*. Academic Press, New York.

DISCUSSION

Hamburgh: You tend to equate the term DNA-like RNA with messenger RNA. The two are not synonymous.

Krawiec: Yes, it is better to say heterogeneous RNA. I call it DNA-like because the U/G ratio is greater than 1.0. Jacob and Mandel named this kind of RNA DNA-like. Scherrer, Latham, and Darnell (1963), Stevenin, Mandel, and Jacob (1969), and Soeiro and Darnell (1970) demonstrated the same U/G ratio for the heterogeneous nuclear RNA and the messenger-like cytoplasmic RNA.

Hamburgh: Out of the total RNA, the component that is DNA-like is probably very small. Looking for a specific messenger RNA is like looking for a needle in a haystack if one uses quantitative determination.

Krawiec: I commented on cerebral RNA polymerase, but we also studied the same phenomenon in the liver. In this tissue, the RNA polymerase II is altered throughout the period studied (from birth until 30 days of life). The RNA polymerase I is not altered at the beginning, but is diminished in the hypothyroid rat at 20 and 30 days of life. Besides, the activity at high ionic strength has the same pattern as the RNA polymerase I. We have no clear explanation for this latter result. We can assume that in liver the process is different from that in brain. In the brain, the alteration is only transitory, between 10 and 13 days, but in the liver it continues and involves not only the RNA with the U/G ratio of 1 but also involves the ribosomal RNA, but in another period.

Geller: There have been reports that adrenocorticoids cause an increase in RNA polymerase in the liver. In a hypothyroid situation you might have increased circulating levels of adrenocorticoids which could be stimulating liver RNA polymerase.

Hamburgh: It will be very exciting if at least some of your DNA-like RNA proves to be messenger RNA. Transcription proceeds from different sites at different stages. The very fact that at a given time, e.g., 10 or 11 days postnatally, RNA levels decrease indicates that certain messengers may be missing. That might be the specific effect we keep hoping to find in hypothyroidism.

Valcana: Dr. Krawiec, how would you explain the high specific activity for uridine or other precursors at 3 days of age in the acid-soluble pool, in the absence of changes in the pool in terms of nucleotides?

Krawiec: There are differences in the radioactivity at 20 min in the rats at 30 days of age. The acid-soluble radioactivity of the hypothyroid brain is twice normal, but only at 20 min. In the other cases, at 10 days and at 30 days, we find no differences.

Valcana: But Geel showed that high specific activity is not associated with differences in the nucleotide pool. Do you have any explanation?

Krawiec: There may be some degradation of RNA and reutilization of the metabolites in the hypothyroid brain. Another reason may be that a decreased cerebral vascularity would diminish the diffusion of precursors out of the brain.

Balázs: I did not quite understand how you corrected for the differences in the amount of precursor entering the brain. Am I right in thinking that the relative specific radioactivity was the ratio of the specific radioactivity of RNA to the total radioactivity in the homogenate? You have been using tritiated precursors; in that case, a significant proportion of the radioactivity in the tissue must be tritiated water. How can you include tritiated water in the correction which, instead of correcting for local uptake will reflect metabolism of the precursor in various organs, followed by distribution of labeled water throughout the body?

Krawiec: That is correct; the expression is disintegrations per minute per milligram of RNA divided by disintegrations per minute per milligram of wet tissue. The most important results occur in a short period of time, and during that short interval the exchange between the radioactive product and the water is minimal. But if this exchange occurs, it will affect normal and hypothyroid pools equally. There is another point: when we performed thin-layer chromatography of the nucleotides, the bulk of the radioactivity was in the uridine nucleotides. We suppose that in 24 hr it is very difficult to eliminate this error.

Balázs: I understand that you must apply a correction. However, when dealing with tritiated precursors you have a problem. If you want to correct for the variation due to the intracerebral injection technique in the simple way you have described, you must use either ^{14}C precursors, in which case the error due to redistribution of label will be smaller or, preferably, you must isolate your precursor from the tissue.

Krawiec: We did it when we studied the uridine metabolism, in which there were no differences, but this was 20 and 60 min after injection.

Sokoloff: We have already discussed the importance of the specific activity of the immediate precursor pool in radioactive studies in terms of protein synthesis (see Discussion, Chapter 16). But, this applies equally to all other reactions studied by radioactivity, including this one. You did not find any effect around 10 days on the polymerase I which makes the ribosomal-like RNA. Yet, this is a period during the development of the brain when there is increasing ribosomal RNA. How do you account for that?

Krawiec: Tata and Widnell (1966) obtained differences only in liver ribosomal RNA. In this case it could be explained because the surgical removal of the thyroid gland was done in adult rats, and the effects may be different in animals radiothyroidectomized at birth. I have no explanation, but our results *in vitro* and *in vivo* coincide. The RNA synthesized *in vivo* which is different in normal and hypothyroid animals is a very rapidly labeled RNA; we must suppose that this is not ribosomal RNA.

Sokoloff: Studies in other tissues show that RNA synthesis in the nucleus proceeds at an enormously greater rate than that which gets out into the rest of the cell. It has been estimated that about 20 times more RNA is synthesized in the nucleus than ever gets out into the cytoplasm. This means that there is within the nucleus an excessive production of RNA which must be degraded there. There is always a problem when you change the rate of a reaction that produces a metabolite far in excess of what is being used: what possible implication could this have on cellular function outside the nucleus? There may be in hypothyroidism an effect on the transport of nucleic acid out of the nuclei into the cytoplasm where it does its work. Perhaps there are some important regulatory changes occurring in that process in dysthyroid states.

Krawiec: Twenty-four hours after the injection, the radioactivity of nuclear RNA in the hypothyroid rats is twice that in the controls. In this case the catabolic mechanisms may be altered in the hypothyroid brain. The other possibility might be that the posttranscriptional processes and migration of RNA from the nucleus might be delayed in the hypothyroid animal.

DISCUSSION REFERENCES

Scherrer, K., Latham, H., and Darnell, J. E. (1963): Demonstration of an unstable RNA and of a precursor to ribosomal RNA in HeLa cells. *Proc. Natl. Acad. Sci. (USA)*, 49:240.

Soeiro, R., and Darnell, J. E. (1970): A comparison between heterogeneous nuclear RNA and polysomal messenger RNA in HeLa cells by RNA-DNA hybridization. *J. Cell Biol.*, 44:467.

Stevenin, J., Mandel, P., and Jacob, M. (1969): Relationship between nuclear giant size dRNA and microsomal dRNA of the rat brain. *Proc. Natl. Acad. Sci. (USA)*, 62:490.

Tata, J. R., and Widnell, C. C. (1966): Ribonucleic acid synthesis during the early action of thyroid hormones. *Biochem. J.*, 98:604–620.

Thyroid Hormones and Brain Development,
edited by Gilman D. Grave. Raven Press,
New York, 1977.

Thyroid Hormone, Undernutrition, and Cyclic AMP: Relation to Cell Division and Thymidine Kinase Activity During Cerebellar Development

Morton E. Weichsel, Jr.*

Recent morphological and biochemical studies have elucidated the developmental changes in the neonatal rat cerebellum in the normal state (Altman, 1966, 1969), as well as in neonatal endocrinopathies (Hamburgh, Mendoza, Burkart, and Weil, 1971; Cotterell, Balázs, and Johnson, 1972; Nicholson and Altman, 1972; Gourdon, Clos, Coste, Dainat, and Legrand, 1973). Because the developing rat cerebellum undergoes a multifold increase in content of DNA over a 3-week period, these studies have led to our interest in this organ as a model for the study of endocrine and other environmental influences that affect enzyme systems critical to the synthesis of DNA in the brain. Because the rat cerebellum both accelerates and decelerates its rate of DNA synthesis at a postnatal time when it is accessible for anatomic dissection, it can serve as a model for study of DNA biosynthesis *in vivo* in brain as well as other body organs which are otherwise accessible in mammals only toward the end of the active stage of cell proliferation.

Our studies of enzymes critical to DNA biosynthesis involve the *de novo* and salvage pathways for pyrimidine biosynthesis (Fig. 1). The *de novo* pathway utilizes the simple substrates, CO_2, ATP, and glutamine with the enzyme carbamyl phosphate synthetase, to form carbamyl phosphate. The enzymes which follow are aspartate transcarbamylase and dihydroorotase. All three enzymes are now known to copurify (Levine, Hoogenraad, and Kretchmer, 1974). The ultimate product, after three more enzymatic steps, is uridine monophosphate, which is converted into a range of pyrimidine nucleotides by a series of pathways that appear to be under complex metabolic control. The salvage pathway or reutilization pathway uses preformed pyrimidines or pyrimidine nucleosides from exogenous sources and from endogenous breakdown of nucleic acids (Levine et al., 1974).

Figure 2 demonstrates the activity of aspartate transcarbamylase in rat cerebellar cortex and cerebellum. The obvious relationship of this *de novo* pathway enzyme to cerebral and cerebellar histological development pro-

---

* Division of Pediatric Neurology, Department of Pediatrics, Harbor General Hospital, UCLA School of Medicine, Torrance, California 90509.

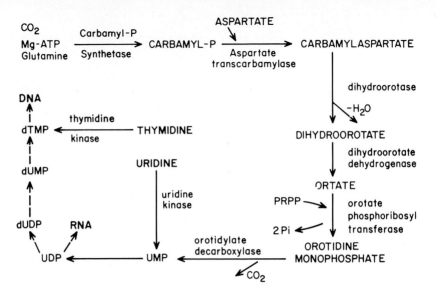

FIG. 1. Pathways for *de novo* and salvage incorporation of pyrimidines into nucleic acids in eukaryocytic cells.

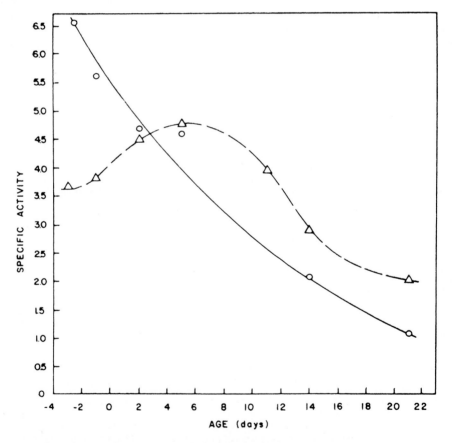

FIG. 2. Developmental curves for aspartate transcarbamylase from cerebellum ($\triangle$———$\triangle$) and cerebral cortex (O———O). One U enzymatic activity = 1 μM carbamyl aspartate formed/min/mg of protein. (From Weichsel et al., 1972.)

vided the first suggestion of a relationship between brain cell replication in the rat and the *de novo* pyrimidine pathway (Weichsel, Hoogenraad, Levine, and Kretchmer, 1972).

Figure 3 demonstrates the parallel rise and fall in carbamyl phosphate synthetase and aspartate transcarbamylase (the first two enzymes of the *de novo* pathway), which were felt to represent enzymatic markers for cerebellar cell division (Weichsel et al., 1972). The activity of uridine kinase, a salvage pathway enzyme, appears to peak later in development and is felt to be of more importance in the sustenance of nondividing cells.

Shortly after these studies, Yamagami, Mori, and Kawakita (1972) and Sung (1971) showed a peak in the activity of the salvage pathway enzyme, thymidine kinase, at 6 days of extrauterine life, just prior to the period of most rapid cerebellar cell replication, determined by incorporation

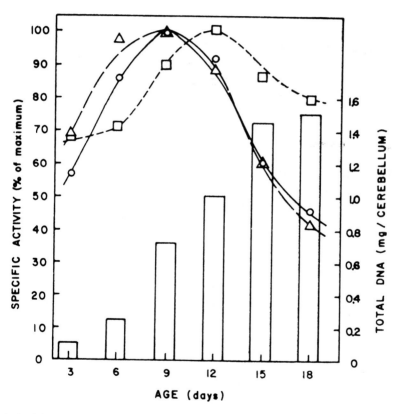

FIG. 3. Activity of pyrimidine nucleotide biosynthetic enzymes carbamyl phosphate synthetase (CPS) (O———O), aspartate transcarbamylase (ATC) (△———△), and uridine kinase (UK) (□———□) in cerebellum of developing rat. The data are reported as percentage of maximal activity and compared with total content of DNA in cerebellum (histograms). The maximal activities (100%) in μM/min/mg of protein were CPS 1.56×10^{-2}; ATC 823; and UK 0.34. (From Weichsel et al., 1972.)

of radioactively labeled thymidine. Because of the reported inhibition of that incorporation by thyroxine (T_4), and the prolonged uptake of labeled thymidine in the cerebella of hypothyroid rat pups, these studies were undertaken to determine if a relationship might exist between hormones, cerebellar DNA synthesis, and the activity of thymidine kinase.

METHODS

Sprague-Dawley rat pups from second pregnancies were used in all instances. Hyperthyroidism was created by injecting 4 animals from each litter of 8 with 0.4 μg of T_4/g of body weight daily, from the day of birth through weaning. At least 6 litters were used at each experimental age. Entire litters were rendered hypothyroid by daily injection of 50 mg of propylthiouracil into the stomachs of the mothers, starting at 18 days gestation, and using other litters of 8 pups as controls. At least 4 pups from 5 treated and control litters were used at each experimental age.

In all experiments, individual cerebella from control and treated animals were homogenized in a solution containing magnesium and ATP. From each crude homogenate, an aliquot was removed for DNA determination, and the remaining homogenate spun at 35,000 $\times$ g for 15 min. The supernatant fraction was then assayed for thymidine kinase by an adaptation of the methods of Yamagami et al. (1972) and Breitman (1963), and the resultant enzyme activity was expressed as activity per milligram of protein in the supernatant fraction. Expression of activity on the basis of enzyme per unit of DNA produced similar results.

In studies involving hyper- and hypothyroidism, paired t-testing was used to demonstrate significant differences between groups of hyperthyroid animals and their control littermates; group t-tests were used to demonstrate significance between data from hypothyroid animals and controls.

RESULTS

In experimental hyperthyroidism, body weights (Fig. 4) of T_4-treated pups were slightly less than controls, the difference becoming significant at age 3 days.

Cerebellar wet weight in treated animals was significantly decreased only after age 9 days (Fig. 5).

In Fig. 6 the cerebellar DNA from T_4-treated animals and controls are compared. Values in treated animals are significantly greater than in controls by paired t-test from age 2 through 6 days, with a peak difference of 118% of control values at age 4 days. By 9 days, there is no significant difference, and at ages 12 and 15 days, values in treated animals are significantly less than in controls. The figure further compares the normal developmental curve for cerebellar thymidine kinase activity with activity of the

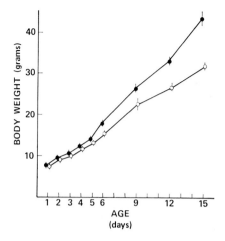

FIG. 4. Developmental curves for body weight of rat pups treated from birth with 0.4 μg of thyroxine/g of body weight/day (O———O) and body weight of littermate controls (●———●). Vertical bars represent confidence limits ($p < 0.05$). (From Weichsel, 1974.)

enzyme in the T_4-treated rat pups. The control curve for thymidine kinase activity peaks at 5 days and subsequently declines to become marginal at about 18 days. Thymidine kinase in treated animals is significantly greater than that of controls by 1 day of age. This elevation of enzyme activity becomes statistically significant 1 day prior to the significant elevation of cerebellar DNA in treated animals. Enzyme activity falls significantly below control values by day 9, prior to the significant decrease in cerebellar DNA synthesis noted in treated animals. The early increase in rate of cerebellar DNA synthesis therefore is accelerated in the hyperthyroid state, with a concomitant shift to the left in the developmental curve for thymidine kinase.

Figure 7 shows the effect of perinatal hypothyroidism on body weights of rats through 22 days of age. Treated animals gain far less weight than con-

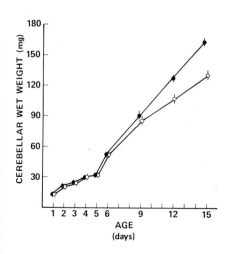

FIG. 5. Developmental curves for cerebellar wet weight of rat pups treated from birth with 0.4 μg of thyroxine/g of body weight/day (O———O), and cerebellar wet weights of littermate controls (●———●). Vertical bars represent confidence limits ($p < 0.05$). (From Weichsel, 1974.)

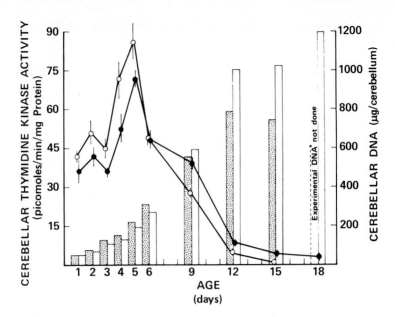

FIG. 6. Stippled bars = total cerebellar DNA of rat pups treated from birth with 0.4 μg of thyroxine/g of body weight. Clear bars = cerebellar DNA in littermate controls. (O———O) = thymidine kinase activity in cerebella of treated animals; (●———●) = littermate controls. Enzyme activity is reported as pM/min/mg of protein. Vertical linear bars represent confidence limits ($p < 0.05$). (From Weichsel, 1974.)

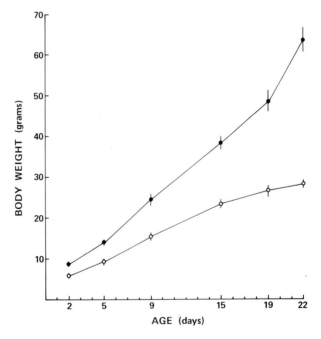

FIG. 7. Developmental curves for body weight of propylthiouracil-treated rat pups (O———O) and controls (●———●). Vertical bars represent confidence limits of $p < 0.05$. $N = 20$ or more at each experimental age.

trols, with a significant difference by age 2 days. Cerebellar wet weight (Fig. 8) is significantly less in hypothyroid animals by age 2 days, and remains so thereafter. The effect of hypothyroidism on cerebellar DNA is shown in Fig. 9. The maximum deficit in the treated animals occurs at 9 days of age and becomes less pronounced at later ages. The work of others (Gourdon et al., 1973) has shown that DNA in treated animals will eventually approach that of controls. The figure compares the normal developmental curve for thymidine kinase with activity of the enzyme in the hypothyroid rat pups from ages 2 through 22 days. Again, the developmental curve for thymidine kinase in control animals peaks at 5 days and falls thereafter. Activity in the cerebellum of treated animals is significantly below control values at ages 2 and 5 days, and becomes elevated above control values by 15 days of age. The enzyme continues to be active in the cerebellum of the treated animals at least 4 days after it has disappeared in controls. Thus, in hypothyroidism, the developmental curve for both DNA and thymidine kinase is shifted to the right, in contrast to hyperthyroidism where the shifts were to the left.

In hyperthyroid rats, cerebellar DNA synthesis was accelerated for about 5 days and terminated early, thus documenting an early induction of DNA synthesis by T_4 and supporting the observations of others (Hamburgh et al.,

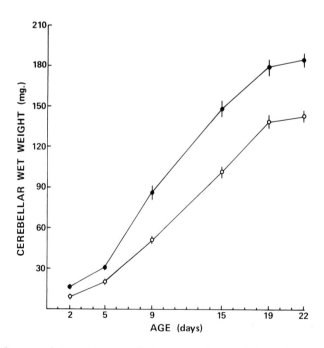

FIG. 8. Developmental curves for cerebellar weight of propylthiouracil-treated rat pups (O———O) and controls (●———●). Vertical bars represent confidence limits $p < 0.05$. $N = 20$ or more at each experimental age.

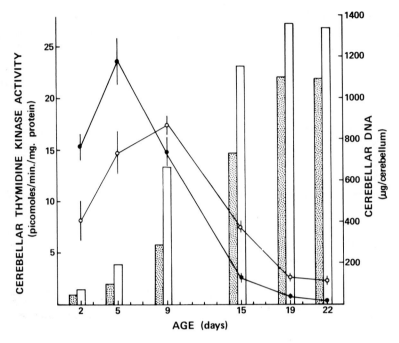

FIG. 9. Stippled bars = total cerebellar DNA of propylthiouracil-treated rat pups. Clear bars = cerebellar DNA in littermate controls. (O————O) = thymidine kinase activity in the cerebellum of treated animals; ●————● = controls. Enzyme is reported as pM/min/mg of protein. $N = 20$ or more at each experimental age. Vertical linear bars represent confidence limits, $p < 0.05$.

1971) that T_4 accelerates the transition from the state of cell replication to cell differentiation. These findings are in contrast to the developmental delay of cerebellar DNA synthesis in the hypothyroid state.

The reciprocal relationships between thymidine kinase and DNA synthesis in hyper- and hypothyroidism support the conclusion that the rat cerebellum is highly sensitive to T_4 during development and that thymidine kinase may be an important regulatory enzyme in cerebellar cell division (Weichsel, 1974).

DISCUSSION

The mechanisms by which thyroid hormones regulate cell division and enzyme biosynthesis are not well understood, and our data in relation to thymidine kinase support the probability that a hormone may function by one mechanism in early development and another at later stages, with multiple sites of action, depending on the developmental stage (Tata, 1971). Others have pointed out that the influence of T_4 on enzyme synthesis may be at the level of genetic transcription, by primary action on other hormones, or through mediation by adenyl cyclase (Pitot and Yatvin, 1973). In our experiments involving hyperthyroidism, we elected to administer a pharmacologic dose of T_4, which resulted in minimal mortality of the treated animals. Future experiments with altered dosage schedules and concomitant measurement of T_4 and other circulating hormones should clarify the interrelationships between hormones which affect neonatal cerebellar cell division.

During the course of our work with neonatal endocrinopathies, we have noted that treated animals often gain much less weight than controls, thus raising the question of the relative contribution of undernutrition in the experimental results. In the past, we have had difficulty raising undernourished rats which are as low in weight as our hypothyroid animals; therefore we attempted to establish undernourished weight-matched controls. Oversized litters of 16 to 20 pups were established to be studied at age 5 days, corresponding to the age of peak cerebellar thymidine kinase activity, as well as at age 12 days when activity in hypothyroid animals was elevated, and at age 19 days, when the activity normally disappeared. Eight such oversized litters as well as 8 control litters of 8 pups were established at each of the 3 experimental ages, at which time the heaviest, middle, and lightest animal was selected from each large litter to be studied along with a pup randomly selected from each control litter. The middle-sized undernourished subgroup was omitted at age 19 days. Comparisons were made for biochemical measurements between the control and each of the three undernourished subgroups, by group *t*-test. The undernourished subgroups from within the oversized litters at each age were compared by paired *t*-test. Body weights of the lightest subgroup of undernourished animals at each age were slightly less than the experimental hypothyroid pups mentioned previously.

Figure 10 shows the body weights of controls and each subgroup of undernourished pups, referred to as undernourished high, middle, and low. The weights of all groups were significantly different from controls and from each other at each of the three experimental ages.

Cerebellar DNA values for all groups at each age are compared in Fig. 11. At age 5 days, there is no difference between DNA in controls and the undernourished high group, suggesting that if cerebellar DNA is a marker for undernutrition, these animals would not be considered undernourished even though their body weights were significantly reduced. At age 12 days, DNA from all undernourished subgroups was significantly below control values. At age 19 days, neither subgroup showed a significantly decreased DNA value compared with controls, although the undernourished low subgroup had 12% less DNA than controls.

Figure 12 shows thymidine kinase activity in the control and the undernourished subgroups at each age. Thymidine kinase in the undernourished-low group was significantly below the control value at age 5 days, and

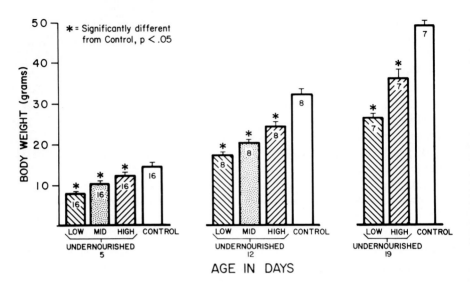

FIG. 10. Body weights from control and undernourished subgroups of rat pups, ages 5, 12, and 19 days. *N* for each subgroup is shown within bars. * = significant difference from control by group *t*-test, *p* < 0.05.

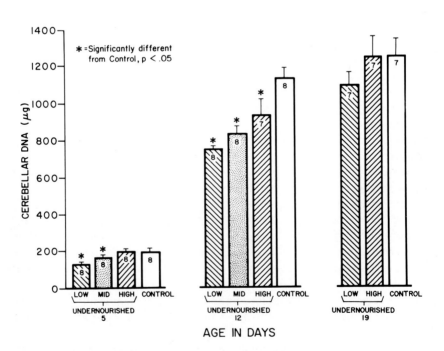

FIG. 11. Cerebellar DNA from control and undernourished subgroups of rat pups, ages 5, 12, and 19 days. *N* for each subgroup is shown within bars. * = significant difference from controls by group *t*-test, *p* < 0.05.

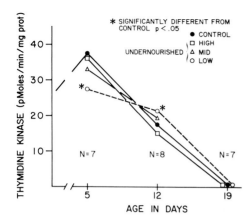

FIG. 12. Thymidine kinase activity reported as pM/min/mg of protein from control and undernourished subgroups of rat pups, ages 5, 12, and 19 days. Controls = ●———●; undernourished-high □———□; undernourished-middle △———△; undernourished-low ○———○. * = significant difference from controls by group t-test, $p < 0.05$.

significantly greater than the control value at age 12 days, whereas there was no significant activity in any group at age 19 days. The other subgroups of undernourished pups were not significantly different from the control group at ages 5 and 12 days, although when data from within the undernourished litters are compared by paired t-test, there is a stepwise decrease of thymidine kinase activity with undernutrition at 5 days and a stepwise increase in activity at age 12 days, with these directional changes resembling the changes seen in hypothyroidism. Such results suggest that a severe degree of undernutrition may affect the activity of thymidine kinase during cerebellar development and that, at a given degree of undernutrition, a critical enzyme may be selectively affected. These results also suggest that data selection may be critical in such measurements, and that results are likely to be subject to numerous biological variables.

Treated animals from hypothyroid experiments had delayed eye opening and suckled well in spite of a cretinoid body habitus and rather sluggish body movements. They were noted to maintain stomachs full of milk as frequently as controls. In the undernourished groups, the lack of cerebellar thymidine kinase activity at 19 days, as well as their small but otherwise normal appearance, suggest that the processes of hypothyroidism and undernutrition are not the same although they share a number of common features and may have an interrelationship that is not yet clear. Rosman and Malone (1974) have shown an intermediate state of brain myelination in undernourished rat pups between control and hypothyroid animals, but further studies will be necessary to delineate the components of each process as it affects the other (Muzzo, Blas, Brasel, and Gardner, 1973).

Among the mechanisms that control cell division under hormonal stimuli, cellular regulations might be influenced by the actions of cyclic AMP and cyclic GMP. Goldberg, Haddox, Estensen, Lopez, and Hadden (1976) have proposed a "dualism" theory by which cellular processes that are bidirectionally controlled might be regulated by the ratio of the intracellular con-

centration of cyclic GMP to cyclic AMP. Accordingly, the early acceleration of cerebellar DNA synthesis secondary to T_4 administration should be
accompanied by an increase in the ratio of these two nucleotides. Because
regulation of cerebellar cell division by T_4 appears to be subject to such
bidirectional control, and because the majority of studies supporting Goldberg's hypothesis have been conducted *in vitro,* we questioned if the elevation of cyclic AMP *in vivo* might retard cerebellar cell division during
development by affecting the hypothetical intracellular cyclic nucleotide
relationships secondary to the increase in cell division produced by administration of T_4.

In a study performed in collaboration with Dr. James E. Trosko of Michigan State University, 5 litters of Sprague-Dawley rats born within a 12-hr
period were reduced to 9 pups each. Two pups randomly selected were
treated with 0.4 μg of T_4/g of body weight subcutaneously in the right flank.
Two pups received dibutyryl cyclic AMP, 0.12 mg/g of body weight in the
left flank, followed 10 min later by a dose of T_4 in the right flank. The remaining 2 pups in each litter were used as saline-injected controls.

At 5 days of age all pups were decapitated and the whole brain and
cerebellum weighed on a torsion balance. Each cerebellum was then
homogenized and aliquots removed for determination of DNA. Statistical
analysis was applied by paired *t*-test, comparing the mean value of each
pair or trio of treated animals with the mean value of the controls from each
of the 5 litters, and with means from all other treated groups. In addition,
the mean and standard error of the mean (SEM) were calculated for all
animals from each treatment group.

In Fig. 13 the body weights for the different treatment groups are compared. Body weights of animals treated with cyclic AMP and both drugs
were significantly decreased to 92 and 90% of controls, respectively.

Cerebellar wet weight in the four groups is compared in Fig. 14. T_4-

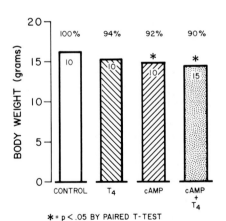

FIG. 13. Body weights from 5 litters of 5-
day-old rat pups, each litter divided into
treatment groups consisting of thyroxine,
dibutyryl cyclic AMP, both drugs, and littermate controls (see text). *N* for each
treatment is shown within bars. * = statistical significance between treated and
control groups by paired *t*-test, $p < 0.05$.

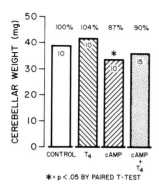

FIG. 14. Cerebellar wet weight from 5 litters of 5-day-old rat pups, each litter divided into treatment groups consisting of thyroxine, dibutyryl cyclic AMP, both drugs, and littermate controls (see text). *N* for each treatment group is shown within bars. * = statistical significance between treated and control groups by paired *t*-test, $p < 0.05$.

treated animals showed no statistical difference in cerebellar weight (104% of controls), whereas cerebellar weight from dibutyryl cyclic AMP-treated animals was 87% that of controls. The mean cerebellar weight of animals receiving both drugs was 90% that of controls but did not differ significantly from mean cerebellar weight of controls or dibutyryl cyclic AMP-treated animals.

Cerebellar DNA from T_4-treated pups (Fig. 15) is elevated to 117% of control values, whereas the level of cerebellar DNA from cyclic AMP-treated pups is significantly decreased to 89% of control values. DNA from pups receiving both T_4 and cyclic AMP did not differ from control values, although this value was significantly different from each of the other two groups.

The significant deficit in cerebellar DNA in animals receiving cyclic AMP alone suggests that this drug exerts a selective effect on cerebellar cell division at the time of maximum cell division when the organ is most subject to the effects of biochemical stimuli.

The deficits in cerebellar DNA and cerebellar wet weight were greater than the deficit in total body weight, a situation somewhat opposed to that of neonatal protein-calorie undernutrition, where a deficiency in body weight of an animal must be relatively great in order to produce an effect on cerebellar

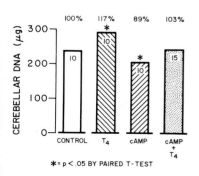

FIG. 15. Cerebellar DNA from 5 litters of 5-day-old rat pups, each litter divided into treatment groups consisting of thyroxine, dibutyryl cyclic AMP, both drugs, and littermate controls (see text). *N* for each treatment group is shown within bars. * = statistical significance between treated and control groups by paired *t*-test, $p < 0.05$.

growth. The reversal of the T_4-induced increase in cerebellar cell division by prior injection of dibutyryl cyclic AMP gives rise to speculation that the effect of T_4 on cell division may be mediated by the intracellular balance between cyclic GMP and cyclic AMP, and that this balance may have been distorted by elevation of intracellular cyclic AMP levels *in vivo*. Such speculations are supported by a number of experiments *in vitro* showing that endogenously or artificially increased concentrations of cyclic AMP are correlated with contact inhibition of the growth of several species of fibroblasts, and that high concentrations of cyclic AMP in mouse fibroblasts inhibit proliferation and promote differentiation (Otten, Johnson, and Pastan, 1971; Sheppard, 1972; Anderson, Russel, Carchman, and Pastan, 1973; Kolata, 1973; Millis, Forrest, and Pious, 1974).

The present study presents a potential experimental model for the study of intracellular cyclic nucleotide relationships *in vivo* during development, and suggests further that the developing rat cerebellum might provide a good model for further investigation of intracellular events that mediate the relationships between hormones and cell division.

ACKNOWLEDGMENTS

The author gratefully acknowledges the technical assistance of Mrs. Lila Dawson. This research was supported by Michigan State University General Research Support Grants 71–0993 and 71–0903 and by National Institutes of Health Grant HD-07275–01 and HD 09277–01 from the U.S. Public Health Service. Computing assistance was obtained from the Health Sciences Computing Facility, UCLA, sponsored by NIH Grant FR-3.

REFERENCES

Altman, J. (1966): Autoradiographic and histologic studies of postnatal neurogenesis. II. A longitudinal investigation of the kinetics, migration, and transformation of cells incorporating tritiated thymidine in infant rat, with special reference to postnatal neurogenesis in some brain regions. *J. Comp. Neurol.,* 128:431–474.

Altman, J. (1969): Autoradiographic and histological studies of postnatal neurogenesis. III. Dating the time of production and onset of differentiation of cerebellar microneurons in rats. *J. Comp. Neurol.,* 136:269–294.

Anderson, W. B., Russel, T. R., Carchman, R. A., and Pastan, I. (1973): Interrelationship between adenylate cyclase activity, adenosine 3':5'cyclic monophosphate levels, and growth of cells in culture. *Proc. Natl. Acad. Sci. (USA),* 70:3802–3805.

Breitman, T. R. (1963): The feedback inhibition of thymidine kinase. *Biochim. Biophys. Acta,* 67:153–155.

Cotterell, M., Balázs, R., and Johnson, A. L. (1972): Effects of corticosteroids on the biochemical maturation of rat brain: Postnatal cell formation. *J. Neurochem.,* 19:2151–2167.

Goldberg, N. D., Haddox, M. D., Estensen, R., Lopez, C., and Hadden, J. W. (1976): Evidence for a dualism between cyclic GMP and cyclic AMP in the regulation of cell proliferation and other cellular processes. In: *Cyclic AMP in Immune Response and Tumor Growth,* edited by L. M. Lichtenstein, et al. Springer-Verlag, New York.

Gourdon, J., Clos, J., Coste, C., Dainat, J., and Legrand, J. (1973): Comparative effects of hypothyroidism, hyperthyroidism, and undernutrition on the protein and nucleic acid contents of the cerebellum in the young rat. *J. Neurochem.,* 21:861–871.

Hamburgh, M., Mendoza, L. A., Burkart, J. W., and Weil, F. (1971): The thyroid as a time clock in the developing nervous system. In: *Cellular Aspects of Neural Growth and Differentiation,* UCLA Forum Med. Sci., edited by D. C. Pease, pp. 321–328. University of California Press, Los Angeles.

Kolata, G. B. (1973): Cyclic GMP: Cellular regulatory agent? *Science,* 182:149–151.

Levine, R. L., Hoogenraad, N. J., and Kretchmer, N. (1974): A review: Biological and clinical aspects of pyrimidine metabolism. *Pediatr. Res.* 8:724–734.

Millis, A. J. T., Forrest, G. A., and Pious, D. A. (1974): Cyclic AMP-dependent regulation of mitosis in human lymphoid cells. *Exp. Cell Res.,* 83:335–343.

Muzzo, S. J., Blas, F., Brasel, J. A., and Gardner, L. I. (1973): The effects of hormones and malnutrition on mitochondrial oxygen consumption and DNA synthesis in rat brain. In: *Endocrine Aspects of Malnutrition: Marasmus, Kwashiorkor, Psychological Deprivation,* Kroc Foundation Symposia #1, edited by L. Gardner and P. Amacher. Kroc Foundation, Santa Ynez, Calif.

Nicholson, J. L., and Altman, J. (1972): The effects of early hypo- and hyperthyroidism on the development of rat cerebellar cortex. I. Cell proliferation and differentiation. *Brain Res.,* 44:13–23.

Otten, J., Johnson, G. S., and Pastan, I. (1971): Cyclic AMP levels in fibroblasts: Relationships to growth rate and contact inhibition of growth. *Biochem. Biophys. Res. Commun.,* 44:1192–1198.

Pitot, H. C., and Yatvin, M. D. (1973): Interrelationships of mammalian hormones and enzyme levels *in vivo. Physiol. Rev.,* 53:228–325.

Rosman, N. P., and Malone, M. S. (1974): Myelin development in hypothyroidism and malnutrition: A comparative morphological and biochemical study. *Neurology,* 24:377 (abstract).

Sheppard, J. R. (1972): Difference in the cyclic adenosine 3′:5′ monophosphate levels in normal and transformed cells. *Nature New Biol.,* 236:14–16.

Sung, S. C. (1971): Thymidine kinase in the developing rat brain. *Brain Res.,* 35:268–271.

Tata, J. R. (1971): Cell structure and biosynthesis during hormone-mediated growth and development. In: *Hormones in Development,* edited by M. Hamburgh and E. J. W. Barrington, pp. 19–39. Appleton-Century-Crofts, New York.

Weichsel, M. E., Jr. (1974): Effect of thyroxine on DNA synthesis and thymidine kinase activity during cerebellar development. *Brain Res.,* 78:455–465.

Weichsel, M. E., Jr., Hoogenraad, N. J., Levine, R. L., and Kretchmer, N. (1972): Pyrimidine biosynthesis during development of rat cerebellum. *Pediatr. Res.,* 6:682–686.

Yamagami, S., Mori, K., and Kawakita, Y. (1972): Changes of thymidine kinase in the developing rat brain. *J. Neurochem.,* 19:369–376.

DISCUSSION

Lauder: At what age did you study the animals treated with T_4 and cyclic AMP?

Weichsel: At 5 days. You might wonder why we did not assay thymidine kinase. We did, but I think we chose the wrong day. At 4 days of age we might have shown a difference in thymidine kinase activity, but we did not find one at 5 days.

Valcana: From the rapid calculation I just made, you are using a dose of T_4 that is 250 times higher than needed to return a hypothyroid rat to a euthyroid state. Why this high dose of T_4? Have you tried lower doses without finding an effect?

Weichsel: I am amazed that your calculation came out exactly like mine, although I calculated it for people.

We chose the dose arbitrarily. We are among the few to give a pharmacologic dose. We felt the need to do this because we were working among a group of pharmacologists, and I dared not just give a fixed dose and then raise it 3 days later. We administered the T_4 per gram of body weight, which seemed most appropriate scientifically. The animals were clinically very jittery, but we lost only a few of them during the study.

Timiras: If you gave such a high dose because, as you say, you were close to pharmacologists, you should move your laboratory close to physiologists.

Kollros: I was intrigued by the data relating to the nutritional level, because a cold-blooded beast like the frog could have some very different problems. It is possible, by regulating food and temperature, for example in *Rana pipiens,* to get an animal to metamorphose at 15 mm length at one end of the scale and 35 mm at the other. So, we get tremendous differences at the time of metamorphosis, and so far as I know nobody knows whether these will grow up to the same size adult. As one illustration of a great difference in these nutritional studies, I have published a study in which we starved tadpoles and then matched them exactly with controls that had been fed very well. Our measure of development was the cell population in the peripheral layers of the optic lobe, the layer to which the optic nerve sends its fibers. The starved animals had up to 2.5 times as many cells in that layer than well-fed controls. They had a longer time to accumulate this cell population, since they took a long time to grow to exactly the same appearance as controls. This is a different kind of result from what one finds in mammals.

Weichsel: I attempted these undernutritional experiments because I knew that any reviewer might ask, "How do you know the results were not caused by malnutrition?" Prior to this I had been pretty sure that all my undernourished animals would not have their cerebellar thymidine kinase affected. I was chagrined to find that at 5 days it was affected, but not in the partially undernourished animals. At 12 days, we found a step-up effect which I cannot explain. Again, at 19 days we found no activity of this enzyme.

Balázs: At first, there is evidence that the activity of certain enzymes very closely reflects whether the cells are in the replicating or non-replicating phase of existence. Such a group of enzymes includes, besides thymidine kinase, ribonucleotide reductase, DNA polymerase II, and thymidine synthetase. Thus, it seems justifiable to use any of these enzymes as an index of the proliferative capacity of the tissue. One would expect, therefore, that the normal age curve for thymidine kinase should parallel that of a different estimate of cell proliferation, e.g., the rate of labeled thymidine incorporation into DNA *in vivo.* When I looked at your age curves of thymidine kinase activity, I noticed that this expectation has not been realized. However, the discrepancy may only be apparent.

This brings me to the troublesome question of how to express developmental estimates. When the proliferative capacity of an organ is assessed, the relevant information is the total activity per organ, rather than the concentration of the marker of replication or its specific activity. The latter estimate can be misleading, since protein concentration in the brain changes during development. For example, in the first week after birth, the protein concentration of the cerebellum is about 60% of that at 21 days. Thus, when the results are expressed in terms of protein, the specific activities at an early age are boosted artificially. It would be interesting to recalculate the thymidine kinase activity in terms of the weight of the whole cerebellum to appreciate whether the pattern of the age curve becomes more similar to that of overall DNA synthesizing capacity.

My other comment refers to the experiments on undernutrition. Altman et al. (1971) compared different techniques of undernutrition. Inadvertently, we used their method, which happens to generate the most reproducible results. I am also grateful to John Dobbing, who advised us to adopt this technique, in which the mother is underfed. We have never come across the formidable variation in growth retardation in the young that Dr. Weichsel did. Of course, it is a great experimental advantage to work with whole litters of uniformly growth-retarded animals, rather than to introduce a selection of animals from overcrowded litters which are characterized by different degrees of growth retardation.

Finally, a brief question: how long did you treat the animals with cyclic AMP and T_4?

Weichsel: From birth through 5 days of age, never longer. The animals given cyclic AMP subcutaneously, by the way, were perfectly healthy and could not be detected from the controls, except by the numbers on their backs. We injected the cyclic AMP first and T_4 10 min later; in one litter of a prior study we reversed that order. The pups injected with T_4 first all died. I presume that T_4 must have saturated the binding sites because the animals suddenly rolled over and died within about 2 hr, whereas 4 littermates injected with cyclic AMP first survived.

Sokoloff: Does dibutyryl cyclic AMP get into brain cells?

Weichsel: It is supposed to. That is why we chose it as the particular cyclic AMP derivative to use. Also, we had much difficulty in finding that dose of dibutyryl cyclic AMP that would neither kill all the rats nor be ineffective. It took 3 weeks to do this, and we finally found the optimal dose. In fact, in a preliminary experiment we found a dose which did not affect the body weight at all but knocked the cerebellar DNA down 8% and the cerebellar weight down 10%, at which time I told my psychiatric colleagues that at last I had shrunk a brain.

Balázs: The experiments with exogenous cyclic AMP are definitely worth pursuing. I have vested interest in this topic, since in a recent review paper (Balázs, 1974) I suggested that cyclic nucleotide systems may be involved, even in the brain, in the regulation of cell proliferation. I am glad that your results indicate that this view is probable. It is especially important that your experiments were done *in vivo,* since most of the relevant results on the effects of cyclic nucleotides on proliferation and differentiation of cells in nervous tissues have been obtained *in vitro;* e.g., tissue culture of tumor cells of nervous origin.

Bass: You have documented the poor model of undernutrition which involves overcrowding the litter. I hope that everyone will remember your results, because you have done much work to emphasize its weaknesses. The fierce competition and the random assortment of degrees of undernutrition in the overcrowded model make it totally inadequate. If you pool brains from these animals, the true consequences of malnutrition will be diluted by brains from animals which are barely malnourished.

Seven years ago Dr. Altman and I discussed undernutrition and found exactly what Dr. Balázs described. You can achieve a uniform result if you starve the whole litter by taking the mother away for limited periods of time. However, that brings up the problem that psychologists complain about, i.e., that you are changing the psychological environment of the pups, and, of course, that is true.

DISCUSSION REFERENCES

Altman, J., Das, G. D., Sudarshan, K., and Anderson, J. B. (1971): The influence of nutrition on neural and behavioural development. II. Growth of body and brain in infant rats using different techniques of undernutrition. *Dev. Psychobiol.,* 4:55–70.

Balázs, R. (1974): Influence of metabolic factors on brain development. *Br. Med. Bull.,* 30:126–134.

Thyroid Hormones and Brain Development,
edited by Gilman D. Grave. Raven Press,
New York, 1977.

Some Factors Controlling the Activity of Cerebral tRNA Sulfurtransferase

Ting-Wa Wong, Susan L. Harris, and Mariel A. Harris*

Transfer RNA contains a number of minor nucleotides in addition to those derived from the four major bases, among which are the thionucleotides (Lipsett, 1965; Baczynskyj, Biemann, and Hall, 1968; Burrows, Armstrong, Skoog, Hecht, Boyle, Leonard, and Occolowitz, 1968; Carbon, David, and Studier, 1968; Kimura-Harada, Saneyoshi, and Nishimura, 1971). The usual role postulated for these minor constituents is that they regulate the secondary structure and consequently the functioning of tRNA. Earlier work suggested that the amino acid-accepting ability of several species of bacterial and mammalian tRNA is controlled by thionucleotides; the latter must remain in the reduced form for the tRNA molecules to function as amino acid acceptors (Carbon, Hung, and Jones, 1965; Goehler and Doi, 1968). More recent studies have revealed the presence of thionucleotides in the anticodon region of certain tRNAs of *E. coli,* yeast, and rat liver (Ohashi, Saneyoshi, Harada, Hara, and Nishimura, 1970; Yoshida, Takeishi, and Ukita, 1971; Kimura-Harada et al., 1971); further, there are indications that they are crucial to precise codon recognition by tRNA (Saneyoshi and Nishimura, 1971; Nishimura, 1972; Agris, Söll, and Seno, 1973). Desulfuration of the thionucleotides in the anticodon of certain *E. coli* tRNAs by chemical means leads to inability to recognize the usual codons (Saneyoshi and Nishimura, 1971; Agris et al., 1973). Similarly, tRNA molecules isolated from *E. coli* grown in a sulfur-deficient medium (and hence lacking their usual complement of sulfur in the anticodon nucleotides) show ambiguity in codon recognition (Agris et al., 1973). Because of the central role played by tRNA in protein synthesis, the manner by which these unusual nucleotides come to be present in the tRNA molecules presents a challenging riddle. Two basic mechanisms may be visualized for the biosynthesis of minor nucleotides in a tRNA molecule: (1) insertion during nucleotide polymerization, or (2) modification of nucleotides after polymerization. Investigations in bacterial systems have indicated that the sulfur of thionucleotides originates from biochemical alteration occurring after polynucleotide assembly, through enzymatic transfer of the sulfur moiety of cysteine or β-mercaptopyruvate to the tRNA molecule (Hayward and Weiss, 1966; Lipsett and Peterkofsky, 1966; Wong, Weiss, Eliceiri, and

---

* Department of Pathology, The University of Chicago, Chicago, Illinois 60637.

Bryant, 1970). The sulfur in *E. coli* tRNA has been shown to be derived from cysteine. Soluble extracts of *E. coli* capable of catalyzing such reactions were first described by Hayward and Weiss (1966) and by Lipsett and Peterkofsky (1966). Alkaline hydrolysis and chromatography of the *in vitro* thiolated tRNA indicated that the major product was 4-thioUMP, which was known to occur naturally in the tRNA of *E. coli* (Lipsett, 1965). More recently, we have isolated another *in vitro* sulfurtransferase system from *B. subtilis* which, in contrast to the *E. coli* system, does not produce 4-thioUMP as the major product, but other thiopyrimidine nucleotides that are not yet identified (Wong et al., 1970). The *B. subtilis* enzyme is capable of transferring the labeled sulfur from either [^{35}S]cysteine or [^{35}S]β-mercaptopyruvate to tRNA. The substitution of [^{14}C]cysteine or [^{14}C]β-mercaptopyruvate for the corresponding [^{35}S]substrate leads to no labeled product, indicating that only the sulfur moiety of cysteine or β-mercaptopyruvate, and not their carbon skeleton, is transferred to tRNA in the reaction. Of the two sulfur donors, β-mercaptopyruvate is by far the more efficient and exhibits a K_m 200 to 300 times smaller than the K_m for cysteine. Further, there are indications that when cysteine functions as the sulfur donor, it is first converted to β-mercaptopyruvate as an intermediate (Wong et al., 1970).

While tRNA sulfurtransferases had been isolated from two bacterial systems, no such enzymes had been reported in mammals. Nonetheless, the finding of thiolated tRNA in mammalian species (Eliceiri, 1970; Kimura-Harada et al., 1971) implies that such enzymes must exist in mammals. Recently, we have isolated a tRNA sulfurtransferase system from the rat brain that is capable of thiolating tRNA *in vitro* by catalyzing the transfer of sulfur from β-mercaptopyruvate to tRNA (Wong, Harris, and Jankowicz, 1974). It is the purpose of this chapter to describe the properties of this mammalian tRNA sulfurtransferase and some of the factors that control its activity.

MATERIALS AND METHODS

Enzyme preparation. The enzyme used was derived from the cerebral hemispheres of 35- to 36-day old male Buffalo rats. A 10% whole homogenate in chilled 0.14 M KCl–0.02 M Tris (pH 7.4) was centrifuged successively at $1,600 \times g$ for 10 min, at $33,000 \times g$ for 20 min, and at $160,000 \times g$ for 60 min. The $160,000 \times g$ supernatant obtained was further subjected to ammonium sulfate fractionation (40 to 70% saturation) and CM-cellulose treatment as described in our previous publication (Wong et al., 1974). The resulting cerebral tRNA sulfurtransferase preparation, still relatively crude, was used in much of the studies described in this chapter.

Determination of tRNA sulfurtransferase activity. The tRNA sulfurtransferase activity of an enzyme fraction is measured by the amount of ^{35}S transfer from the sulfur donor to the acceptor tRNA which it catalyzes. The extent of ^{35}S transfer is determined by the quantity of [^{35}S]tRNA formed, according to the following reaction scheme:

$$[^{35}\text{S}]\text{sulfur-donor} + \text{tRNA} \xrightarrow{\text{tRNA sulfurtransferase}} [^{35}\text{S}]\text{tRNA}$$

Assay procedure. The *in vitro* transsulfuration reaction utilized the cerebral tRNA sulfurtransferase as enzyme, [^{35}S]β-mercaptopyruvate as sulfur donor, and tRNA as sulfur acceptor. The standard assay mixture was 0.5 ml in volume and contained 5 nmoles of ammonium [^{35}S]β-mercaptopyruvate, 0.5 mg of yeast tRNA, 0.02 to 0.04 ml of rat brain tRNA sulfurtransferase, 50 μmoles of Tris (pH 7.4), 1 μmole of ATP, 3 μmoles of MgCl$_2$, and 1 μmole of β-mercaptoethanol. The standard control consisted of the above mixture with 25 μmoles of EDTA added. This control is based on the fact that the reaction requires magnesium ion; in the presence of EDTA, which binds magnesium ion, the reaction cannot take place.

When the ability of the various types of tRNAs to serve as ^{35}S acceptors was tested, tRNA other than that from yeast, rRNA, mRNA, and synthetic ribohomopolymers were each used in place of yeast tRNA in the assay mixture. Similarly, various other components of the standard reaction mixture were omitted or varied individually to determine their effects on the tRNA sulfurtransferase activity.

The assay mixture was incubated at 37°C for 20 min. Thereafter, the tRNA was recovered for determination of its ^{35}S-labeling by scintillation counting as described previously (Wong et al., 1974).

Radioactive and nonradioactive substrates. Ammonium [^{35}S]β-mercaptopyruvate, ranging from 150 to 650 mCi/mmole in specific activity, was purchased from New England Nuclear Corp. Authentic nonradioactive ammonium β-mercaptopyruvate was a generous gift from Dr. Ernest Kun (1957).

Preparation of nucleic acids for use as ^{35}S acceptors. Yeast tRNA was purchased from Schwarz-Mann and served as the sulfur acceptor for most of the experiments described here. Prior to use, it was purified by phenol extraction and ethanol precipitation. *E. coli* B tRNA, rat liver tRNA, and rabbit liver tRNA were purchased from General Biochemicals and purified in the same manner. Synthetic ribohomopolymers (poly U, poly C, poly A, and poly G) were procured from Miles Laboratory, Inc. Ribosomal RNA from *E. coli* B was prepared from isolated ribosomes by phenol extraction and precipitated with 1 M NaCl (Gierer and Schramm, 1956). Messenger RNA from the bacteriophage MS2 was also obtained by phenol extraction.

Isolation of [^{35}S]tRNA for product analysis. For those studies dealing with product analysis, the homologous rat liver tRNA was used as the sulfur acceptor. The [^{35}S]tRNA was prepared by the standard assay procedure and first purified by phenol extraction and ethanol precipitation. It was then chromatographed on a Sephadex G-25 column to remove all unreacted [^{35}S]β-mercaptopyruvate and other low-molecular-weight contaminants, according to the procedure described previously (Wong et al., 1974). The [^{35}S]tRNA recovered from this chromatography was resuspended in water or other solutions for further use.

DEAE-cellulose chromatography of alkaline hydrolysate of [^{35}S]tRNA. To analyze the nature of the [^{35}S]thionucleotides formed, approximately 3 mg of [^{35}S]tRNA, obtained from the Sephadex G-25 chromatography described above, were hydrolyzed in 0.5 ml of 0.3 M KOH at 37°C for 18 hr. The hydrolysate obtained was first neutralized with Dowex 50 (H$^+$ form) to pH 10 and then with 0.01 M HCl to pH 8.6. About 8 A$_{320}$ units of nonradio-active 4-thio-2'(3')-UMP were then added as marker, and the entire mixture was adjusted to 0.01 M NH$_4$HCO$_3$ (pH 8.6) in a volume of 100 ml. This solution was applied to a 30 × 1 cm DEAE-cellulose column and eluted with a linear gradient consisting of 180 ml of 0.05 M NH$_4$HCO$_3$ (pH 8.6) in 7 M urea and 180 ml of 0.25 M NH$_4$HCO$_3$ (pH 8.6) in 7 M urea, as described by Lipsett (1965). Fractions (4 ml each) were collected, and their A$_{260}$, A$_{280}$, A$_{320}$, and radioactivity were determined.

Paper electrophoresis of nucleotides derived from [^{35}S]tRNA. The [^{35}S]tRNA obtained from Sephadex G-25 chromatography was suspended in 0.01 M NH$_4$HCO$_3$ (pH 8.6) and treated with RNase (50 μg of pancreatic RNase and 10 μg of T$_1$ RNase/0.2 ml of reaction) by incubating at 37°C for 2 hr. Afterwards, one-half of the RNase-treated material was incubated with crystalline *E. coli* alkaline phosphatase (29 μg/0.1 ml of reaction) at 37°C for 1 hr. The RNase digests, with and without alkaline phosphatase treatment, were adjusted to contain 0.05 M NH$_4$HCO$_3$ (pH 8.6) and 0.0014 M β-mercaptoethanol. That amount of each digest sufficient to give 6,000 to 8,000 cpm was spotted on Whatman No. 3MM paper and electrophoresed in the same buffer at 400 V for 7 hr in the cold. Afterwards, the paper was air-dried, cut into small strips, placed in glass vials, and counted with 0.5 ml of water and 10 ml of scintillation fluid.

Isolation of subcellular fractions from the cerebral hemispheres and determination of their tRNA sulfurtransferase activity. To determine the distribution of tRNA sulfurtransferase activity in the various subcellular fractions, the cerebral hemispheres derived from 10 male Buffalo rats (35 to 36 days old) were homogenized in 0.14 M KCl–0.02 M Tris (pH 7.4) in the amount of 10 ml/g of tissue. The homogenate was then subjected to dif-ferential centrifugations according to the method of Ivanova, Rubel, and Semenova (1967), with the exception that the sucrose–CaCl$_2$ buffer in the reported procedure was replaced by 0.14 M KCl–0.02 M Tris (pH 7.4) in all steps. The nuclear fraction obtained from the above method, which was contaminated with cell debris and unbroken cells, was further purified by centrifugation in 2.05 M sucrose–0.02 M Tris (pH 7.4)–0.001 M MgCl$_2$.

Afterwards, all particulate fractions were leached with 0.02 M Tris (pH

7.4). The supernatants from these leached particulate fractions as well as the supernatant from the whole homogenate were assayed for their tRNA sulfurtransferase activity with the standard assay mixture, from which the total activity of each subcellular fraction was calculated.

Effects of age and propylthiouracil-induced hypothyroidism on the tRNA sulfurtransferase activity of the cerebral hemispheres. For this study, male suckling Buffalo rats 0 to 35 days old were used. This age range encompasses the entire process of cerebral development, since by 35 days, the rat brain is considered to have matured completely (Balázs, Kovács, Teichgräber, Cocks, and Eayrs, 1968). The animals were divided into three groups: (1) normal controls, (2) a hypothyroid group, and (3) a similar hypothyroid group receiving thyroxine replacement therapy.

Hypothyroidism was induced in the suckling rats by feeding the mothers 0.2% propylthiouracil in Purina chow beginning from day 12 of a 21-day pregnancy and continuing this diet throughout the lactating period until the study was terminated. Since propylthiouracil crosses the placental barrier freely and is also excreted in the milk (Williams, Kay, and Jandorf, 1944), this is a convenient way of inducing hypothyroidism in the late fetal and postnatal suckling period. The mothers of the control rats were fed Purina laboratory chow throughout. Following delivery, all female offspring were eliminated and only the males were saved. They were allowed to remain with their mothers throughout the entire experiment. Beginning on the second day after birth, one group of hypothyroid rats received replacement therapy in the form of daily subcutaneous injections of sodium L-thyroxine in sterile saline at a dose of 2 μg/100 g of body weight. The normal controls and the remaining hypothyroid group were uninjected.

On days 0–1, 7, 14, 21, 28, and 35, four animals randomly chosen from each group were killed by decapitation. A 160,000 $\times$ g supernatant was prepared from the cerebral hemispheres of each rat for determination of tRNA sulfurtransferase activity. The 160,000 $\times$ g supernatant was used directly without further purification because quantitative recovery of enzyme activity is essential for such comparative studies. In this way, the enzyme loss that accompanies purification procedures is avoided.

To assess thyroid function, blood was collected from each rat during decapitation for determination of the serum total thyroxine concentration (TT$_4$) and the free thyroxine index (FT$_4$I); the latter is a measure of (and bears a linear relationship to) the concentration of free, unbound thyroxine in the serum (Robin, Hagen, Callaço, Refetoff, and Selenkow, 1971). Both the TT$_4$ and FT$_4$I were determined by competitive protein binding analysis (Robin et al., 1971).

Miscellaneous materials. Buffalo rats were obtained from Simonsen Laboratories, Inc. Propylthiouracil was purchased from Sigma Chemical Co. and sodium L-thyroxine (as Synthroid®) from Flint Laboratories. Nonradioactive 4-thio-2'(3')-UMP was isolated from the alkaline hydrolysate of *E. coli* B tRNA by the method of Lipsett (1965). 4-Thiouridine was obtained from Sigma Chemical Co. Pancreatic RNase, pancreatic DNase, and *E. coli* alkaline phosphatase were procured from Worthington Biochemical Corp. T_1 RNase was purchased from Calbiochem. Hexokinase (Type III yeast) was obtained from Sigma Chemical Co.

RESULTS

Properties of the transsulfuration reaction. The general characteristics of the transsulfuration reaction catalyzed by the cerebral tRNA sulfurtransferase are summarized in Table 1. Radioactive label is incorporated into tRNA when $[^{35}S]\beta$-mercaptopyruvate is incubated in a complete reaction mixture with the enzyme. Incorporation is reduced to baseline levels when enzyme is omitted or when heated enzyme is used. ^{35}S transfer to tRNA also requires the presence of ATP and magnesium ion. When ATP or magnesium ion is omitted, or when the magnesium ion is bound by the addition of EDTA, no ^{35}S transfer occurs. Formation of labeled product requires tRNA, and does not take place in its absence. Adding RNase abolishes transsulfuration, but adding DNase has no such effect, indicating that the ^{35}S is incorporated into tRNA. When authentic, nonradioactive β-mercaptopyruvate is added to the reaction mixture in amounts onefold or tenfold that of $[^{35}S]\beta$-mercaptopyruvate, the decrease in percentage of ^{35}S incorporation into tRNA reflects almost exactly the dilution of the radioactive substrate. This finding

TABLE 1. *Requirements of transsulfuration reaction with $[^{35}S]\beta$-mercaptopyruvate as sulfur donor and yeast tRNA as sulfur acceptor*

Reaction mixture	^{35}S incorporated into tRNA (pmoles)
Complete	24.4
No enzyme	1.4
Heated enzyme	1.0
No ATP	1.6
No $MgCl_2$	1.3
Add EDTA	1.1
No tRNA	1.0
Add RNase	1.3
Add DNase	23.4
Add nonradioactive β-mercaptopyruvate (onefold)	13.2
Add nonradioactive β-mercaptopyruvate (tenfold)	2.9

The complete reaction mixture was as described under Assay Procedure. Where indicated, one of the following was also present: (1) 0.04 ml of heated enzyme (5 min at 100°C) in place of the same amount of unheated enzyme, (2) 25 μmoles of EDTA, (3) 50 μg of pancreatic RNase and 10 μg of T_1 RNase, (4) 50 μg of pancreatic DNase, and (5) 5 nmoles or 50 nmoles of nonradioactive β-mercaptopyruvate.

indicates that $[^{35}S]\beta$-mercaptopyruvate, and not some radioactive contaminant, is the actual sulfur donor.

The extent of transsulfuration is dependent on the concentration of the sulfur donor, $[^{35}S]\beta$-mercaptopyruvate, the K_m for which is 6×10^{-6} M (Fig. 1). The reaction is also dependent on the concentration of the enzyme, tRNA sulfurtransferase (Fig. 2), and on the concentration of the sulfur acceptor, yeast tRNA (Fig. 3).

The ability of various types of RNA to serve as ^{35}S acceptors is shown in Table 2. All tRNAs tested, whether from rat liver, rabbit liver, *E. coli* B, or yeast, can serve as ^{35}S acceptors. Because yeast tRNA has a reasonably high ^{35}S-accepting capacity among the tRNAs tested and is readily available commercially, we have found it convenient to use yeast tRNA in all the standard assays. Table 2 also shows that ribosomal RNA from *E. coli* B, messenger RNA from the bacteriophage MS2, and synthetic ribohomopolymers such as poly U, poly C, poly A, and poly G are ineffective as ^{35}S

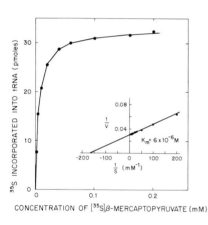

FIG. 1. ^{35}S incorporation into tRNA as a function of the concentration of the sulfur donor, $[^{35}S]\beta$-mercaptopyruvate.

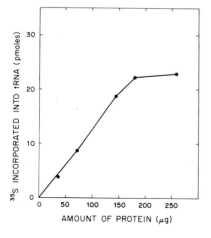

FIG. 2. ^{35}S incorporation into tRNA as a function of enzyme concentration (in μg of protein/0.5 ml of reaction mixture).

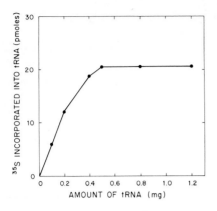

FIG. 3. [35]S incorporation as a function of the concentration of the sulfur acceptor, yeast tRNA.

acceptors. These findings indicate that among the different kinds of RNA, only tRNA has the required structural attributes to accept sulfur.

The dependence of sulfurtransferase activity on ATP concentration is shown in Fig. 4. The K_m for ATP is 5×10^{-4} M. The ability of ATP to function as the activating nucleotide in the transsulfuration reaction is highly specific, since ATP cannot be replaced by other nucleotides such as GTP, UTP, or CTP (Table 3). The ^{35}S transfer obtained with ADP is apparently due to the formation of ATP by the following reaction: 2 ADP $\rightleftarrows$ ATP + AMP. This reaction is catalyzed by adenylate kinase, with which the tRNA sulfurtransferase preparation appears to be contaminated. The correctness of this speculation is confirmed by the following observation: when hexokinase and glucose are added to the reaction mixture to consume all ATP

TABLE 2. *Ability of various RNAs to serve as acceptors in the transsulfuration reaction*

Type of RNA used as acceptor	[35]S incorporated into RNA (pmoles)
None	0.8
Rat liver tRNA	22.7
Rabbit liver tRNA	18.8
Yeast tRNA	22.3
E. coli B tRNA	24.1
E. coli B rRNA	0.3
MS2 RNA	0.4
Poly U	0.1
Poly C	0.2
Poly A	0.2
Poly G	0.5

The reaction mixture was the same as given under Assay Procedure. Where indicated, yeast tRNA was either omitted or replaced by 0.5 mg of each of the RNAs or ribohomopolymers shown.

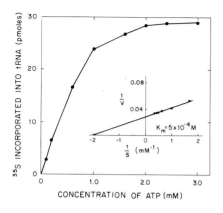

FIG. 4. ^{35}S incorporation into tRNA as a function of ATP concentration.

present via the reaction, glucose + ATP $\xrightarrow{\text{hexokinase}}$ glucose-6-phosphate + ADP, no ^{35}S transfer occurs. Hexokinase or glucose individually has no effect on the sulfurtransferase activity (Table 3). AMP is totally ineffective as the activating nucleotide.

TABLE 3. *Specificity of nucleotide requirement for sulfurtransferase activity*

Nucleotide present in reaction mixture	^{35}S incorporated into tRNA (pmoles)
None	1.4
ATP	23.0
GTP	1.1
UTP	0.8
CTP	1.0
ADP	16.0
ADP + hexokinase + glucose	1.0
ATP + hexokinase	22.8
ATP + glucose	23.1
AMP	1.0

The reaction mixture was as given under Assay Procedure. Where indicated, ATP was omitted or replaced by GTP, UTP, CTP, ADP, or AMP (1 μmole each). In three instances, 20 units of hexokinase (52.8 μg) and/or 20 μmoles of glucose were added.

The transsulfuration reaction also requires activation by a divalent metal ion. Either MgCl$_2$ or MnCl$_2$ may fulfill this role (Fig. 5). Of the two, MgCl$_2$ is the more effective. Maximal sulfur transfer occurs at a concentration of 6 mM for magnesium ion and 3 mM for manganese ion. Higher concentrations lead to suppression of ^{35}S incorporation into tRNA. Other divalent metal ions such as calcium and cadmium ions are incapable of activating the transsulfuration reaction (Fig. 5).

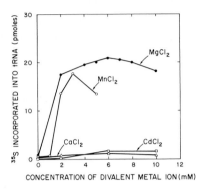

FIG. 5. Effect of divalent metal ion concentration on tRNA sulfurtransferase activity.

Optimal formation of [^{35}S]tRNA requires the presence of some reducing agent such as β-mercaptoethanol. In the absence of this thiol, [^{35}S]tRNA formation is about one-half to one-third of the maximum (Fig. 6). Above a certain concentration, β-mercaptoethanol has an inhibitory effect on the reaction. The stimulatory effect of this thiol is probably due in part to its ability to maintain the substrate, [^{35}S]β-mercaptopyruvate, in the reduced form.

The extent of ^{35}S incorporation into tRNA is dependent on the time and temperature of incubation (Fig. 7). The transsulfuration reaction can take place over a fairly broad pH range, but maximal sulfur transfer occurs at pH 7.4 (Fig. 8).

Nature of the labeled product of transsulfuration. It has already been indicated that the product of the transsulfuration reaction behaves like RNA, judging from its sensitivity to RNase (Table 1). When the labeled product is chromatographed on Sephadex G-100, almost all the radioactivity is excluded in a position coincident with tRNA; a small amount of ^{35}S appears much later in a region known to exclude ATP and other low-molecular-weight compounds (Fig. 9A). When the ^{35}S-labeled product is treated with RNase prior to Sephadex chromatography, the radioactivity and ultraviolet-absorbing material are no longer seen in the position for elution of tRNA but

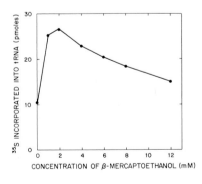

FIG. 6. Effect of β-mercaptoethanol concentration on tRNA sulfurtransferase activity.

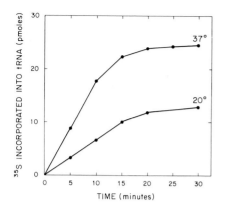

FIG. 7. Effect of time and temperature of incubation on ^{35}S incorporation into tRNA.

are now excluded in the same region as the low-molecular-weight substances (Fig. 9B).

When the *in vitro* labeled product is exposed to alkali under conditions that hydrolyze RNA and then chromatographed on DEAE-cellulose, the bulk of the radioactivity distributes itself in several peaks in the region where the major nucleotides are found (Fig. 10). Little label is seen to elute with the 4-thio-2′(3′)-UMP that was added as a marker prior to chromatography. A small amount of labeled material elutes after 4-thio-2′(3′)-UMP; similar material has been observed by Eliceiri (1970) on DEAE-cellulose chromatography of alkaline hydrolysate derived from *in vivo* labeled ^{35}S]tRNA of mouse lymphoma cells.

Figure 11 shows the electrophoretic patterns of the hydrolysate of *in vitro* labeled ^{35}S]tRNA with and without additional alkaline phosphatase treatment. The hydrolysate contains a major product that migrates toward the anode at a slightly slower rate than 4-thio-2′(3′)-UMP (Fig. 11A). Treatment with alkaline phosphatase retards significantly its rate of anodal migration, as would be expected if the ^{35}S is associated with a nucleotide, but again the dephosphorylated ^{35}S]product does not coincide with 4-thiouri-

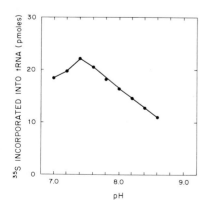

FIG. 8. Effect of pH on tRNA sulfurtransferase activity. The pH of the reaction mixture was varied with Tris buffers.

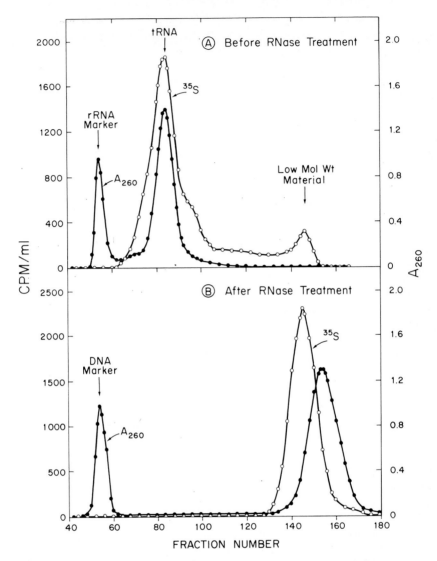

FIG. 9. Sephadex G-100 chromatography of *in vitro* labeled rat liver [³⁵S]tRNA before and after RNase treatment. The [³⁵S]tRNA was prepared in a standard reaction mixture and purified by phenol extraction, ethanol precipitation, and Sephadex G-25 chromatography to remove the vast amount of unreacted [³⁵S]β-mercaptopyruvate. The [³⁵S]tRNA was then used in the following experiments: In **A**, approximately 3 mg of [³⁵S]tRNA (114,000 cpm), mixed with 0.6 mg of marker *E. coli* B rRNA, were chromatographed on a 90 × 2.4 cm column of Sephadex G-100; elution was carried out with 0.05 M NH₄HCO₃ (pH 8.6)– 0.0014 M β-mercaptoethanol, and 3-ml fractions were collected. In **B**, approximately 3 mg of [³⁵S]tRNA (110,000 cpm) were incubated with 50 μg of pancreatic RNase and 10 μg of T₁ RNase in a volume of 0.5 ml at 37°C for 2 hr; then 0.6 mg of heat-denatured calf thymus DNA was added as a marker, and the entire mixture was chromatographed on Sephadex G-100 as described for **A**. ●————● A₂₆₀; ○————○ ³⁵S.

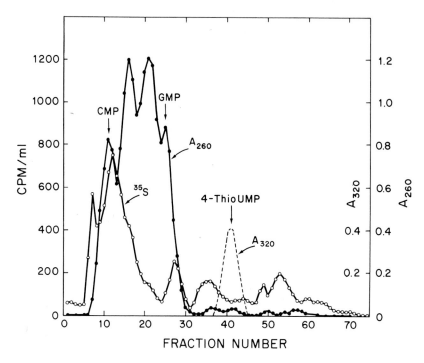

FIG. 10. DEAE-cellulose chromatography of alkaline hydrolysate of *in vitro* labeled rat liver [^{35}S]tRNA. The procedures for [^{35}S]tRNA preparation, isolation, alkaline hydrolysis, and DEAE-cellulose chromatography were as described under Materials and Methods. About 3 mg of [^{35}S]tRNA (108,000 cpm) were used in the preparation of the alkaline hydrolysate, and 8 A$_{320}$ units of 4-thio-2'(3')-UMP were added as marker. ●———● A$_{260}$; - - - - A$_{320}$; ○———○ ^{35}S.

dine (Fig. 11B). In addition to this major product, several minor, slower-moving ^{35}S-containing nucleotides also appear to be present (Fig. 11A).

Distribution of tRNA sulfurtransferase activity in the various subcellular fractions of the cerebral hemispheres. Assays performed with the leaching fluids obtained from the nuclear, mitochondrial, and microsomal fractions, as well as the supernatant of the whole homogenate indicate that the bulk of the tRNA sulfurtransferase activity is present in the supernatant fraction (Table 4). A minute quantity of the activity is also found in the leaching fluids from the mitochondrial and microsomal fractions. Without further purification by sucrose gradient, it is impossible to state whether such low levels of enzyme activities are the result of contamination of the mitochondrial and microsomal fractions by the cell sap or whether they represent true activities residing in these cell organelles. In view of the report of thionucleotides in the mitochondrial tRNA of chicken liver (Lalyre-G. and Titchener, 1971), however, these activities, though low, may be meaningful.

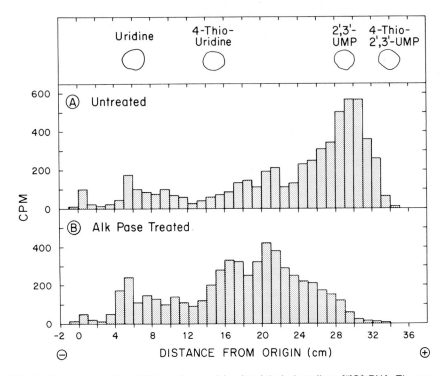

FIG. 11. Electrophoresis of RNase digest of *in vitro* labeled rat liver [³⁵S]tRNA. The conditions for [³⁵S]tRNA preparation, hydrolysis with RNase, treatment of the RNase digest with alkaline phosphatase, and electrophoresis were as described under Materials and Methods. In **A,** the RNase digest was electrophoresed directly. In **B,** the RNase digest was further treated with alkaline phosphatase before electrophoresis. Total cpm spotted was about 6,000 in each instance. Nonradioactive markers including 4-thio-2′(3′)-UMP, 2′(3′)-UMP, 4-thiouridine, and uridine were electrophoresed simultaneously.

TABLE 4. *Distribution of sulfurtransferase activity in various subcellular fractions of rat cerebral hemispheres*

Subcellular fraction	% Sulfurtransferase activity
Nuclei	0.0 ± 0.0
Heavy mitochondria	0.5 ± 0.3
Light mitochondria	0.4 ± 0.1
Microsomes	0.6 ± 0.2
Supernatant	98.5 ± 0.4

Preparation of the various subcellular fractions and assay for sulfurtransferase activity were as described under Materials and Methods. The above data represent the average ± 1 SD from three separate experiments on fractionation. For each experiment, 10 male Buffalo rats 35 to 36 days old were used.

The influence of age and thyroid function on the tRNA sulfurtransferase activity of the maturing cerebral hemispheres. The specific activity of tRNA sulfurtransferase in the rat cerebral hemispheres, determined at weekly intervals from 0 to 35 days of age, is presented in Table 5. An increase in the specific activity of this enzyme was observed from birth to 21 days. Thereafter, it plateaued to an adult level. The greatest increase in activity occurred from day 7 to day 14, coinciding with a period when the TT_4 and FT_4I rose sharply to their peak values (Table 5), therefore suggesting an inductive effect of thyroid hormone on the enzyme.

Animals made hypothyroid in the late fetal and postnatal period with propylthiouracil showed a decrease in tRNA sulfurtransferase activity that was slight at birth but worsened with time. While the tRNA sulfurtransferase activity rose approximately 250% in normal rats in the first 21 days of postnatal life, it increased only 50% in the hypothyroid animals during the same period (Table 5). This discrepancy was sustained subsequently.

Thyroxine replacement beginning from day 2 of life brought about a rapid return of the enzyme activity to the normal levels, so that by day 7, the enzyme levels in the thyroxine-replaced animals were indistinguishable from those of the controls (Table 5).

DISCUSSION

A sulfurtransferase system has been partially purified from the whole homogenate of rat cerebral hemispheres that is capable of transferring the sulfur from β-mercaptopyruvate to tRNA *in vitro*. In addition to the sulfur donor, enzyme, and tRNA as acceptor, the *in vitro* system requires ATP and magnesium ion for activation and a thiol such as β-mercaptoethanol for optimal sulfur transfer.

Among the different kinds of RNA, only tRNA is capable of accepting sulfur in this mammalian sulfurtransferase system. Both homologous and heterologous tRNAs are effective in this respect, but rRNA, mRNA, and synthetic ribohomopolymers are ineffective. This specificity implies that certain structural attributes peculiar to tRNA are requisite for the ability to accept sulfur.

Chromatography of the ^{35}S-labeled enzymatic product on Sephadex G-100 before and after RNase treatment indicates that the radioactive sulfur is an integral part of tRNA or its RNase digest. The electrophoretic properties of the [^{35}S] products formed after hydrolysis of the *in vitro* labeled rat liver tRNA, and their behavior after exposure to alkaline phosphatase, suggest that they are sulfur-containing nucleotides. DEAE-cellulose chromatography of the alkaline digest of *in vitro* labeled rat liver tRNA reveals the formation of several thionucleotides, none of which is 4-thioUMP, the major thionucleotide of *E. coli*. This observation is in accord with that of Lipsett (1965), who found no 320 nm-absorbing material in unfractionated rat liver

TABLE 5. *tRNA sulfurtransferase activity in the developing rat cerebral hemispheres and its regulation by thyroid hormone*

Group	Age (days)	Thyroid function		Body weight (g)	Weight of cerebral hemispheres (mg)	Specific activity of cerebral tRNA sulfurtransferase in pmoles ^{35}S incorporated/ mg protein
		TT$_4$(μg/100 ml)	FT$_4$I			
Control	0–1	2.40 ± 0.27	2.78 ± 0.11	5.46 ± 0.24	198 ± 12	17.81 ± 0.36
Hypothyroid	0–1	1.94 ± 0.19	2.21 ± 0.24	4.95 ± 0.40	178 ± 16	17.01 ± 0.44
Hypothyroid + T$_4$	0–1	1.90 ± 0.20	2.15 ± 0.19	4.86 ± 0.36	175 ± 15	16.90 ± 0.47
Control	7	3.68 ± 0.46	4.31 ± 0.54	13.73 ± 0.71	554 ± 36	22.77 ± 0.12
Hypothyroid	7	2.04 ± 0.20	2.43 ± 0.22	10.43 ± 1.43	470 ± 18	19.17 ± 0.67
Hypothyroid + T$_4$	7	3.60 ± 0.26	4.40 ± 0.28	12.47 ± 0.93	531 ± 25	23.67 ± 1.13
Control	14	6.33 ± 0.36	7.87 ± 0.64	24.77 ± 0.93	892 ± 30	42.45 ± 1.61
Hypothyroid	14	2.38 ± 0.38	2.97 ± 0.22	17.13 ± 1.20	760 ± 29	25.76 ± 1.63
Hypothyroid + T$_4$	14	6.30 ± 0.38	7.75 ± 0.37	24.23 ± 1.06	864 ± 48	40.96 ± 0.96
Control	21	4.99 ± 0.68	7.28 ± 0.79	36.51 ± 2.76	1028 ± 21	44.07 ± 2.86
Hypothyroid	21	1.72 ± 0.26	2.18 ± 0.38	24.40 ± 2.78	850 ± 22	26.42 ± 0.83
Hypothyroid + T$_4$	21	4.78 ± 0.61	7.06 ± 0.69	36.38 ± 3.56	1012 ± 11	43.95 ± 3.93
Control	28	4.46 ± 0.61	6.28 ± 0.71	62.57 ± 1.24	1088 ± 26	44.27 ± 2.19
Hypothyroid	28	1.65 ± 0.28	1.75 ± 0.21	26.27 ± 2.50	847 ± 45	26.00 ± 0.96
Hypothyroid + T$_4$	28	4.52 ± 0.52	6.46 ± 0.49	61.40 ± 3.61	1070 ± 35	43.60 ± 3.16
Control	35	4.21 ± 0.36	5.89 ± 0.40	97.79 ± 5.76	1121 ± 22	44.95 ± 4.12
Hypothyroid	35	1.51 ± 0.11	1.51 ± 0.12	26.07 ± 5.61	853 ± 40	26.25 ± 2.17
Hypothyroid + T$_4$	35	4.10 ± 0.63	5.82 ± 0.61	96.20 ± 6.36	1101 ± 29	44.80 ± 2.19

Thyroxine replacement was begun from day 2 of age and consisted of daily subcutaneous injections of sodium L-thyroxine at a dose of 2 μg/100 g of body weight. For determination of tRNA sulfurtransferase activity, a 160,000 × g supernatant was prepared from the cerebral hemispheres of each rat. The specific activity was calculated from ^{35}S incorporation data obtained with the standard assay and protein concentration determined by the method of Lowry, Rosebrough, Farr, and Randall (1951). All values given above represent the mean ± SD for four animals.

tRNA. It is also in agreement with the report of Eliceiri (1970), who found no 4-thioUMP in the alkaline hydrolysate of *in vivo* labeled [^{35}S] tRNA isolated from mouse lymphoma cells.

The mechanism by which sulfur is transferred from β-mercaptopyruvate to the acceptor tRNA is not known. The specific requirement for ATP in the transsulfuration reaction suggests the formation of an activated intermediate, either of the sulfur donor or of specific bases in the acceptor tRNA. Kinetic data from the study of Abrell, Kaufman, and Lipsett (1971) with *E. coli* tRNA sulfurtransferase using cysteine as the sulfur donor indicate that ATP may be involved in activating tRNA, but the nature of the intermediate has not yet been elucidated, nor have attempts at demonstrating phosphate or pyrophosphate exchange with ATP been successful.

Fractionation of the subcellular components of the rat cerebral hemispheres indicates that the tRNA sulfurtransferase activity is localized predominantly in the soluble portion of the cytoplasm. It is of interest that another group of enzymes involved in the biosynthesis of minor nucleotides, the tRNA methylases, are also localized predominantly in the cell supernatant (Burdon, Martin, and Lal, 1967; Culp and Brown, 1968).

The reason for studying the tRNA sulfurtransferase in the brain is twofold: First, to find out whether thiolated tRNA, and consequently the enzyme responsible for its formation, plays a role in regulating protein synthesis, the brain is an organ of choice for study because of its profound growth and maturation in the immediate postnatal period and the considerable protein synthesis accompanying this process (Davison and Dobbing, 1968; Geel and Timiras, 1970; Roberts, Zomzely, and Bondy, 1970; Sokoloff, 1970; Balázs, 1971; Gómez, 1971). The steep rise in specific activity of cerebral tRNA sulfurtransferase observed in the first 21 days of life when the rat brain is maturing biochemically, morphologically, and physiologically, suggests that this enzyme may be important in cerebral differentiation. Second, there is some indication from recent reports that abnormal metabolism of β-mercaptopyruvate may be responsible for certain instances of genetically determined mental retardation (Ampola, Effron, Bixby, and Meshorer, 1969; Crawhall, Parker, Sneddon, and Young, 1969). Since β-mercaptopyruvate is a substrate for tRNA sulfurtransferase, studies of the factors controlling the action of this enzyme may have some bearing in understanding the manifestations of such a genetic abnormality.

The finding that intact thyroid function is necessary for the maintenance of normal tRNA sulfurtransferase activity during the critical period of cerebral development suggests that one way thyroxine may regulate the differentiation of the brain is by controlling the levels of tRNA sulfurtransferase, which in turn may govern the availability of thiolated tRNA in the translational processes of protein synthesis.

It is now known that such structural modifications as thiolation can profoundly affect the functioning of tRNA molecules in protein synthesis. The

studies of Carbon et al. (1965) and Goehler and Doi (1968) indicate that
certain species of tRNA from rabbit liver, *E. coli,* and *B. subtilis* lose their
ability to accept amino acids following oxidation with dilute iodine solutions.
Because this inactivation is readily reversible by reduction of the iodine-
exposed tRNAs with thiosulfate or glutathione, the phenomenon was interpreted as potentially due to disulfide bond formation involving thionucleotides in the tRNA molecules (Carbon et al., 1965).

   More recent studies have disclosed the presence of 2-thiouridine derivatives in the first position of the anticodon of tRNA^{Glu} from such diverse
sources as yeast, *E. coli,* and rat liver; further, there are indications that
these strategically placed thionucleotides play a role in precise codon recognition by tRNA through imposition of strict base-pairing between codon and
anticodon and consequently prevention of wobbling (Ohashi et al., 1970;
Kimura-Harada et al., 1971; Yoshida et al., 1971). Sekiya, Takeishi, and
Ukita (1969) were the first to draw attention to the fact that one species of
glutamic acid-accepting tRNA from yeast, tRNA$_3^{Glu}$, specifically recognizes
GAA from the two known code words for glutamic acid, GAA and GAG, in
trinucleotide-stimulated ribosome binding assays. Such specificity in codon
recognition is contrary to the prediction of the wobble hypothesis of Crick
(1966). The subsequent discovery of 2-thiouridine-5-acetic acid methyl
ester in the first position of the anticodon of yeast tRNA$_3^{Glu}$ readily explained this specificity in codon recognition, since the 2-thiouridine derivative in the first position of the anticodon could only form a stable base pair
with A in the third position of the codon but not with G (Yoshida et al.,
1971). Parallel studies by others (Ohashi et al., 1970; Kimura-Harada et al.,
1971; Agris et al., 1973) with tRNA^{Glu} from *E. coli* and rat liver further confirmed the correlation between the existence of a 2-thiouridine derivative
in the first position of the anticodon and preferential recognition of A in the
third position of the codon for glutamic acid. The 2-thiouridine derivative
in *E. coli* tRNA$_2^{Glu}$ has been identified as 5-methylaminomethyl-2-thiouri-
dine (Carbon et al., 1968; Ohashi et al., 1970) and that in rat liver tRNA$_3^{Glu}$
as 5-methyl-2-thiouridine (Kimura-Harada et al., 1971). Desulfuration of
the tRNA$_2^{Glu}$ from *E. coli* with cyanogen bromide leads to loss of the ability
to recognize the usual codon GAA (Agris et al., 1973). Similarly, tRNA$_2^{Glu}$
isolated from a cysteine-requiring relaxed mutant of *E. coli* grown in a sulfur-
deficient medium, and therefore lacking its usual complement of sulfur in the
anticodon nucleotides, shows imprecision and error in codon recognition,
in that it recognizes GAG in addition to the usual codon GAA; moreover, it
recognizes GAG far better than GAA (Agris et al., 1973).

   Another thionucleoside, 6-(3-methyl-2-butenylamino)-2-methylthio-9-β-
D-ribofuranosylpurine (Burrows et al., 1968), which is found adjacent to the
3′-end of the anticodon of *E. coli* tRNA^{Tyr} (Harada, Gross, Kimura, Chang,
Nishimura, and RajBhandary, 1968), has been shown to affect the efficiency

of binding of the particular tRNA to ribosome-mRNA complexes. When this nucleoside is not thiolated (as occurred in a species of suppressor tRNA^{Tyr} isolated from *E. coli* infected with the defective transducing phage $\phi80$ dsu^+_{III}), the tRNA molecule is capable of being charged but incapable of binding to ribosome-mRNA complexes and consequently unable to support protein synthesis *in vitro* (Gefter and Russell, 1969).

An increasing body of evidence suggests that tRNA may play a regulatory role at a variety of levels in the cell, including transcription (Singer, Smith, Cortese, and Ames, 1972), translation (Anderson and Gilbert, 1969; Sharma, Mays, and Borek, 1971; Wainwright, 1971), and expression of enzyme activity (Jacobson, 1971). Proper modifications of the tRNA molecule with the formation of specific minor nucleotides have been found to be requisite for a number of these functions. These include repression of transcription (Singer et al., 1972), reaction with aminoacyl synthetases (Shugart, Novelli, and Stulberg, 1968), codon response (Capra and Peterkofsky, 1968), prevention of wobble (Ohashi et al., 1970; Kimura-Harada et al., 1971; Yoshida et al., 1971; Agris et al., 1973), and binding to ribosome-mRNA complexes (Gefter and Russell, 1969). Quantitative and qualitative changes in tRNA have been shown to accompany embryological differentiation (Lee and Ingram, 1967; Yang and Comb, 1968), bacterial sporulation (Doi, Kaneko, and Igarashi, 1968), hormonal stimulation (Turkington, 1969; Busby and Hele, 1970; Mäenpää, 1972) and deprivation (Yang and Sanadi, 1969; Sharma and Borek, 1970), viral infection (Sueoka and Kano-Sueoka, 1964; Hsu, Foft, and Weiss, 1967; Weiss, Hsu, Foft, and Scherberg, 1968), and neoplastic transformation (Yang and Novelli, 1968; Srinivasan, Srinivasan, Grunberger, Weinstein, and Morris, 1971; Grunberger, Weinstein, and Mushinski, 1975; Wong, Harris, and Morris, 1975). At least in some of these situations, thiolated tRNA is directly involved (Hsu et al., 1967; Weiss et al., 1968; Wong et al., 1975). An enzyme such as tRNA sulfurtransferase, which governs the formation of thiolated tRNA, could therefore exert a regulatory influence on growth processes by controlling the extent of tRNA thiolation. The observation that this enzyme rises sharply during cerebral maturation and is dependent on thyroxine for maintenance of normal activity unveils yet another facet of the action of thyroid hormones in controlling the myriads of events associated with growth and differentiation.

ACKNOWLEDGMENTS

This study was supported by Grant HD-06477 from the National Institute of Child Health and Human Development, and by Grant CA-19265 from the National Cancer Institute. M.A.H. was a predoctoral trainee supported by Training Grant HD-00001 from the National Institute of Child Health and Human Development.

REFERENCES

Abrell, J. W., Kaufman, E. E., and Lipsett, M. N. (1971): The biosynthesis of 4-thiouridylate. Separation and purification of two enzymes in the transfer ribonucleic acid-sulfurtransferase system. *J. Biol. Chem.*, 246:294–301.

Agris, P. F., Söll, D., and Seno, T. (1973): Biological function of 2-thiouridine in *Escherichia coli* glutamic acid transfer ribonucleic acid. *Biochemistry*, 12:4331–4337.

Ampola, M. G., Effron, M. L., Bixby, E. M., and Meshorer, E. (1969): Mental deficiency and a new aminoaciduria. *Am. J. Dis. Child.*, 117:66–70.

Anderson, W. F., and Gilbert, J. M. (1969): tRNA-dependent translational control of *in vitro* hemoglobin synthesis. *Biochem. Biophys. Res. Commun.*, 36:456–462.

Baczynskyj, K., Biemann, K., and Hall, R. H. (1968): Sulfur-containing nucleoside from yeast transfer ribonucleic acid: 2-Thio-5(or 6)-uridine acetic acid methyl ester. *Science*, 159:1481–1483.

Balázs, R. (1971): Biochemical effects of thyroid hormones in the developing brain. *UCLA Forum Med. Sci.*, 14:273–320.

Balázs, R., Kovács, S., Teichgräber, P., Cocks, W. A., and Eayrs, J. T. (1968): Biochemical effects of thyroid deficiency on the developing brain. *J. Neurochem.*, 15:1335–1349.

Burdon, R. H., Martin, B. T., and Lal, B. M. (1967): Synthesis of low molecular weight ribonucleic acid in tumor cells. *J. Mol. Biol.*, 28:357–371.

Burrows, W. J., Armstrong, D. J., Skoog, F., Hecht, S. M., Boyle, J. T. A., Leonard, N. J., and Occolowitz, J. (1968): Cytokinin from soluble RNA of *Escherichia coli*: 6-(3-Methyl-2-butenylamino)-2-methylthio-9-β-D-ribofuranosylpurine. *Science*, 161:691–693.

Busby, W. F., Jr., and Hele, P. (1970): Estrogen-induced variation of lysine transfer ribonucleic acid isoacceptors in chicken liver. *Biochim. Biophys. Acta*, 224:413–422.

Capra, J. D., and Peterkofsky, A. (1968): Effect of *in vitro* methylation on the chromatographic and coding properties of methyl-deficient leucine transfer RNA. *J. Mol. Biol.*, 33:591–607.

Carbon, J., David, H., and Studier, M. H. (1968): Thiobases in *Escherichia coli* transfer RNA: 2-Thiocytosine and 5-methylaminomethyl-2-thiouracil. *Science*, 161:1146–1147.

Carbon, J. A., Hung, L., and Jones, D. S. (1965): A reversible oxidative inactivation of specific transfer RNA species. *Proc. Natl. Acad. Sci. (USA)*, 53:979–986.

Crawhall, J. C., Parker, R., Sneddon, W., and Young, E. P. (1969): β-Mercaptolactate-cysteine disulfide in the urine of a mentally retarded patient. *Am. J. Dis. Child.*, 117:71–82.

Crick, F. H. C. (1966): Codon-anticodon pairing: The wobble hypothesis. *J. Mol. Biol.*, 19:548–555.

Culp, L. A., and Brown, G. M. (1968): Transfer ribonucleic acid methylases of Hela cells. *Arch. Biochem. Biophys.*, 124:483–492.

Davison, A. N., and Dobbing, J. (1968): The developing brain. In: *Applied Neurochemistry*, edited by A. N. Davison and J. Dobbing, pp. 253–286. Blackwell Scientific Publications, Oxford.

Doi, R. H., Kaneko, I., and Igarashi, R. T. (1968): Patterns of valine transfer ribonucleic acid of *Bacillus subtilis* under different growth conditions. *J. Biol. Chem.*, 243:945–951.

Eliceiri, G. L. (1970): Incorporation of ³⁵S into mammalian 4-S RNA. *Biochim. Biophys. Acta*, 209:387–395.

Geel, S. E., and Timiras, P. S. (1970): The role of hormones in cerebral protein metabolism. In: *Protein Metabolism of the Nervous System*, edited by A. Lajtha, pp. 335–354. Plenum Press, New York.

Gefter, M. L., and Russell, R. L. (1969): Role of modifications in tyrosine transfer RNA: A modified base affecting ribosome binding. *J. Mol. Biol.*, 39:145–157.

Gierer, A., and Schramm, G. (1956): The infectiousness of nucleic acid from tobacco mosaic virus. *Z. Naturforsch.*, 11B:138–142.

Goehler, B., and Doi, R. H. (1968): Presence and function of sulfur-containing transfer ribonucleic acid of *Bacillus subtilis*. *J. Bacteriol.*, 95:793–800.

Gómez, C. J. (1971): Hormonal influences of the biochemical differentiation of the rat cerebral cortex. In: *Hormones in Development*, edited by M. Hamburgh and E. J. W. Barrington, pp. 417–435. Appleton-Century-Crofts, New York.

Grunberger, D., Weinstein, I. B., and Mushinski, J. F. (1975): Deficiency of the Y base in a hepatoma phenylalanine tRNA. *Nature*, 253:66–67.

Harada, F., Gross, H. J., Kimura, F., Chang, S. H., Nishimura, S., and RajBhandary, U. L. (1968): 2-Methylthio-N⁶-(Δ²-isopentenyl) adenosine: A component of *E. coli* tyrosine transfer RNA. *Biochem. Biophys. Res. Commun.*, 33:299–306.

Hayward, R. S., and Weiss, S. B. (1966): RNA thiolase: The enzymatic transfer of sulfur from cysteine to sRNA in *Escherichia coli* extracts. *Proc. Natl. Acad. Sci. (USA)*, 55:1161–1168.

Hsu, W.-T., Foft, J. W., and Weiss, S. B. (1967): Effect of bacteriophage infection on the sulfur-labeling of sRNA. *Proc. Natl. Acad. Sci. (USA)*, 58:2028–2035.

Ivanova, T. N., Rubel, L. N., and Semenova, N. A. (1967): The phosphorus turnover of phosphatidylcholine, plasmalogen and diacyl phosphatidylethanolamines of the brain of rats of different ages, in various areas and some microstructures of the brain. *J. Neurochem.*, 14:653–659.

Jacobson, K. B. (1971): Role of an isoacceptor transfer ribonucleic acid as an enzyme inhibitor: effect on tryptophan pyrrolase of *Drosophila. Nature New Biol.*, 231:17–19.

Kimura-Harada, F., Saneyoshi, M., and Nishimura, S. (1971): 5-Methyl-2-thiouridine: A new sulfur-containing minor constituent from rat liver glutamic acid and lysine tRNAs. *FEBS (Fed. Eur. Biochem. Soc.) Lett.*, 13:335–338.

Kun, E. (1957): The reaction of β-mercaptopyruvate with lactic dehydrogenase of heart muscle. *Biochim. Biophys. Acta*, 25:135–137.

Lalyre-G., Y., and Titchener, E. B. (1971): Four-thiouracil content of chicken liver mitochondrial transfer ribonucleic acid. *Biochem. Biophys. Res. Commun.*, 42:926–931.

Lee, J. C., and Ingram, V. M. (1967): Erythrocyte transfer RNA: Change during chick development. *Science*, 158:1330–1332.

Lipsett, M. N. (1965): The isolation of 4-thiouridylic acid from the soluble ribonucleic acid of *Escherichia coli. J. Biol. Chem.*, 240:3975–3978.

Lipsett, M. N., and Peterkofsky, A. (1966): Enzymatic thiolation of *E. coli* sRNA. *Proc. Natl. Acad. Sci. (USA)*, 55:1169–1174.

Lowry, O. H., Rosebrough, N. J., Farr, A. L., and Randall, R. J. (1951): Protein measurement with the Folin phenol reagent. *J. Biol. Chem.*, 193:265–275.

Mäenpää, P. H. (1972): Seryl transfer RNA alterations during estrogen-induced phosvitin synthesis. Quantitative assay of the hormone-responding species by ribosomal binding. *Biochem. Biophys. Res. Commun.*, 47:971–974.

Nishimura, S. (1972): Minor components in transfer RNA: Their characterization, location, and function. *Prog. Nucleic Acid Res. Mol. Biol.*, 12:49–85.

Ohashi, Z., Saneyoshi, M., Harada, F., Hara, H., and Nishimura, S. (1970): Presumed anticodon structure of glutamic acid tRNA from *E. coli:* A possible location of a 2-thiouridine derivative in the first position of the anticodon. *Biochem. Biophys. Res. Commun.*, 40:866–872.

Roberts, S., Zomzely, C. E., and Bondy, S. C. (1970): Protein synthesis in the nervous system. In: *Protein Metabolism of the Nervous System*, edited by A. Lajtha, pp. 3–37. Plenum Press, New York.

Robin, N. I., Hagen, S. R., Collaço, F., Refetoff, S., and Selenkow, H. A. (1971): Serum tests for measurement of thyroid function. *Hormones*, 2:266–279.

Saneyoshi, M., and Nishimura, S. (1971): Selective inactivation of amino acid acceptor and ribosome-binding activities of *Escherichia coli* tRNA by modification with cyanogen bromide. *Biochim. Biophys. Acta*, 246:123–131.

Sekiya, T., Takeishi, K., and Ukita, T. (1969): Specificity of yeast glutamic acid transfer RNA for codon recognition. *Biochim. Biophys. Acta*, 182:411–426.

Sharma, O. K., and Borek, E. (1970): Hormonal effect on transfer ribonucleic acid methylases and on serine transfer ribonucleic acid. *Biochemistry*, 9:2507–2513.

Sharma, O. K., Mays, L. L., and Borek, E. (1971): Enhancement of the synthesis of a hormone-induced protein by transfer ribonucleic acids. *J. Biol. Chem.*, 248:7622–7624.

Shugart, L., Novelli, G. D., and Stulberg, M. P. (1968): Isolation and properties of under-methylated phenylalanine transfer ribonucleic acids from a relaxed mutant of *Escherichia coli. Biochim. Biophys. Acta*, 157:83–90.

Singer, C. E., Smith, G. R., Cortese, R., and Ames, B. N. (1972): Mutant tRNA^His ineffective in repression and lacking two pseudouridine modifications. *Nature New Biol.*, 238:72–74.

Sokoloff, L. (1970): The mechanism of action of thyroid hormones on protein synthesis and its relationship to the differences in sensitivities of mature and immature brain. In: *Protein Metabolism of the Nervous System,* edited by A. Lajtha, pp. 367–382. Plenum Press, New York.

Srinivasan, D., Srinivasan, P. R., Grunberger, D., Weinstein, I. B., and Morris, H. P. (1971): Alterations in specific transfer ribonucleic acids in a spectrum of hepatomas. *Biochemistry,* 10:1966–1973.

Sueoka, N., and Kano-Sueoka, T. (1964): A specific modification of leucyl-sRNA of *Escherichia coli* after phage T2 infection. *Proc. Natl. Acad. Sci. (USA),* 52:1535–1540.

Turkington, R. W. (1969): Hormonal regulation of transfer ribonucleic acid and transfer ribonucleic acid-methylating enzymes during development of the mouse mammary gland. *J. Biol. Chem.,* 244:5140–5148.

Wainwright, S. D. (1971): Stimulation of hemoglobin synthesis in developing chick blastodisc blood islands by a minor alanine-specific transfer RNA. *Cancer Res.,* 31:694–696.

Weiss, S. B., Hsu, W.-T., Foft, J. W., and Scherberg, N. H. (1968): Transfer RNA coded by the T4 bacteriophage genome. *Proc. Natl. Acad. Sci. (USA),* 61:114–121.

Williams, R. H., Kay, G. A., and Jandorf, B. J. (1944): Thiouracil. Its absorption, distribution, and excretion. *J. Clin. Invest.,* 23:613–627.

Wong, T.-W., Harris, M. A., and Jankowicz, C. A. (1974): Transfer ribonucleic acid sulfurtransferase isolated from rat cerebral hemispheres. *Biochemistry,* 13:2805–2812.

Wong, T.-W., Harris, M. A., and Morris, H. P. (1975): The presence of an inhibitor of tRNA sulfurtransferase in Morris hepatomas. *Biochem. Biophys. Res. Commun.,* 65:1137–1145.

Wong, T.-W., Weiss, S. B., Eliceiri, G. L., and Bryant, J. (1970): Ribonucleic acid sulfurtransferase from *Bacillus subtilis* W168. Sulfuration with β-mercaptopyruvate and properties of the enzyme system. *Biochemistry,* 9:2376–2386.

Yang, S. S., and Comb, D. G. (1968): Distribution of multiple forms of lysyl transfer RNA during early embryogenesis of sea urchin, *Lytechinus variegatus. J. Mol. Biol.,* 31:139–142.

Yang, S. S., and Sanadi, D. R. (1969): Changes in the distribution of transfer ribonucleic acid species specifically induced by thyroxine. *J. Biol. Chem.,* 244:5081–5083.

Yang, W. K., and Novelli, G. D. (1968): Isoaccepting tRNA's in mouse plasma cell tumors that synthesize different myeloma protein. *Biochem. Biophys. Res. Commun.,* 31:534–539.

Yoshida, M., Takeishi, K., and Ukita, T. (1971): Structural studies on a yeast glutamic acid tRNA specific to GAA codon. *Biochim. Biophys. Acta,* 228:153–166.

DISCUSSION

Sokoloff: Thank you, Dr. Wong, for a classically beautiful biochemical study of another reaction that those of us who are interested in the maturation of the brain and the action of thyroid hormones will now have to concern ourselves with. We are running short of time, but I think we can entertain a few comments or questions.

Balázs: We know that tRNA sulfurtransferase normally introduces sulfur into the critical position in the anticodon region, but does this enzyme ever introduce sulfur into the wrong positions in a tRNA molecule?

Wong: Before answering this question, I would like to clarify the term "tRNA sulfurtransferase." Whereas I have sometimes referred to the crude enzyme preparation isolated from the rat brain imprecisely as tRNA sulfurtransferase (in the singular), such a crude preparation in fact contains several tRNA sulfurtransferases, as evidenced by the fact that the *in vitro* labeled [^{35}S]tRNA yields several radioactive thionucleotides on hydrolysis. When the crude enzyme preparation is subjected to further purification, as for example in the case of *E. coli,* several tRNA sulfurtransferases can eventually be separated, each of which will only lead to the formation of one particular thionucleotide at a specific location of the tRNA molecule. So far as we know, the tRNA sulfurtransferases isolated from normal tissues are highly specific in the sense that they always produce the same thionucleotides in the same locations of the tRNA molecule; they do not indiscriminately introduce sulfur into the wrong positions. But whether such abnormal thiolation occurs under pathological conditions is an entirely different and intriguing question which awaits further study.

Balázs: Do I understand you to say that the critical point with respect to tRNA function is the introduction of sulfur into the anticodon region?

Wong: There are two locations where the introduction of sulfur has been shown to be crucial to precise functioning of tRNA. One is at the first position of the anticodon, and the other is at the position immediately adjacent to the 3'-end of the anticodon. The former has been shown to be essential for all classes of organisms examined so far, including bacteria, yeast, and mammals. The latter has been shown to be important for bacteria only.

Sokoloff: May we turn it around and say that in the absence of thiolation, the tRNA molecule may be nonfunctional in protein synthesis or ambiguous in its recognition of the codon?

Wong: Yes.

Balázs: What sort of tRNA was used as sulfur acceptor in the *in vitro* transsulfuration reaction?

Wong: In our routine assays, we used unfractionated tRNA from yeast.

Balázs: Isn't the tRNA already thiolated as it is isolated from this organism?

Wong: The unfractionated tRNA isolated from yeast and for that matter from any other organism generally contains some tRNA molecules that are fully thiolated, others that are partly thiolated, and still others that are not thiolated at all.

Sokoloff: In fact, it is possible that in the cell tRNA exists in a mixed population, some thiolated and some not.

Wong: Most certainly, and it is the partly thiolated and unthiolated tRNA molecules that are the actual sulfur acceptors in the *in vitro* transsulfuration reaction.

Sokoloff: Is there any possibility that the *in vitro* transsulfuration reaction you described actually represents an exchange reaction?

Wong: This important question was studied by Dr. E. B. Titchener at the University of Illinois, using a cysteine-requiring, relaxed mutant of *E. coli*. When grown in a normal, sulfur-rich medium, this organism produces normally thiolated tRNA. When cultured in a sulfur-deficient medium, however, it produces tRNA which is under-thiolated. The normally thiolated tRNA and under-thiolated tRNA isolated from these two types of cultures were compared for their ability to incorporate ^{35}S in the *in vitro* transsulfuration reaction. If the reaction is essentially exchange in nature, that is, if the enzyme merely accomplishes an exchange of the radioactive sulfur in $[^{35}S]\beta$-mercaptopyruvate with the nonradioactive sulfur already present in native tRNA, one would expect to find more ^{35}S in the normally thiolated tRNA than in the under-thiolated tRNA at the end of the reaction, since the normally thiolated tRNA has more nonradioactive sulfur available for exchange to begin with. But in the experiment, the reverse was observed; considerably more ^{35}S was found incorporated into the under-thiolated tRNA than into the normally thiolated tRNA, indicating that there was a net transfer or addition of ^{35}S from $[^{35}S]\beta$-mercaptopyruvate into the tRNA molecules, rather than an exchange of sulfur between the radioactive substrate and the tRNA molecules.

Sokoloff: I have one question which may have some relevance to the organized pattern of changes that occur during the biochemical maturation of the brain. If the thionucleotide in the first position of the anticodon is dethiolated, does the tRNA lose its specificity for the usual codon?

Wong: Yes.

Sokoloff: Is the specificity lost in a reproducible way, or does it just become random and make nonsense proteins? Is it possible that the same messenger RNA, depending on whether the tRNA is thiolated or not, might make different species of proteins?

Wong: I will answer this question by using glutamic acid-accepting tRNA as an example. The two known code words for glutamic acid are GAA and GAG. The species of tRNA^{Glu} which has a 2-thiouridine derivative in the first position of the anticodon normally recognizes only GAA but not GAG. When this tRNA^{Glu} is chemically dethiolated, it will lose its ability to recognize the usual codon entirely, whereas the same tRNA^{Glu} isolated from a cysteine-requiring, relaxed mutant of *E. coli* grown in a sulfur-poor medium, which is deficient in sulfur in the anticodon region, shows ambiguity and error in codon recognition, in that it recognizes both GAA and GAG, and in fact prefers the codon GAG to the usual codon GAA. Inability to recognize a prescribed codon in a messenger RNA can lead to interruption of protein synthesis or the formation of incomplete proteins.

Sokoloff: This in turn could lead to alterations of enzymes during maturation. We now have another possible explanation for the reduced or altered protein synthesis in hypothyroidism, but we still do not know how the thyroid hormone works in the maturation of the brain. We did not really expect that this conference would solve that problem, but we have learned a great deal more than we knew before, especially from the morphologists, who seem to be making more progress in elucidating the action of T$_4$ than the biochemists and the physiologists.

We have learned the strengths and the weaknesses of each others' disciplinary approaches. That is important because this problem will require the combined application of many specialists working collaboratively. To repeat what used to be a favorite saying of an eminent physiologist of the last generation, Axel Johann Karlson, "Now is the time for less talk and more dogs." We owe the National Institute of Child Health and Human Development, the Developmental Biology and Nutrition Branch, particularly Dr. Gilman Grave, a great debt of gratitude for having organized a beautiful meeting.

Subject Index

Actinomycin D, and RNA synthesis in
brain, 322
Adenohypophysis
hypothalamic regulation of hormones in,
1
ultrastructure in hypothyroidism, 21-23,
27-29
Adenosine triphosphate, and cerebral
tRNA sulfurtransferase activity, 352
Adrenal weight, in neonatal
hypothyroidism, 21
Age
and accumulation of triiodothyronine in
rat brain, 7-9
and cell proliferation in hypothyroid
cerebellum, 299
and cerebellar cell enzyme activity in
hypothyroidism, 97-99
and cerebral tRNA sulfurtransferase
activity, 349, 359
and cortical evoked responses in
cerebral regions, 259-261
and critical periods of development, 33
and degradation of triiodothyronine,
11-14
and dendritic spine development in
cerebral cortex, 261-263
and development of M-V cells in
amphibians, 131-132
and effects of thyroid hormone in brain,
76, 85-86
and effects of thyroid hormone therapy
in ataxia, 101
and β-hydroxybutyrate activity in brain,
in hyperthyroidism, 308
and iodide levels, 12
and leucine incorporation into proteins,
38-39
and protein binding of thyroid
hormones, 18
and uridine incorporation into RNA,
39-42
α-Amanitin, and RNA synthesis in brain,
322
Amino acid levels, thyroid states
affecting, 272
γ-Aminobutyric acid
accumulation in glial cells, 102
neurotransmitter function of, 100-101
γ-Aminobutyric acid transaminase activity,
cerebellar, in hypothyroidism, 93-102,
104-105

AMP, cyclic, and cerebellar DNA levels,
337-340, 341
Amphibians
brain growth affected by thyroid states,
2
cerebellar maturation in,
thyroid-induced, 107-117
deiodination of thyroid hormones in
metamorphosis, 139-148
mesencephalic fifth nucleus size affected
by thyroid hormones, 119-136
nutritional studies of, 342
tail disk studies of thyroxine effects,
65-68, 71-72
thiourea affecting metamorphosis,
130-131
thyroid hormone role in metamorphosis,
73, 75, 107-117, 137-150
Androgen, and triiodothyronine
accumulation in rat brain, 10
Anura, *see* Amphibians
Arcuate nucleus, neuron changes in
neonatal hypothyroidism, 23-24, 29
Aspartate transcarbamylase activity, in
brain, 327-329
Ataxia, cerebellar, in hypothyroidism, 101,
102

Basket cells, cerebellar
chronology in formation of, 296
in hyperthyroidism, 242
in hypothyroidism, 242-243, 292, 296
Behavioral patterns
after postnatal thyroid replacement
therapy, 205, 208
maternal, hypothyroidism affecting,
53-55
thyroid states affecting, 7
Bergmann cells
in hyperthyroidism, 243
in hypothyroidism, 90, 97-99, 101, 102,
195, 243, 296
uptake of GABA in, 101, 105
Brainstem, triiodothyronine accumulation
in, age affecting, 9

Carbamyl phosphate synthetase, activity
in brain, 327, 329
Castration, and triiodothyronine
accumulation in neonatal rat brain,
9-10